Milestones in Drug Therapy
MDT

Macrolide Antibiotics

Edited by W. Schönfeld and H. A. Kirst

Springer Basel AG

Editors
Wolfgang Schönfeld
PLIVA Research
Antiinfective Research
Prilaz baruna Filipovića 25
10000 Zagreb
Croatia

Herbert A. Kirst
Elanco Animal Health Research & Development
2001 West Main Street
P.O. Box 708
Greenfield, Indiana 46140
USA

Library of Congress Cataloging-in-Publication Data
Macrolide antibiotics / edited by W. Schönfeld and H.A. Kirst.
p. cm. – (Milestones in drug therapy)
Includes bibliographical references and index.
ISBN 978-3-0348-9438-8 ISBN 978-3-0348-8105-0 (eBook)
DOI 10.1007/978-3-0348-8105-0
1. Macrolides antibiotics. I. Schönfeld, W. (Wolfgang), 1956– II. Kirst, Herbert A. III. Series.

Deutsche Bibliothek Cataloging-in-Publication Data
Macrolides antibiotics / ed. by W. Schönfeld and H.A. Kirst. – Basel ; Boston ; Berlin : Birkhäuser, 2002
(Milestones in drug therapy)
ISBN 978-3-0348-9438-8

ISBN 978-3-0348-9438-8

Originally published by Birkhäuser Verlag in 2002
Softcover reprint of the hardcover 1st edition 2002

Cover Illustration: Erythromycin – the macrolide core and its most important derivatives
Printed on acid-free paper produced from chlorine-free pulp. TCF ∞

ISBN 3-7643-6186-7

9 8 7 6 5 4 3 2 1

www.birkhäuser-science.com

Contents

List of contributors

Jacques F. Acar, Hôpital Saint Joseph, Laboratoire de Microbiologie Médicale, 185 rue Raymond Losserand, 75674 Paris Cedex 14, France

Takashi Adachi, Medicinal Research Laboratories, Taisho Pharmaceutical Co., Ltd., 403 Yoshino-cho 1-chome, Saitama-shi, Saitama 330–8530, Japan; e-mail: takashi.adachi@po.rd.taisho.co.jp

Adel Ben Ali, Hôpital Saint Joseph, Laboratoire de Microbiologie Médicale, 185 rue Raymond Losserand, 75674 Paris Cedex 14, France; e-mail: adel_ben_ali@hotmail.com

Norris E. Allen, Animal Science Discovery and Development Research, Elanco Animal Health, 2001 West Main Street, Greenfield, IN 46140, USA; e-mail: allen_norris_e@lilly.com

Luiz E. Bermudez, Kuzell Institute for Arthritis and Infectious Diseases, California Pacific Medical Center Research Institute, 2200 Webster Street, Suite 305, San Francisco, CA 94115, USA; e-mail: luizb@cooper.cpmc.org

André Bryskier, Aventis Pharma Research Center, 102, route de Noisy, 93230 Romainville, France; e-mail: andre.bryskier@aventis.com

Eric Cundliffe, Department of Biochemistry, University of Leicester, Adrian Bldg., University Road, Leicester LE1 7RH, United Kingdom; e-mail: ec13@le.ac.uk

Alexis Denis, Aventis Pharma Research Center, 102, route de Noisy, 93230 Romainville, France; e-mail: alexis.denis@aventis.com

Fred W. Goldstein, Hôpital Saint Joseph, Laboratoire de Microbiologie Médicale, 185 rue Raymond Losserand, 75674 Paris Cedex 14, France

Margaret R. Hammerschlag, Division of Infectious Diseases, Department of Pediatrics, SUNY Health Science Center at Brooklyn, 450 Clarkson Ave., Brooklyn, NY 11203–2098, U.S.A.; e-mail. mhammerschlag@pol.net

Vito R. Iacoviello, Harvard Medical School, Mount Auburn Hospital, 330 Mount Auburn Street, Cambridge, MA 02238, USA

Leonard Katz, Kosan Biosciences Inc., 3832 Bay Center Place, Hayward, CA 94611, USA; e-mail: katz@kosan.com

Herbert A. Kirst, Elanco Animal Health Research & Development, 2001 West Main Street, Greenfield, IN 46140–0708, USA; e-mail: Kirst_Herbert_A@Lilly.com

Marie-Thérèse Labro, INSERM U479, CHU X. Bichat-Cl. Bernard, 46 rue Henri Huchard, 75018 Paris, France; e-mail: labro@bichat.inserm.fr

Roland Leclerq, Department of Microbiology, CHU, Côte de Nacre, Av. Côte de Nacre, 14033 Caen, France; e-mail: leclercq-r@chu-caen.fr

Zhenkun Ma, Abbott Laboratories, 200 Abbott Park Road, Abbott Park, IL 60064–3537, USA; e-mail: zhenkun.ma@abbott.com
Holly M. Mattoes, Department of Pharmacy Research, Hartford Hospital, University of Connecticut, 80 Seymour Street, Hartford, CT 06102–5037, USA
Francis Mégraud, Laboratoire de Bactériologie, Hôpital Pellegrin, Place Amélie Raba-Léon, 33076 Bordeaux cedex, France; e-mail: francis.megraud@chu-bordeaux.fr
Shigeo Morimoto, Medicinal Research Laboratories, Taisho Pharmaceutical Co., Ltd., 403 Yoshino-cho 1-chome, Saitama-shi, Saitama 330–8530, Japan; e-mail: shigeo.morimoto@po.rd.taisho.co.jp
Stjepan Mutak, Antiinfective Research, PLIVA d.d., Prilaz Baruna Filipovicá 25, 10000 Zagreb, Croatia; e-mail: stjepan.mutak@pliva.hr
Charles H. Nightingale, Department of Pharmacy Research, Office of Research Administration, Hartford Hospital, University of Connecticut, 80 Seymour Street, Hartford, CT 06102–5037, USA; e-mail: cnighti@harthos.org
Ly T. Phan, Enanta Pharmaceuticals, Inc., 500 Arsenal Street, Watertown, MA 02472, USA; e-mail: phan@enanta.com
Geoffrey L. Ridgway, Department of Clinical Microbiology, University College London Hospitals, Grafton Way, London WC1E 6DB, UK, e-mail: geoff.ridgway@uclh.org
Wolfgang Schönfeld, PLIVA Research, Antiinfective Research, Prilaz Baruna Filipovicá 25, 10000 Zagreb, Croatia; e-mail: wolfgang.schoenf@hotmail.com
Joyce A. Sutcliffe, Rib-X Pharmaceuticals, 25 Science Park, Room 561, New Haven, CT 06511, USA; e-mail: sutcliffe@rib-x.com
Lowell S. Young, Kuzell Institute for Arthritis and Infectious Diseases, California Pacific Medical Center Research Institute, 2200 Webster Street, Suite 305, San Francisco, CA 94115, USA; e-mail: kiaid@cooper.cpmc.org
Stephen Zinner, Harvard Medical School, Mount Auburn Hospital, 330 Mount Auburn Street, Cambridge, MA 02238, USA

Preface

There are only very few chemical classes of antibiotics in medical use, and these have originated over a span of more than 60 years of research. Almost half a century ago, the first member of the macrolides, erythromycin, was introduced as a treatment option for bacterial infections. Erythromycin is a very complex fermentation product obtained from the soil bacterium *Saccharopolyspora erythraea* (originally named *Streptomyces erythreus*). The success of erythromycin, based on its efficacy and tolerability, stimulated researchers throughout the world to undertake intense efforts to understand the biology and chemistry of macrolides and to use this experience to improve the properties of this compound class. The second generation of macrolides, based on chemical modifications of erythromycin, is currently being in broad use, especially for treatment of respiratory tract infections. We presently foresee the introduction of a new generation of macrolides, i.e. the ketolides, which have the potential to overcome rising resistance problems.

This monograph is intended to give the interested reader an overview on "macrolide experience", covering important areas from basic research to clinical use.

Starting from a historic overview, the essential basic parameters – efficacy, pharmacokinetics, pharmacodynamics, and pharmacology – are highlighted in order to introduce the reader to the rationale for clinical use of macrolides.

The following group of chapters cover the complex chemistry of the macrolactone structures, giving historic background, basic structure-activity relationships of various derivatization strategies, and perspectives for future discovery of new semisynthetic macrolide antibiotics.

Our current understanding of the biosynthesis of the natural macrolide scaffolds is summarized in the following two chapters. This area rapidly emerged during the last few years as a result of the enormous progress in understanding the metabolic pathways by which macrolides are assembled in microorganisms and developing new technologies to exploit this knowledge to create novel analogs.

In the next chapters, the authors give detailed overviews of the antibacterial properties of macrolides, which are the basis for their clinical use. General profiles allowing the physician to evaluate the potency and usefulness of individual compounds for treatment of defined bacterial infections are combined with epidemiological data indicating the status of resistance among important bacteria.

Finally, the molecular mode of action of macrolides and the molecular basis of bacterial resistance mechanisms are thoroughly described in the last two chapters.

This book is intended to give the readers – whether they are professionals in the pharmaceutical industry, physicians treating infections, or microbiologists at hospitals, health institutes, or universities – a detailed and up-to-date knowledge base about current research activities and also a sound, stimulating overview and perspective about the class of macrolide antibiotics.

We are very grateful to all authors who took the additional effort on top of their daily multiple obligations to prepare this book. Without their enthusiasm and outstanding expertise, this monograph would not be available.

In addition, we highly appreciate the great help from the team of our publishing team, Karin Neidhart and Detlef Klüber, who gave us the professional support needed to successfully publish this book.

Herbert Kirst
Wolfgang Schönfeld

Summer 2001

Macrolide Antibiotics
ed. by W. Schönfeld and H. A. Kirst

Introduction to the macrolide antibiotics

Herbert A. Kirst

Elanco Animal Health Research & Development, 2001 West Main Street, Greenfield, IN 46140–0708, USA

Historical developments and classification of naturally-occurring macrolides

Macrolide antibiotics are an old and well-established class of antimicrobial agents that have long played a significant role in the chemotherapy of infectious diseases [1–3]. Among the most important characteristics of the macrolide class are a moderately broad spectrum of antimicrobial activity, an orally effective route of administration, and a relatively high margin of safety (high therapeutic index). Although macrolides have been the primary antibiotic of choice for a few indications, they have also played a very critical role as an alternative drug of choice, particularly as an alternative to the penicillins. Over the past two decades, the macrolide class has undergone a remarkable resurgence that has been characterized by 1) the discovery and commercial development of several important new semi-synthetic derivatives exhibiting a variety of improved features and 2) clinical efficacy in the treatment of several infectious diseases not originally associated with macrolide therapy. The subsequent chapters of this book will 1) document the clinical progress that has been made thus far in utilizing the more recent semi-synthetic macrolides, 2) update our knowledge and understanding about the biosynthetic origins of the macrolides and the mechanisms involved in their antibacterial activity and in microbial resistance to them, and 3) look toward the future emergence of additional new macrolides potentially arising from the discovery and development pipelines of several pharmaceutical research organizations.

The prototype for the macrolide class is erythromycin, a structurally complex secondary metabolite isolated in 1952 from the culture broth *of Saccharopolyspora erythraea* (originally named *Streptomyces erythreus*), a microorganism first isolated from a soil sample from the Philippines [4]. Erythromycin A is the major factor obtained from the fermentation and is the principal component of the antibiotic called erythromycin. The structure of erythromycin A (Fig. 1) consists of a highly substituted 14-membered lactone (named erythronolide A), to which is attached 1) an amino sugar (D-desosamine) via a β-glycosidic linkage to the 5-hydroxyl group and 2) a neutral sugar (L-cladinose) via an α-glycosidic bond to the 3-hydroxyl group [5]. Despite its continuous use since the 1950s, erythromycin still remains the most important macrolide antibiotic world-wide, whose principal applications have been to treat infections in the respiratory tract, skin and

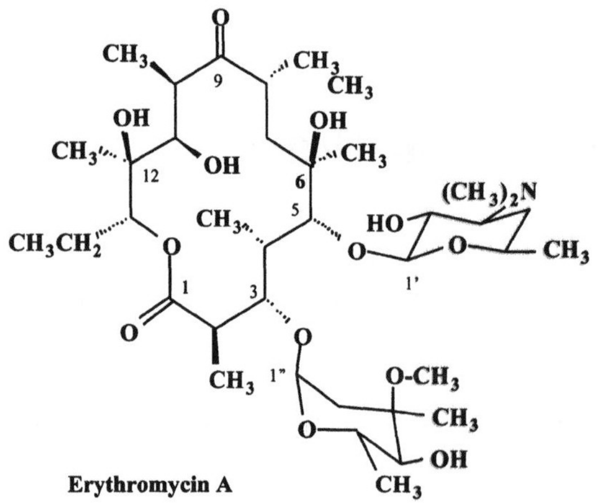

Figure 1. Structure of erythromycin A.

soft tissues, and genital tract [2, 6, 7]. During the past several decades that have been devoted to the discovery and investigation of antibiotics, many additional members of the macrolide class have been isolated from culture broths produced from a large number and wide variety of microorganisms [8]. Among the numerous naturally occurring macrolides, the most clinically useful ones are readily divided into two large families: 14-membered and 16-membered macrolides. This classification is based upon the size of the aglycone (lactone without sugar substituents). Erythromycin A is the principal representative of the 14-membered family. Oleandomycin is the other 14-membered macrolide that has achieved some clinical utility [9].

The 16-membered family generally is divided into two sub-families based upon differences in the substitution patterns of their aglycones: the tylosin sub-family and the leucomycin-spiramycin sub-family [8, 10]. Many of these 16-membered macrolides contain a substituted disaccharide moiety [4'-O-(α-L-mycarosyl)-β-D-mycaminosyl] attached to the 5-hydroxyl group of the aglycone. The most widely used member of the leucomycin series is josamycin (identical to leucomycin A_3) (Fig. 2) [11, 12], although a few other naturally occurring members of the leucomycin series also have been developed commercially in certain countries [9]. Spiramycin (Fig. 2) differs from the leucomycins by the presence of a second amino sugar substituent (D-forosamine) attached to the 9-hydroxyl group via a β-glycosidic bond [13]. Spiramycin has found a variety of applications in both human and veterinary medicine as well as in food animal production [14–17]. Tylosin is another important 16-membered macrolide antibiotic, first introduced in 1961, that has been used exclusively in veterinary medicine and for growth enhancement of food animals [17–19]. In addition to the typical disaccharide substituent on the 5-hydroxyl group, tylosin has a second neutral sugar (β-D-mycinose) attached to its 23-hydroxyl group (Fig. 3) [13, 20, 21].

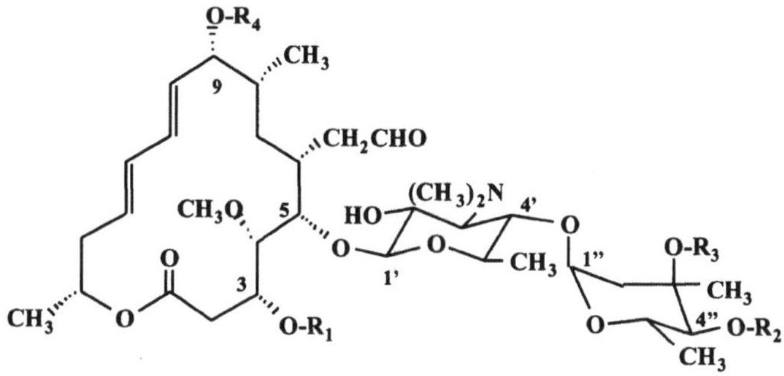

	R_1	R_2	R_3	R_4
Josamycin (Leucomycin A_3)	**acetyl**	**isovaleryl**	**H**	**H**
Leucomycin A_5	**H**	**n-butyryl**	**H**	**H**
Rokitamycin	**H**	**n-butyryl**	**propionyl**	**H**
Midecamycin A_1	**propionyl**	**propionyl**	**H**	**H**
Miocamycin	**propionyl**	**propionyl**	**acetyl**	**acetyl**
Spiramycin I	**H**	**H**	**H**	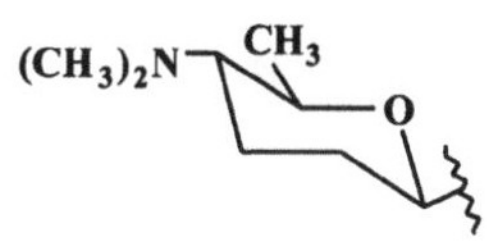

Figure 2. Structures of 16-membered clinical macrolides.

Semi-synthetic derivatives of erythromycin

Several limitations of erythromycin were identified early in its history, which included chemical instability (especially under acidic conditions), low degree of oral bioavailability, bitter taste, low antibiotic concentrations in serum, short *in vivo* half-life, high inter- and intra-patient variability, and gastrointestinal pain and discomfort. In order to overcome many of these inter-related problems and limitations, many formulations and product presentations of erythromycin have been investigated over several decades, such as enteric-coated, acid-resistant tablets and granules designed to protect the antibiotic from degradation during its passage through the acidic environment of the stomach until it reaches the more alkaline upper intestine where absorption occurs [22, 23].

An alternative approach to overcome these limitations has encompassed the preparation of numerous semi-synthetic derivatives of erythromycin, an on-going effort in medicinal chemistry that also was begun soon after the antibiotic's discovery. The initial focus of many derivatization efforts centered on modifications of the amino sugar (desosamine), involving either esterification of the 2'-hydroxyl group and/or formation of acid-addition salts with the 3'-dimethylamino group [23–26]. The more successful approaches have utilized either 2'-esters

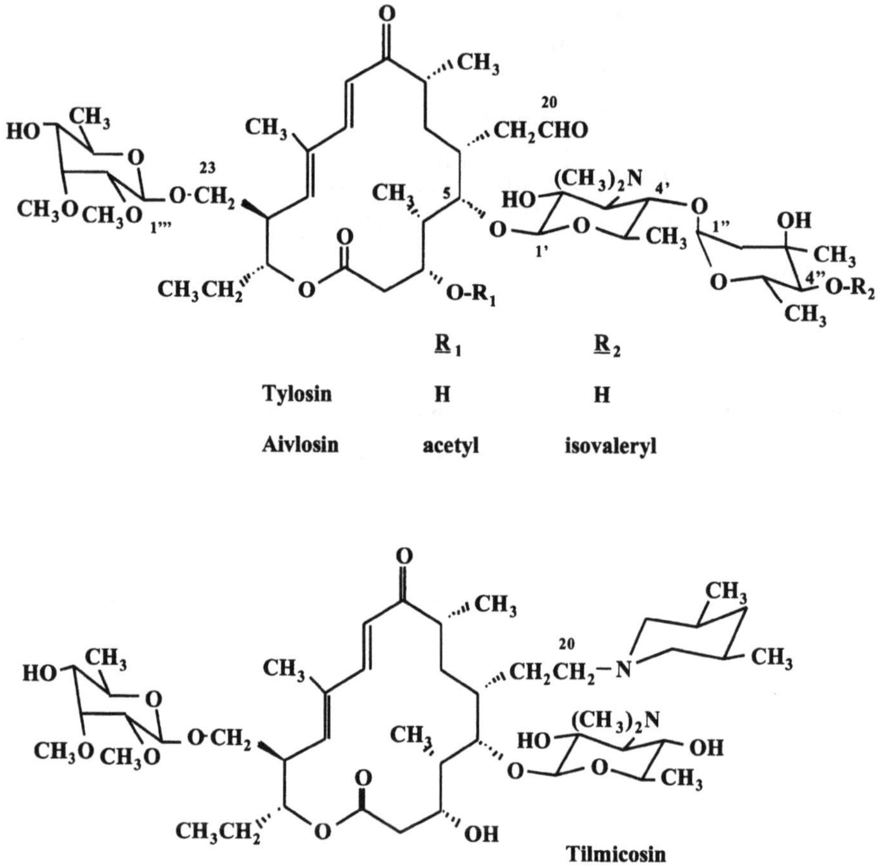

Figure 3. Structures of 16-membered veterinary macrolides.

prepared from short-chain organic acids, such as acetate, propionate, ethyl carbonate, and ethyl succinate, and/or highly lipophilic acid-addition salts, such as stearate and lauryl sulphate. These more lipophilic derivatives are postulated to further diminish the aqueous solubility of erythromycin such that it is less degraded in the stomach and passes intact to a greater degree into the more alkaline intestine; although this hypothesis has been difficult to prove and has not been accepted universally, absorption of these more highly lipophilic derivatives has been reported to occur to a higher and less-variable extent [22, 26]. In contrast, acid-addition salts with hydrophilic acids produce more water-soluble derivatives that are better suited for parenteral administration of erythromycin [23, 26]. All these esters and salts serve as pro-drugs that must be hydrolyzed or neutralized to liberate erythromycin free base, which is the active antimicrobial entity [27–29].

Studies of its chemical instability and loss of antimicrobial activity under acidic conditions revealed that erythromycin decomposed initially *via* a set of intramolecular cyclizations, resulting in formation of the 8,9-anhydro-6,9-hemiketal and

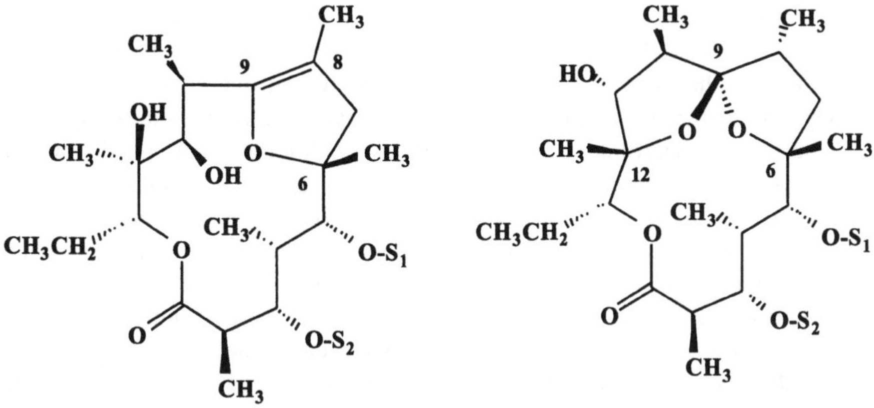

**8,9-Anhydroerythromycin A
6,9-hemiketal**

**Anhydroerythromycin A
6,9; 9,12-spiroketal**

Figure 4. Structures of initial decomposition products of erythromycin A.

6,9; 9,12-spiroketal derivatives (Fig. 4) [30–32]. One early structural modification of the lactone was the 11,12-carbonate derivative (Fig. 5), which stabilized the molecule in its 6,9-hemiketal form and prevented irreversible dehydration to the inactive anhydro-hemiketal moiety [33, 34]. The 1980s witnessed a major renaissance of research on macrolides, from which emerged several new semi-synthetic derivatives of erythromycin, beginning with roxithromycin and subse-

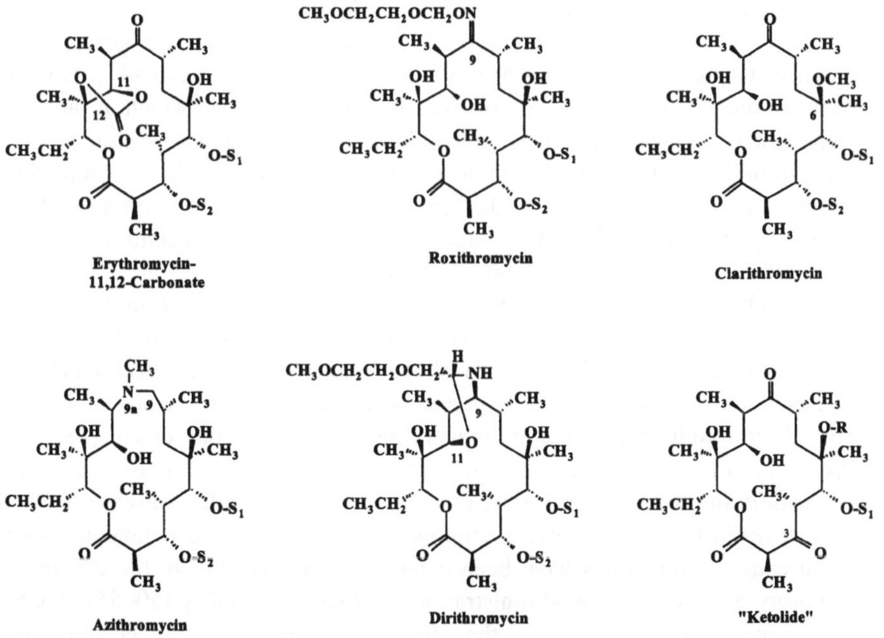

Figure 5. Structures of semi-synthetic derivatives of erythromycin A.

quently progressing to clarithromycin, azithromycin, and dirithromycin (Fig. 5). The semi-synthetic derivative azithromycin is formed from a ring expansion of erythromycin that produces a 15-membered macrolide; this unique ring system having a basic nitrogen atom inserted into the aglycone was the first example of a new series of macrolides termed "azalides". Although each of the newer derivatives of erythromycin exhibits some unique characteristics, and each derivative does not possess the identical set of attributes as the others, as a whole, this new group of semi-synthetic macrolides has broadened the antimicrobial spectrum, improved pharmacodynamic features, and increased oral bioavailability compared with older macrolides [35–40]. An extremely large number of reviews, summaries, monographs, and perspectives have been published over the past decade that have described all aspects of the therapeutic advancements resulting from these newer macrolides. Although even a partial list of these published reviews is too numerous to cite individually, the reader is directed to several of the following chapters in this book that will provide recent additional information about these important newer antimicrobial agents.

Semi-synthetic derivatives of 16-membered macrolides

In addition to the substantial progress that has been accomplished with all of the semi-synthetic derivatives of erythromycin, some important and successful efforts also should be mentioned regarding the discovery of new semi-synthetic derivatives of 16-membered macrolide antibiotics. For human medicine, the two most important semi-synthetic 16-membered macrolides are miocamycin and rokitamycin (Fig. 2). Miocamycin (also spelled miokamycin) is the 9,3"-di-O-acetyl derivative of midecamycin A_1, one of the naturally occurring components produced during the fermentation of *Streptomyces mycarofaciens* [41]. Rokitamycin is the 3"-O-propionyl derivative of leucomycin A_5, which is another component of the leucomycin complex (kitasamycin) that was originally produced from fermentation of *Streptomyces kitasatoensis* [42]. Both compounds exhibit many favorable features that are similar to other macrolides, such as efficacy against susceptible microorganisms, good tissue concentrations, oral bioavailability, and patient tolerability [43–47].

Although veterinary antibiotics are not covered extensively in this book, analogous advances have occurred with veterinary macrolides. Aivlosin (3-O-acetyl-4"-O-isovaleryltylosin, Fig. 3) showed activity against certain tylosin-resistant strains of bacteria and *Mycoplasma* and gave higher serum concentrations of antibiotic from oral administration of comparable doses [48, 49]. Tilmicosin (Fig. 3) is a second semi-synthetic derivative of tylosin that has significantly improved control or treatment of bovine respiratory diseases caused by *Pasteurella haemolytica* when administered *via* a single subcutaneous injection to cattle; applications have been extended more recently to the control of respiratory diseases by oral administration to swine and poultry [50–55]. Analogous to many other macrolides, the efficacy of tilmicosin may be attributed partially to its high intracellular accumulation, prolonged tissue concentrations, and long *in vivo* bioavailability; its intriguing anti-inflammatory effects also may contribute significantly to its beneficial *in vivo* activity [56–59]. A new series of derivatives of tylosin has been prepared more recently during a medicinal chemistry program designed to optimize activity against *Pasteurella* species for the treatment of bovine respiratory disease, but no results from field trials have been reported yet [60–62]. In addition to these semi-synthetic derivatives of tylosin, another important recent veterinary development is the recognition of the bacterium *Lawsonia intracellularis* as the causative agent of an infectious disease in pigs called porcine proliferative enteropathy (PPE; also called ileitis) and the demonstration of efficacy of tylosin against this disease [63, 64]. These recent advancements involving veterinary macrolides have paralleled closely the advances recorded for macrolides used in human medicine.

The ketolide era

Despite the many significant improvements in various features of macrolides that have resulted from the newer semi-synthetic derivatives described above, these compounds have all exerted their antimicrobial activity by the same general mechanism of action as their parent macrolides, although some differences have been well documented between 14- and 16-membered macrolides. However, when microbial resistance to erythromycin has developed, all derivatives of erythromycin generally have exhibited cross-resistance with their parent antibiotic [65]. Consequently, the recent heightened concerns about microbial resistance to antibiotics also have included the macrolides [65–68].

Because of this high concern about microbial resistance, the initial report describing a new macrolide series having activity against certain strains of bacteria resistant to the conventional macrolide-lincosamide-streptogramin B (MLS_B) group of antibiotics generated a substantial amount of interest and subsequent research effort [69]. This new group of semi-synthetic derivatives was termed "ketolides" because they are prepared from erythromycin by first removing the neutral sugar (cladinose) normally found on the 3-hydroxyl group and then oxidizing the 3-hydroxyl group to a ketone (Fig. 5) [70, 71]. Since these initial reports, efforts have continued both at Hoechst-Marion-Roussel and at other pharmaceutical companies to synthesize new members of the ketolide series [72–74]. In addition to ketolides, several other new series of erythromycin derivatives also have been synthesized and evaluated in the ongoing effort to discover and develop new macrolide antibiotics possessing even more improved features than presently available agents [23, 72–76]. Subsequent chapters in this book will present further recent information and updates on the progress that has been made in the discovery and development of the ketolide family of macrolides.

Future directions and expectations

Medicinal chemistry programs involving synthesis and evaluation of new macrolide derivatives most likely will continue in order to meet the increasing medical need for new antibiotics. These studies of structure-activity relationships will be increasingly coupled to modern tools such as computational chemistry, x-ray crystallography, high-resolution NMR spectroscopy, and molecular modeling, which are becoming even more useful as knowledge increases about molecular details of the interactions between macrolides and the macromolecular entities involved in the mechanisms of biological activity and microbial resistance [77–81]. Knowledge about the molecular details involved in the biosynthesis of macrolides and resistance in antibiotic-producing microorganisms is expanding also [82–84]. This understanding of the molecular and genetic details of the biosynthetic pathways by which macrolides are formed is being applied rapidly to learning techniques to manipulate and alter those biosynthetic pathways [84–89]. As a result of such genetic engineering of the macrolide biosynthetic processes, new macrolide structures are emerging now, many of which are not readily accessible by conventional methodology. The possibility of generating very large numbers of new macrolides by harnessing all available permutations and combinations of structural variability is being pursued vigorously, a technology termed combinatorial biosynthesis [87–89]. If successful, these new technologies will provide medicinal chemists with a prolific wealth of novel starting materials for even further structural modifications.

The increasing attention being paid to the development and spread of microbial resistance has now clearly fostered a heightened awareness that not only are new antimicrobial agents needed but also that all antibiotics must be used worldwide in an optimum manner that maintains their medical value and extends their useful lifetimes as long as possible [90–92]. A large number of studies, analyses, and opinions are now being published that seek to address various aspects of this critical issue and to offer possible solutions. These trends will certainly increase as new strategies continually evolve and are refined to maximize the current and future antibiotic arsenal.

Although it has long been recognized that macrolide antibiotics exhibit a number of intriguing biological effects in addition to their excellent antimicrobial activities [93, 94], substantial progress has been made recently in further understanding some of these apparently independent effects. The first successful example was the separation of the gastrointestinal prokinetic effects of erythromycin from its antimicrobial activity, a saga that has led to the motilide family, such as EM-574, GM-611, and ABT-229 [95–97]. The unrecognized, but critical, infectious role played by *Helicobacter pylori* in gastritis and other gastrointestinal disorders and the therapeutic contributions of the newer macrolides represent another important expansion of the utility of macrolide antibiotics into non-traditional applications.

Macrolides are well known to penetrate a variety of cells and to achieve high intracellular concentrations, a topic discussed in more detail in the chapter by Dr. Labro. Uptake of macrolides into microbial cells is obviously critical if the antibiotics are to reach their antimicrobial target and destroy or cripple microorganisms. The effective intracellular penetration of macrolides into host cells is also clearly essential for activity against many intracellular pathogens. In addition to causing cidal or static effects on microorganisms, macrolides also can exert effects at sub-MIC concentrations on important pathogenic processes such as microbial virulence and adhesion or colonization [18, 98]. Macrolides also interact with cells involved with the host's immune defense system and modulate those activities in a wide variety of ways [99, 100].

The recent flurry of publications concerning anti-inflammatory effects of macrolides and their effects on cytokines and pro-inflammatory mediators have brought this field into greater recent prominence [100–103]. Further research and exploration of this area eventually may produce beneficial effects on such disorders as diffuse panbronchiolitis, asthma, and atherosclerosis, as well as diminishing the inflammatory effects coincident with infectious diseases [59, 101–107]. Positive effects of macrolides on certain tumors *in vitro* and in rodent studies, which may result from immunomodulatory effects [108, 109], also have been reported. More extensive research on all of these intriguing biological activities potentially may lead to novel additional therapeutic applications for the macrolides and thereby increase the therapeutic utility of this class of agents.

References

1 Bryskier AJ, Butzler J-P, Neu HC, Tulkens PM (eds) (1993) *Macrolides: chemistry, pharmacology and clinical uses.* Arnette Blackwell, Paris

2 Steigbigel NH (1995) Macrolides and clindamycin. In: GL Mandell, JE Bennett, R Dolin (eds): *Principles and practice of infectious diseases.* Churchill Livingstone, New York, 334–346

3 Finch RG (1997) Overview of the clinical use of macrolides and streptogramins. In: SH Zinner, LS Young, JF Acar, HC Neu (eds): *Expanding indications for the new macrolides, azalides, and streptogramins.* Marcel Dekker, New York, 3–26

4 McGuire JM, Bunch RL, Anderson RC, Boaz HE, Flynn EH, Powell HM, Smith JW (1952) "Ilotycin," a new antibiotic. *Antibiot & Chemother* 2: 281–284

5 Harris DR, McGeachin SG, Mills HH (1965) The structure and stereochemistry of erythromycin A. *Tetrahedron Lett* 679–685

6 Washington JA II, Wilson WR (1985) Erythromycin: a microbial and clinical perspective after 30 years of clinical use (part I). *Mayo Clin Proc* 60: 189–203

7 Washington JA II, Wilson WR (1985) Erythromycin: a microbial and clinical perspective after 30 years of clinical use (part II). *Mayo Clin Proc* 60: 271–278

8 Kirst HA (1992) Antibiotics (macrolides). In: M Howe-Grant (ed): *Kirk-Othmer encyclopedia of chemical technology*, 4th edition, John Wiley & Sons, New York, 169–213

9 Nakayama I (1984) Macrolides in clinical practice. In: S Omura (ed): *Macrolide antibiotics: chemistry, biology, and practice.* Academic Press, Orlando, FL, 261–300

10 Kirst HA (1994) Semi-synthetic derivatives of 16-membered macrolide antibiotics. In: GP Ellis, DK Luscombe (eds): *Prog Med Chem* 31: 265–295

11 Osono T, Oka Y, Watanabe S, Numazaki Y, Moriyama K, Ishida H, Suzaki K, Okami Y, Umezawa H (1967) A new antibiotic, josamycin. *J Antibiot* (Ser. A) 20: 174–180

12 Omura S, Hironaka Y, Hata T (1970) Chemistry of leucomycin. IX. Identification of leucomycin A_3 with josamycin. *J Antibiot* 23: 511–513

13 Omura S, Nakagawa A, Neszmelyi A, Gero SD, Sepulchre AM, Piriou F, Lukacs G (1975) Carbon-13 nuclear magnetic resonance spectral analysis of 16-membered macrolide antibiotics. *J Am Chem Soc* 97: 4001–4009

14 Rubinstein E, Keller N (1998) Spiramycin renaissance. *J Antimicrob Chemother* 42: 572–576
15 Carbon C (1993) Clinical efficacy and place of spiramycin in the treatment of acute respiratory-tract infections. *Drug Investigation* 6: 35–42
16 Davey P, Pechere J-C, Speller D (eds) (1988) Spiramycin reassessed. *J Antimicrob Chemother* 22 (Suppl B)
17 Prescott JF, Baggot JD (eds) (1993) *Antimicrobial therapy in veterinary medicine*. Iowa State University Press, Ames, IA
18 Kirst HA (1997) Macrolide antibiotics in food-animal health. *Exp Opin Invest Drugs* 6: 103–117
19 Wilson RC (1984) Macrolides in veterinary practice. In: S. Omura (ed): *Macrolide antibiotics: chemistry, biology, and practice*. Academic Press, Orlando, FL, 301–347
20 Omura S, Matsubara H, Nakagawa A, Furusaki A, Matsumoto T (1980) X-ray crystallography of protylonolide and absolute configuration of tylosin. *J Antibiot* 33: 915–917
21 Jones ND, Chaney MO, Kirst HA, Wild GM, Baltz RH, Hamill RL, Paschal JW (1982) Novel fermentation products from *Streptomyces fradiae*: X-ray crystal structure of 5-O-mycarosyltylactone and proof of the absolute configuration of tylosin. *J Antibiot* 35: 420–425
22 Somogyi AA, Bochner F, Hetzel D, Williams DB (1995) Evaluation of the intestinal-absorption of erythromycin in man. *Pharmaceut Res* 12: 149–154
23 Kirst HA (1993) Semi-synthetic derivatives of erythromycin. In: GP Ellis, DK Luscombe (eds): *Prog Med Chem* 30: 57–88
24 Murphy HW (1953) Esters of erythromycin. In: *Antibiotics Annual 1953–1954*. Medical Encyclopedia Inc., New York, 500–513
25 Stephens VC, Conine JW, Murphy HW (1959) Esters of erythromycin IV. *J Amer Pharm Assoc* 48: 620–622
26 Griffith RS (1986) Pharmacology of erythromycin in adults. *Pediatric Infect Dis* 5: 130–140
27 Steffansen B, Bundgaard H (1989) Erythromycin prodrugs: kinetics of hydrolysis of erythromycin and various erythromycin 2'-esters in aqueous solution and human plasma. *Int J Pharmaceutics* 56: 159–168
28 Taskinen J, Ottoila P (1988) Hydrolysis of 2'-esters of erythromycin. *J Antimicrob Chemother* 21 (Suppl D): 1–8
29 Tardrew PL, Mao JHC, Kenney D (1969) Antibacterial activity of 2'-esters of erythromycin. *Appl Microbiol* 18: 159–165
30 Kurath P, Jones PH, Egan RS, Perun TJ (1971) Acid degradation of erythromycin A and erythromycin B. *Experientia* 27: 362
31 Cachet Th, Van den Mooter G, Hauchecorne R, Vinckier C, Hoogmartens J (1989) Decomposition kinetics of erythromycin-A in acidic aqueous solutions. *Int J Pharmaceut* 55: 59–65
32 Vinckier C, Hauchecorne R, Cachet Th, Van den Mooter G, Hoogmartens J (1989) A new mechanism for the decomposition of erythromycin-A in acidic aqueous solutions. *Int J Pharmaceut* 55: 67–76
33 Slawinski W, Bojarska-Dahlig H, Glabski T, Dziegielewska I, Biedrzycki M, Naperty S (1975) The structure of erythromycin A cyclic carbonate. *Rec Trav Chim Pays-Bas* 94: 236–238
34 Bojarska-Dahlig H (1989) Chemical modifications of the macrolide antibiotics. *Prog Indust Microbiol* 27: 299–314
35 Alvarez-Elcoro S, Enzler MJ (1999) The macrolides: erythromycin, clarithromycin, and azithromycin. *Mayo Clin Proc* 74: 613–634
36 Carbon C, Poole MD (1999) The role of newer macrolides in the treatment of community-acquired respiratory tract infection. A review of experimental and clinical data. *J Chemother* 11: 107–118
37 McConnell SA, Amsden GW (1999) Review and comparison of advanced-generation macrolides clarithromycin and dirithromycin. *Pharmacother* 19: 404–415
38 Boswell FJ, Wise R (1998) Advances in the macrolides and quinolones. *Infect Dis Clin North America* 12: 647–670
39 Carbon C (1998) Pharmacodynamics of macrolides, azalides, and streptogramins: effect on extracellular pathogens. *Clin Infect Dis* 27: 28–32
40 Amsden GW (1995) Macrolides versus azalides: a drug interaction update. *Ann Pharmacother* 29: 906–917
41 Omoto S, Iwamatsu K, Inouye S, Niida T (1976) Modifications of a macrolide antibiotic midecamycin (SF-837). *J Antibiot* 29: 536–548

42 Sakakibara H, Okekawa O, Fujiwara T, Otani M, Omura S (1981) Acyl derivatives of 16-membered macrolides. *J Antibiot* 34: 1001–1010

43 Holliday SM, Faulds D (1993) Miocamycin. *Drugs* 46: 720–745

44 Prous JR (ed) (1983) Miokamycin. *Drugs of the Future* 8: 790–792

45 Zhao XJ, Koyama E, Ishizaki T (1999) An *in vitro* study on the metabolism and possible drug interactions of rokitamycin, a macrolide antibiotic, using human liver microsomes. *Drug Metab Dispos* 27: 776–785

46 Benoni G, Cuzzolin L, Puchetti V, Bertrand C, Calvelli C, Mocella S, Fonio W, Mornatti R, Parini J (1992) Rokitamycin plasma kinetics and penetration into bronchial secretions in adult bronchitis patients. *Curr Ther Res* 52: 600–607

47 Prous JR (ed) (1985) TMS-19Q. *Drugs of the Future* 10: 486–489

48 Tsuchiya M, Sawa T, Takeuchi T, Umezawa H, Okamoto R (1982) Binding of 3-O-acetyl-4"-O-isovaleryltylosin to ribosomes from a macrolide-resistant strain of *Staphylococcus aureus. J Antibiot* 35: 673–679

49 Okamoto R, Tsuchiya M, Nomura H, Iguchi H, Kiyoshima K, Hori S, Inui T, Sawa T, Takeuchi T, Umezawa H (1980) Biological properties of new acyl derivatives of tylosin. *J Antibiot* 33: 1309–1315

50 Kirst HA (1996) Expanding the role of macrolide compounds as therapeutic agents. In: M Iqbal Choudhary (ed): *Progress in medicinal chemistry*, Vol 1, Harwood Academic Publishers, Amsterdam, 1–47

51 Vogel GJ, Laudert SB, Zimmermann A, Guthrie CA, Mechor GD, Moore GM (1998) Effects of tilmicosin on acute undifferentiated respiratory tract disease in newly arrived feedlot cattle. *J Am Vet Med Assoc* 212: 1919–1924

52 Huwyler U, Reeve-Johnson L, Korfitsen J, Liesegang A, Wanner M (1999) Efficacy evaluation of the use of oral tilmicosin in pneumonic calves. *Schweiz Arch Tierheilk* 141: 203–208

53 Moore GM, Basson RP, Tonkinson LV (1996) Clinical field trials with tilmicosin phosphate in feed for the control of naturally acquired pneumonia caused by *Actinobacillus pleuropneumoniae* and *Pasteurella multocida* in swine. *Am J Vet Res* 57: 224–228

54 Charleston B, Gate JJ, Aitken IA, Reeve-Johnson L (1998) Assessment of the efficacy of tilmicosin as a treatment for *Mycoplasma gallisepticum* infections in chickens. *Avian Pathol* 27: 190–195

55 Jordan FTW, Forrester CA, Hodge A, Reeve-Johnson LG (1999) The comparison of an aqueous preparation of tilmicosin with tylosin in the treatment of *Mycoplasma gallisepticum* infection of turkey poults. *Avian Diseases* 43: 521–525

56 Modric S, Webb AI, Derendorf H (1998) Pharmacokinetics and pharmacodynamics of tilmicosin in sheep and cattle. *J Vet Pharmacol Therap* 21: 444–452

57 Scorneaux B, Shryock TR (1999) Intracellular accumulation, subcellular distribution, and efflux of tilmicosin in bovine mammary, blood, and lung cells. *J Dairy Sci* 82: 1202–1212

58 Scorneaux B, Shryock TR (1999) The determination of the cellular volume of avian, porcine and bovine phagocytes and bovine mammary epithelial cells and its relationship to uptake of tilmicosin. *J Vet Pharmacol Therap* 22: 6–12

59 Chin AC, Morck DW, Merrill JK, Ceri H, Olson ME, Read RR, Dick P, Buret AG (1998) Anti-inflammatory benefits of tilmicosin in calves with *Pasteurella haemolytica*-infected lungs. *Am J Vet Res* 59: 765–771

60 McFarland JW, Hecker SJ, Jaynes BH, Jefson MR, Lundy KM, Vu CB, Glazer EA, Froshauer SA, Hayashi SF, Kamicker BJ, Reese CP, Olson JA (1997) Repromicin derivatives with potent antibacterial activity against *Pasteurella multocida. J Med Chem* 40: 1041–1045

61 Norcia LJL, Seibel SB, Kamicker BJ, Lemay MA, Lilley SC, Hecker SJ, Bergeron JM, Retsema JA, Hayashi SF (1998) *In vitro* microbiological characterization of novel macrolide CP-163,505 for animal health specific use. *J Antibiot* 51: 136–144

62 Linhares MC, Harran LP, Strelevitz TJ, Gauthier JW, Cole MJ, Hassfurther RL, Risk JE (1998) Disposition and metabolism of the novel macrolide antibiotic CP-163505 in cattle. *J Vet Pharmacol Therap* 21: 99–106

63 McOrist S, Morgan J, Veenhuizen MF, Lawrence K, Kroger HW (1997) Oral administration of tylosin phosphate for treatment and prevention of proliferative enteropathy in pigs. *Am J Vet Res* 58: 136–139

64 Moore GM, Mowrey DH, Veenhuizen MF, Watkins LE (1998) Evaluating a natural outbreak of porcine proliferative enteropathy and treatment with tylosin in the grow-finish phase. *Swine Health Production* 6: 67–72
65 Weisblum B (1998) Macrolide resistance. *Drug Resistance Updates* 1: 29–41
66 Virk A, Steckelberg JM (2000) Clinical aspects of antimicrobial resistance. *Mayo Clin Proc* 75: 200–214
67 Moellering RC Jr (1998) Emerging resistance with gram-positive aerobic infections: Where do we go from here? *Clin Infect Dis* 26: 1177–1178
68 Mitscher LA (1999) Introduction to special issue on multiple drug resistance. *Med Res Rev* 19: 475–476
69 Agouridas C, Bonnefoy A, Chantot JF (1994) Ketolides, a new distinct semi-synthetic class of macrolides: *in vitro* and *in vivo* antibacterial activity. Book of Abstracts of the 34th Intersci Conf Antimicrob Agents Chemother, Oct. 4–7. 1994, Orlando, FL, abstr. F-168, American Society for Microbiology, Washington, D.C.
70 Agouridas C, Benedetti Y, Denis A, Fromentin C, Gouin D'Ambrieres S, Le Martret O, Chantot JF (1994) Ketolides, a new distinct semi-synthetic class of macrolides. Book of Abstracts of the 34th Intersci Conf Antimicrob Agents Chemother, Oct. 4–7. 1994, Orlando, FL, abstr. F-164, American Society for Microbiology, Washington, D.C.
71 Agouridas C, Denis A, Auger JM, Benedetti Y, Bonnefoy A, Bretin F, Chantot JF, Dussarat A, Fromentin C, et al (1998) Synthesis and antibacterial activity of ketolides (6-O-methyl-3-oxoerythromycin derivatives): a new class of antibacterials highly potent against macrolide-resistant and -susceptible respiratory pathogens. *J Med Chem* 41: 4080–4100
72 Kaneko T, McArthur H, Sutcliffe J (2000) Recent developments in the area of macrolide antibiotics. *Exp Opin Ther Patents* 10: 403–425
73 Chu DTW (1999) Recent progress in novel macrolides, quinolones, and 2-pyridones to overcome bacterial resistance. *Med Res Rev* 19: 497–520
74 Chu DTW (1999) Recent developments in macrolides and ketolides. *Curr Opin Microbiol* 2: 467–474
75 Kirst HA (1998) Recent developments with macrolide antibiotics. *Exp Opin Ther Patents* 8: 111–120
76 Chu DTW (1995) Recent developments in 14- and 15-membered macrolides. *Exp Opin Invest Drugs* 4: 65–94
77 Hansen LH, Mauvais P, Douthwaite S (1999) The macrolide-ketolide antibiotic binding site is formed by structures in domains II and V of 23S ribosomal RNA. *Molec Microbiol* 31: 623–631
78 Bertho G, Gharbi-Benarous J, Delaforge M, Lang C, Parent A, Girault JP (1998) Conformational analysis of ketolide conformations of RU 004 in solution and bound to bacterial ribosomes. *J Med Chem* 41: 3373–3386
79 Bertho G, Ladam P, Gharbi-Benarous J, Delaforge M, Girault JP (1998) Solution conformation of methylated macrolide antibiotics roxithromycin and erythromycin using NMR and molecular modelling. *Int J Biol Macromol* 22: 103–127
80 Montenez JP, Van Bambeke F, Piret J, Brasseur R, Tulkens PM, Mingeot-Leclercq MP (1999) Interactions of macrolide antibiotics (erythromycin A, roxithromycin, erythromycylamine [dirithromycin], and azithromycin) with phospholipids: computer-aided conformational analysis on acellular and cell culture models. *Toxicol Appl Pharmacol* 156: 129–140
81 Mordi MN, Pelta MD, Boote V, Morris GA, Barber J (2000) Acid-catalyzed degradation of clarithromycin and erythromycin B: a comparative study using NMR spectroscopy. *J Med Chem* 43: 467–474
82 Cundliffe E (1999) Organization and control of the tylosin-biosynthetic genes of *Streptomyces fradiae*. *Actinomycetologica* 13: 68–75
83 Hopwood DA (1997) Genetic contributions to understanding polyketide synthases. *Chem Rev* 97: 2465–2497
84 Khosla C, Gokhale RS, Jacobsen JR, Cane DE (1999) Tolerance and specificity of polyketide synthases. *Annu Rev Biochem* 68: 219–253
85 Brown MS, Dirlam JP, McArthur HAI, McCormick EL, Morse BK, Murphy PA, O'Connell TN, Pacey M, Rescek DM , Ruddock J, Wax RG (1999) Production of 6-deoxy-13-cyclopropyl-erythromycin B by *Saccharopolyspora erythraea* NRRL 18643. *J Antibiot* 52: 742–747

86 Arisawa A, Tsunekawa H (2001) Direct fermentative production of acyltylosins by genetically engineered strains of *Streptomyces fradiae*. In: HA Kirst, W-K Yeh, M Zmijewski (eds): *Enzyme technologies for pharmaceutical and biotechnological applications*, Marcel Dekker, New York; 89–111

87 Katz L, McDaniel R (1999) Novel macrolides through genetic engineering. *Med Res Rev* 19: 543–558

88 McDaniel RN, Khosla C (2001) Understanding and exploiting bacterial polyketide synthases. In: HA Kirst, W-K Yeh, M Zmijewski (eds): *Enzyme technologies for pharmaceutical and biotechnological applications*, Marcel Dekker, New York; 397–426

89 Weissman KJ, Staunton J (2001) Polyketide synthases: analysis and use in synthesis. In: HA Kirst, W-K Yeh, M Zmijewski (eds): *Enzyme technologies for pharmaceutical and biotechnological applications*, Marcel Dekker, New York; 427–470

90 Polk R (1999) Optimal use of modern antibiotics: emerging trends. *Clin Infect Dis* 29: 264–274

91 Schentag JJ (1999) Antimicrobial action and pharmacokinetics/pharmacodynamics: the use of AUIC to improve efficacy and avoid resistance. *J Chemother* 11: 426–439

92 Burke JP, Pestotnik SL (1999) Antibiotic use and microbial resistance in intensive care units: impact of computer-assisted decision support. *J Chemother* 11: 530–535

93 Kirst H (1991) New macrolides: expanded horizons for an old class of antibiotics. *J Antimicrob Chemother* 28: 787–790

94 Bryskier A, Agouridas C, Chantot J-F (1994) New medical targets for macrolides. *Exp Opin Invest Drugs* 3: 405–410

95 Funabashi Y, Maeshiba Y, Inatomi N, Tanayama S, Harada S, Itoh Z, Omura S (1996) Bioactive metabolites of EM574 and EM523, erythromycin derivatives having strong gastrointestinal motor stimulating activity. *J Antibiot* 49: 794–801

96 Clark MJ, Wright T, Bertrand PP, Bornstein JC, Jenkinson KM, Verlinden M, Furness JB (1999) Erythromycin derivatives ABT 229 and GM 611 act on motilin receptors in the rabbit duodenum. *Clin Exp Pharmacol Physiol* 26: 242–245

97 Khiat A, Boulanger Y (1998) Identification of the motilide pharmacophore using quantitative structure activity relationships. *J Peptide Res* 52: 321–328

98 Shryock TR, Mortensen JE, Baumholtz M (1998) The effects of macrolides on the expression of bacterial virulence mechanisms. *J Antimicrob Chemother* 41: 505–512

99 Van Vlem B, Vanholder R, De Paepe P, Vogelaers D, Ringoir S (1996) Immunomodulating effects of antibiotics: literature review. *Infection* 24: 275–291

100 Khan AA, Slifer TR, Araujo FG, Remington JS (1999) Effect of clarithromycin and azithromycin on production of cytokines by human monocytes. *Int J Antimicrob Agents* 11: 121–132

101 Labro M-T (1998) Immunological effects of macrolides. *Curr Opin Infect Dis* 11: 681–688

102 Wales D, Woodhead M (1999) The anti-inflammatory effects of macrolides. *Eur Respir J* 12: 57–63

103 Ianaro A, Ialenti A, Maffia P, Sautebin L, Rombola L, Carnuccio R, Iuvone T, D'Acquisto F, Di Rosa M (2000) Anti-inflammatory activity of macrolide antibiotics. *J Pharmacol Exp Therapeut* 292: 156–163

104 Howe RA, Spencer RC (1997) Macrolides for the treatment of *Pseudomonas aeruginosa* infections? *J Antimicrob Chemother* 40: 153–155

105 Nakamura H, Fujishima S, Inoue T, Ohkubo Y, Soejima K, Waki Y, Mori M, Urano T, Sakamaki F, Tasaka S et al (1999) Clinical and immunoregulatory effects of roxithromycin therapy for chronic respiratory tract infection. *Eur Respir J* 13: 137–1379

106 Shoji T, Yoshida S, Sakamoto H, Hasegawa H, Nakagawa H, Amayasu H (1999) Anti-inflammatory effect of roxithromycin in patients with aspirin-intolerant asthma. *Clin Exp Allergy* 29: 950–956

107 Cook PJ (1999) Antimicrobial therapy for *Chlamydia pneumoniae*: its potential role in atherosclerosis and asthma. *J Antimicrob Chemother* 44: 145–148

108 Sassa K, Mizushima Y, Fujishita T, Oosaki R, Kobayashi M (1999) Therapeutic effect of clarithromycin on a transplanted tumor in rats. *Antimicrob Agents Chemother* 43: 67–72

109 Hamada K, Mikasa K, Yunou Y, Kurioka T, Majima T, Narita N, Kita E (2000) Adjuvant effect of clarithromycin on chemotherapy for murine lung cancer. *Chemother* 46: 49–61

Macrolide Antibiotics
ed. by W. Schönfeld and H. A. Kirst

Macrolides: a clinical overview

Vito R. Iacoviello and Stephen H. Zinner

Harvard Medical School, Mount Auburn Hospital, 330 Mount Auburn Street, Cambridge, MA 02238, USA

The macrolide antibiotics have played an important role in the therapy of infectious diseases for many decades. Newer formulations have expanded the spectrum of activity, improved tissue penetration, and improved patient acceptance and compliance with reduced side effects and simpler, more convenient dosing regimens. In this chapter we will provide a brief review of some key clinical aspects of the macrolides, including spectrum of activity, emergence of resistance, clinical uses, tolerability and toxicity, pharmacologic considerations for the clinician, and the expanding data regarding the anti-inflammatory properties of the macrolides and their ability to modify selected bacterial virulence factors. Our comments will focus on erythromycin, clarithromycin, azithromycin, and roxithromycin.

Erythromycin remains highly active against group A, beta-hemolytic streptococci (*Streptococcus pyogenes*), penicillin-sensitive *Streptococcus pneumoniae*, and other beta-hemolytic streptococcal strains including groups B, C, F, and G. It is active against most strains of methicillin-sensitive *Staphylococcus aureus, N. meningitidis, N. gonorrhoeae, Bordetella pertussis, Campylobacter jejuni, Treponema pallidum, Ureaplasma urealyticum, Mycoplasma pneumoniae, Legionella pneumophila, Corynebacterium diphtheriae, Corynebacterium minutissimum, Listeria monocytogenes, Entamoeba histolytica*, chlamydia species, and some rickettsial species. It has only weak activity against *Haemophilus influenzae* [1, 2].

In general, clarithromycin expands the spectrum of erythromycin with improved activity against *Haemophilus influenzae* (if its 10-OH metabolite is considered), *Moraxella catarrhalis, Mycobacterium avium-intracellulare* (MAC), and other non-tuberculous or atypical mycobacteria. It has *in vitro* activity against *Toxoplasma gondii, Borrelia burgdorferi*, and *Babesia microti* [1, 3].

Azithromycin provides further expansion with improved activity against *Haemophilus influenzae, Legionella* species, atypical mycobacteria (except *M. leprae*), and probably provides expanded activity against a growing list of pathogens, including *Bartonella henselae, Rhodococcus equi, toxoplasma, cryptosporidium*, and *Plasmodium* species [1, 4–10].

Roxithromycin, like other newer macrolides, penetrates and accumulates within cells, making it much more effective against intracellular pathogens. It has some expanded activity spectrum compared with erythromycin. It has improved activity against *Moraxella catarrhalis*, *Haemophilus* species, *Pasteurella* species, *Eikenella corrodens*, MAC and other atypical mycobacteria, *Mycobacterium leprae* (in the mouse foot pad model), *Rickettsia rickettsii* and *R. conorii*, *Borrelia burgdorferi*, toxoplasma, and cryptosporidium [11, 12, 13].

As with all antibiotics presently in use around the world, resistance to the macrolides is increasing. The macrolides inhibit bacterial growth by interfering with protein synthesis at the level of the bacterial ribosome. As a group they are peptidyl transferase inhibitors. Resistance is acquired by one of three routes: modification of antimicrobial target, antimicrobial inactivation, or active efflux of the antimicrobial agent. In the vast majority of resistant strains, modification of the 23S ribosomal RNA by methylation results in a conformational change and reduced binding [14]. However, recent observations in the U.S. have shown that the efflux mechanism is an increasingly important cause of resistance among *Streptococcus pneumoniae* [15]. The prevalence of macrolide resistance in the U.S. and Europe doubled between 1992 and 1995 [14]. At our institution the rate of erythromycin resistance among all *Streptococcus pneumoniae* isolates was 14% in 1999.

Despite the emergence of resistance, the macrolides continue to be invaluable in the treatment of many infectious diseases, and the spectrum of use appears to be expanding as we gain new information and clinical experience with the newer agents. Erythromycin is the drug of choice for infections caused by *Mycoplasma pneumoniae* and *Legionella pneumophila* and for diphtheria, pertussis, bacillary angiomatosis, and *Chlamydia pneumoniae* pneumonia and conjunctivitis. Erythromycin remains an important alternative to penicillin for a vast array of infections. It has been used in the treatment of *Campylobacter* sp. diarrhea and as an alternative to tetracycline in the treatment of pelvic inflammatory disease in pregnant women [1, 2].

Clarithromycin is indicated in the treatment of acute upper and lower respiratory tract infections caused by susceptible organisms and for the treatment of mild to moderate skin and soft tissue infections. As part of combination therapy it is indicated for treatment of disseminated MAC in patients infected with human immunodeficiency virus (HIV) and has been shown recently to be superior to other macrolide-containing regimens with improved clearance of bacteremia. In addition, it is an important part of combination therapy in the treatment of MAC infections in non-HIV infected individuals as well as in combination therapy for the treatment of other atypical mycobacterial infections including *M. fortuitum*, *M. chelonae* and *M. leprae*. Clarithromycin has been used successfully in the treatment of *Helicobacter pylori* infections and may play a role in the treatment of toxoplasma infections, babesiosis, bacillary angiomatosis, and spirochetal infections. Clarithromycin is approved for use in pediatric patients with sinusitis, acute otitis media, pneumonia, group A streptococcal pharyngitis and tonsillitis, and streptococcal and staphylococcal skin infections. Clarithromycin should not be used during pregnancy [1, 3, 16].

The clinical uses of azithromycin continue to expand. Its spectrum of activity, high tissue and intracellular concentrations, once-a-day dosing, safety in pregnancy, and availability for the treatment of pediatric infections contribute to its usefulness. Azithromycin is indicated for the treatment of adults with the following infections caused by susceptible organisms:

- Acute bacterial exacerbations of chronic obstructive pulmonary disease;
- community acquired pneumonia due to *Chlamydia pneumoniae*, *Haemophilus influenzae*, *Mycoplasma pneumoniae* and *Streptococcus pneumoniae*;
- pharyngitis and tonsillitis caused by *Streptococcus pyogenes* as an alternative to first line therapy;
- uncomplicated skin and soft tissue infections caused by *Staphylococcus aureus*, *Streptococcus pyogenes*, and *Streptococcus agalactiae*;
- and urethritis and cervicitis due to *Chlamydia trachomatis* or *Neisseria gonorrhoeae* and *Haemophilus ducreyi* (chancroid) infections in men.

Azithromycin is also useful in the treatment of lymphogranuloma venereum, pelvic inflammatory disease (in combination with metronidazole), and intravenous treatment of hospitalized patients with mild to moderate pneumonia in areas without highly macrolide-resistant pneumococci. Hook and colleagues have reported that a single 1 g dose was effective in preventing syphilis in persons exposed to infected sexual partners [17]. In pediatric patients, azithromycin is approved for the treatment of acute otitis media, community acquired pneumonia due to the same organisms as in adults, and pharyngitis/tonsillitis as an alternative to first-line therapy [1, 4, 16, 18].

Chia and colleagues recently reported the successful use of azithromycin in the treatment of four patients with Cat-Scratch Disease [5]. Several groups have reported the use of azithromycin, often in combination with other drugs such as pyrimethamine, for the treatment of cerebral toxoplasmosis in AIDS, often in patients who were intolerant or did not respond to conventional therapy. Azithromycin's *in vitro* activity against *Toxoplasma gondii*, including the cyst form; its ability to accumulate within cells; and its wide range of activity against other opportunistic pathogens such as MAC, *Cryptosporidium parvum*, and *Pneumocystis carinii* make it useful in the treatment of patients with AIDS. However, in some studies the relapse rate was unacceptably high. Oral administration may not provide adequate levels and intravenous administration therefore may be necessary. At the present time azithromycin in cerebral toxoplasmosis in patients with AIDS should be used as salvage therapy for those who cannot tolerate or progress on standard therapy [6, 7, 8]. Hoque and colleagues reported the use of azithromycin in a 74-year-old male with continuous ambulatory peritoneal dialysis-associated peritonitis caused by *Rhodococcus equi* [10]. Azithromycin has been used successfully in the treatment of children with Mediterranean Spotted Fever caused by *Rickettsia conorii* [19]. Ferencz described the successful use of azithromycin in the treatment of ulceroglandular tularemia, and Elewski described the effectiveness of intermittent courses of azithromycin (5-day course twice a month) for inflammatory acne vulgaris [20, 21].

Girgis and colleagues described the use of azithromycin in a randomized trial with ciprofloxacin in 64 patients with typhoid fever in Egypt. All isolates demonstrated *in vitro* sensitivity to both agents. Both drugs were equally effective in curing the infection. Of note, the serum levels of azithromycin were below the minimum inhibitory concentration (MIC) of the organism, but the high intracellular concentration of azithromycin against this intracellular pathogen most likely played a role in its effectiveness [22]. Butler and colleagues reported the results of azithromycin versus chloramphenicol in 88 patients with typhoid fever (four patients in each group were excluded because of initial resistance to study drug). Both drugs were highly effective [23]. In areas with rising resistance to chloramphenicol and rising quinolone resistance, azithromycin may be an important drug in our armamentarium against *Salmonella typhi* and S. *paratyphi*. Additionally, it may be an important therapeutic option for the treatment of children and pregnant women with typhoid fever.

Malaria remains a major health problem with 300–500 million infections worldwide each year and growing rates of resistance. Taylor and colleagues described a double-blind, placebo-controlled trial of azithromycin prophylaxis against malaria in Indonesia, an area with high prevalence of malaria as well as high rates of resistance. Unfortunately the protection rate was only 71.6% against *Plasmodium falciparum* for azithromycin compared with 96.3% for doxycycline. It did demonstrate excellent protective efficacy against *Plasmodium vivax*, 96.3% versus 98% for doxycycline. More concerning was the sub-group analysis, which showed only 62.9% effectiveness in the sub-group that more closely resembled non-immune patients. At the present time, azithromycin cannot be considered an acceptable agent for prophylaxis against falciparum malaria [9].

Roxithromycin is indicated for the treatment of upper and lower respiratory tract infections, skin and soft tissue infections, urogenital infections, and orodental infections. It has demonstrated clinical efficacy rates of greater than 90% in the treatment of acute bronchitis; 70% to 96% in the treatment of tonsillitis/sinusitis; 83% to 89% for exacerbations of chronic bronchitis; and efficacy rates similar to amoxicillin/clavulinic acid, azithromycin, clarithromycin, cefaclor, and erythromycin in the treatment of pneumonia. Roxithromycin has shown clinical efficacy in comparative trials in the treatment of skin and soft tissue infections including erysipelas, orodental and odontological infections, and urogenital and gynecological infections. In combination with trimethoprim/ sulfamethoxazole, it is effective in the treatment of Lyme disease, and in combination with omeprazole and bismuth, it has been shown to be effective in the treatment of *Helicobacter pylori* infection. A pilot study demonstrated roxithromycin to be effective in the prevention of toxoplasmosis and pneumocystis infections in patients infected with HIV [24].

The role of *Chlamydia pneumoniae* in athersclerotic heart disease has received much attention. Roxithromycin was evaluated in a pilot study of 202 patients presenting with unstable angina. Patients were treated with conventional therapy and then randomized to receive 150 mg of roxithromycin twice daily or placebo for 30 days. There were reductions in clinical events at 30, 90, and 180 days, some of which reached statistical significance. The authors felt that treatment with roxithromycin appeared to reduce the incidence of reinfarction and death for at least six months following an ischaemic event [25]; however, longer follow-up studies are needed.

Table 1 summarizes the usual dosages of the macrolides in various clinical situations.

Table 1. Common macrolide dosages.

Preparation	**Pediatric**	**Adults**
Erythromycin ethylsuccinate	Mild-mod infections–30–50 mg/kg divided q6, 8, or 12 h Severe infections–60–100 mg/kg divided q6, 8, or 12 h	Usual–1600 mg/D divided q6, 8 or 12 h Severe infections–up to 4 g/D
Erythromycin stearate	Mild-mod infections–30–50 mg/kg divided q6, 8, or 12 h Severe infections–60–100 mg/kg divided q6, 8, or 12 h	Usual–250 q.i.d. or 500 b.i.d Severe infections–up to 4 g/D
Erythromycin base	Mild-mod infections–30–50 mg/kg divided q6, 8, or 12 h Severe infections–60–100 mg/kg divided q 6, 8, or 12 h	250–1000 mg q.i.d., depending on severity
Clarithromycin	15 mg/kg/D divided q 12 h	250–500 mg b.i.d
Azithromycin	Otitis media & community acquired pneumonia– 10 mg/kg/D (D 1); 5 mg/kg/D (D 2–5) Pharyngitis/tonsillitis–12 mg/kg/D	Mild-mod infections–500 mg (D 1); 250 mg (D2–5) Urethritis/cervicitis (*N. gonorrhoeae*)–2 g x 1 dose Chancroid, non-gonococcal urethritis, *Chlamydia trachomatis*–1 g x 1 dose Pneumonia–500 mg IV/PO 1–2 D then 500 QD to complete 7–10 D Pelvic inflammatory disease–500 mg IV/PO 1–2 D then 250 QD to complete 7 D MAC prophylaxis 1200 mg 1 x wk
Roxithromycin	5–8 mg/kg/D divided q 12 h	300 mg QD or 150 mg b.i.d

The major side effects associated with the use of erythromycin remain gastrointestinal and include nausea, vomiting, abdominal cramps, and diarrhea. Rare side effects include rash, eosinophilia, and agranulocytosis. The estolate form of erythromycin has been associated with cholestasis, hepatitis, and acute pancreatitis. Transient hearing loss has been associated with high doses of erythromycin in patients with impaired renal function. Ventricular tachycardia and QT_c prolongation have been observed with intravenous erythromycin [1, 2, 26]. Recently, the Centers for Disease Control and Prevention in the U.S. have reported a significantly increased risk of hypertrophic pyloric stenosis in infants associated with erythromycin therapy. This occurred among seven infants, aged 2–7 days, who received erythromycin as prophylaxis against pertussis. As there are no data to support alternatives to erythromycin in the prophylaxis of neonates exposed to pertussis, which may cause significant morbidity and mortality in infants, the report recommends that health care providers prescribe erythromycin with caution, carefully defining those patients who need prophylaxis, and inform parents about the risks of erythromycin and the signs of hypertrophic pyloric stenosis [27].

Side effects reported with clarithromycin, usually at a much lower rate than erythromycin, include nausea, abdominal pain, diarrhea, metallic taste, and headache. Leukopenia, liver function test abnormalities, and isolated cases of pancreatitis, hepatitis, and fulminant hepatic failure also have been reported [1, 3]. Azithromycin is associated with mild to moderate gastrointestinal side effects, and a case of intrahepatic cholestasis also has been reported [1, 4, 28]. Roxithromycin is also generally well-tolerated with an incidence of side effects of 4%; 75% to 80% of which are gastrointestinal. Rash is infrequently reported; there have been a few reports of cholestatic hepatitis and some case reports of agranulocytosis and fulminant acute hepatitis [24, 26, 29].

Dosage adjustments with renal and hepatic insufficiency differ somewhat among the macrolides. Erythromycin is primarily metabolized by the liver; however, if renal function is normal, then no dosage adjustments are recommended. There does appear to be an increased incidence of erythromycin-induced hearing loss in individuals with both renal and hepatic insufficiency. As with erythromycin, no dose adjustments are recommended for clarithromycin in patients with hepatic dysfunction as long as renal function is normal. In those with a creatinine clearance less than 30 cc/min, a 50% reduction in clarithromycin dosage is necessary. There is no suggested dosage adjustment for clarithromycin in patients undergoing dialysis. There are no recommended dosage adjustments for azithromycin in patients with renal or hepatic insufficiency. Roxithromycin requires no dosage adjustment for renal impairment, but a 50% dosage reduction is recommended for patients with severe hepatic insufficiency. The relation of roxithromycin to hearing loss is not clear [24, 30].

Pharmacologic interactions among simultaneously prescribed medications are a major concern and clearly may be associated with unpleasant as well as dangerous adverse drug events. Erythromycin is a potent inhibitor of the hepatic isoenzyme CYP3A. It has significant interactions with astemizole, carbamazepine, cisapride, cyclosporin, digoxin, disopyrimide, lovastatin, tacrolimus, terfenadine, theophylline, triazolam, and warfarin. Clarithromycin is also metabolized by the CYP3A system and has predictable effects when co-administered with the following drugs: 20% increase in theophylline levels, 350% increase in midazolam levels, 99% increase in rifabutin levels, 33% increase in cyclosporin levels, 300% increase in cisapride levels, and 77% increase in ritonavir levels. Azithromycin is not metabolized by the CYP3A system but is cleared by biliary excretion; therefore, these interactions are not predicted. Roxithromycin has very little CYP3A activity, and no significant interactions with theophylline or warfarin have been described [31].

An exciting area of the use of macrolides in clinical medicine is their potential role as anti-inflammatory agents as well as agents that alter bacterial virulence factors. It was recognized decades ago that erythromycin improved the status of patients with severe steroid-dependent asthma. Initially it was felt that part of this benefit was due to drug interactions with theophylline and a steroid sparing effect. However, recent data argue that direct effects on host-cell function contribute to this improvement. One of the most well-described and successful non-bacterial uses of erythromycin is in the treatment of diffuse pan-bronchiolitis (DPB). This illness is especially prevalent in Japan. It is a disease of adults characterized by chronic inflammation of the respiratory bronchioles with chronic inflammatory cell infiltration. Other such conditions where macrolides have shown clinical benefit include bronchiectasis, cystic fibrosis, atheroma, cancer, and arthritis [32].

The postulated mechanisms by which the macrolides exert their anti-inflammatory effects include reduced production of endothelin-1, a potent vasoconstrictor that also is postulated to stimulate mucus secretion and cause mucosal edema; inhibition of the neutrophil oxidative burst; inhibition of neutrophil chemotaxis; reduced production of interleukin (IL)-6, IL-8, and IL-1beta; reduced soluble intercellular adhesion molecules; reduced production of tumor necrosis factor (TNF) alpha; suppression of granulocyte-macrophage colony stimulating factor; and reduced production of defensin. The data leading to these proposals have been variable and at times contradictory. Varied results have been observed with different macrolides, different test systems, and different durations of drug exposure. In one animal model system, short-term use of macrolides led to enhanced immune responses, as measured by production of IL-1, IL-2, and TNF-alpha, while longer-term exposure led to decreased responses. Limited human studies revealed that five-day courses of erythromycin increased IL-1 alpha and TNF production by stimulated blood monocytes and that short course azithromycin (500 mg/day for 3 days) increased the amounts of IL-2 receptor after stimulation of mononuclear cells. In four patients with cystic fibrosis, four-week courses of erythromycin led to decreased IL-8 in sputum; in two patients individual post-treatment levels of IL-8 produced by IL-1beta-stimulated alveolar macrophages were lower than pre-treatment levels. In patients with diffuse pan-bronchiolitis, long term erythromycin use decreased the production of IL-1beta and IL-8 in bronchoalveolar lavage fluid [32, 33].

Equally exciting have been the effects of macrolides on bacterial virulence factors. Erythromycin reduces the adherence of *Moraxella catarrhalis* to ciliated epithelial cells at physiologically obtainable doses. Erythromycin also has been shown to decrease the adherence of *Neisseria meningitidis* as well as its ability to produce pili. Also, it interferes with the binding of fibronectin to *Staphylocacccus aureus*, the first step in adherence to host cells. Both *Streptococcus pneumoniae* and *Staphylococcus aureus* have shown decreased adherence to cells in the presence of erythromycin. Clarithromycin has been shown to impair the ability of *Bordetella pertussis* to adhere to human epithelial cells, postulated to be due to interference with adhesin production by the bacteria. It has also been shown to interfere with the adherence of *Staphylococcus aureus* to buccal mucosa cells. Azithromycin has been observed to decrease production of pili and attachment to epithelial cells by *Neisseria gonorrhoeae*. Azithromycin also decreases adherence of *Staphylococcus* sp. and *Escherichia coli* to buccal mucosa cells [34].

Of particular interest are the effects of the macrolides on *Pseudomonas aeruginosa*. It has been proposed that some of the beneficial effects seen in DPB and possibly much of the potential benefit in cystic fibrosis and bronchiectasis may be due to the actions of the macrolides on virulence factors of *P. aeruginosa*. There are two proposed mechanisms by which these events may take place: an effect on the immune system to modify the inflammatory response or a direct effect on the organism. The macrolides inhibit endotoxin A, total protease, elastase, phospholipase C, DNAase, lecithinase, gelatinase, lipase, pyocyanin and bacterial motility. Erythromycin reduces the adherence of pseudomonas to cilitated human epithelial cells and decreases pili production.

Of particular interest with pseudomonas are the effects the macrolides have on biofilm. Biofilm is an important virulence factor for pseudomonas, not only allowing attachment to respiratory epithelium but also providing a protective environment for the bacteria to evade host defenses and antibiotics. The macrolide effect is at least partially mediated by inhibition of alginate production. The results of further clinical trials of low-dose macrolides in the treatment of cystic fibrosis and bronchiectasis as well as other conditions complicated by chronic pseudomonas colonization and infection will be eagerly anticipated [32, 33, 34, 35].

The use of macrolides in clinical practice undoubtedly will continue to evolve. The activity of the newer agents with fewer side effects, fewer drug-drug interactions, more convenient dosing, and high intracellular concentrations will allow their use in an expanding spectrum of infectious diseases. Unfortunately, the emergence of resistance is also likely to continue and will require careful monitoring. Macrolides might become less effective in certain clinical conditions such as community acquired pneumonia caused by *Streptococcus pneumoniae* in areas of high penicillin and macrolide-resistance. We await with interest the potential expansion of macrolide use into other areas of clinical practice, both infectious and non-infectious, as we gather more data and knowledge concerning the role of macrolides as anti-inflammatory agents and modifiers of bacterial virulence factors.

References

1 Alvarez-Elcoro, S Enzler MJ (1999) The macrolides: erythromycin, clarithromycin, and azithromycin. *Mayo Clin Proc* 74: 613–634

2 Erythromycin (2000) In: *Physicians desk reference 54th edition.* Medical Economics Co., Inc., Montvale, NJ, 439–448

3 Clarithromycin (2000) In: *Physicians desk reference 54th edition.* Medical Economics Co., Inc., Montvale, NJ, 409–417

4 Azithromycin (2000) In: *Physicians desk reference 54th edition.* Medical Economics Co., Inc., Montvale, NJ, 2389–2399

5 Chia JK, Nakata MM, Lami JL, Park SS, Ding JC (1998) Azithromycin for the treatment of Cat-Scratch disease. *Clin Infect Dis* 26: 193–194

6 Wiselka MJ, Read R, Finch RG (1996) Response to oral and intravenous azithromycin in a patient with toxoplasma encephalitis and AIDS. *J Infect* 33: 227–229

7 Nasta P, Chiodera S (1997) Azithromycin for relapsing cerebral toxoplasmosis in AIDS. *AIDS* 11: 1188

8 Ramos JT, Saavedra J, Ruiz-Contreras J (1997) Cryptosporidium in patients infected with human immunodeficiency virus: azithromycin revisited. *J Pediatr* 130: 1009–1010

9 Taylor WRJ, Richie TL, Fryauff DJ, Picarima H, Ohrt C, Tang D, Braitman D, Murphy GS, Widjaja H, Tjitra E et al (1999) Malaria prophylaxis using azithromycin: a double-blind, placebo-controlled trial in Irian Jaya, Indonesia. *Clin Infect Dis* 28: 74–81

10 Hoque S, Weir A, Fluck R, Cunningham J (1996) Rhodococcus equi in CAPD-associated peritonitis treated with azithromycin. *Nephrol Dial Transplant* 11: 2340–2341

11 Bryskier A (1998) Roxithromycin: review of its antimicrobial activity. *J Antimicrob Chemother* 41(Suppl. B): 1–21

12 Uip DE, Lima AL, Amato VS, Boulos M, Neto VA, Bem David D (1998) Roxithromycin treatment of diarrhoea caused by *Cryptosporidium* spp. in patients with AIDS. *J Antimicrob Chemother* 41(Suppl B): 93–97

13 Durant J, Hazime F, Carles M, Pechere JC, Dellamonica P (1995) Prevention of *Pneumocystis carinii* pneumonia and of cerebral toxoplasmosis by roxithromycin in HIV-infected patients. *Infection* 23(Suppl 1): S33–S37

14 Boswell FJ, Wise R (1998) Advances in the macrolides and quinolones. *Infect Dis Clin North Am* 12: 647–670

15 Shortridge VD, Doern GV, Brueggmann AB, Beyer JM, Flamm RK (1999) Prevalence of macrolide resistance mechanisms in *Streptococcus pneumoniae isolates* from a multicenter antibiotic resistance surveillance study conducted in the United States in 1994–1995. *Clin Infect Dis* 29: 1186–1188

16 Wiedemann BL (1998) Macrolides: clarithromycin and azithromycin. *Pediatr Rev*; 19: 238–239

17 Hook EW, Stephens J, Ennis DM (1999) Azithromycin compared with penicillin G benzathine for treatment of incubating syphilis. *Ann Int Med* 131: 434–437

18 Morles CA, Hernandez I, Ferreiro MC (1997) Donovanosis: treatment with azithromycin. *International J STD & AIDS* 8: 54–56

19 Meloni G, Meloni T (1996) Azithromycin vs. doxycycline for Mediterranean Spotted Fever. *Pediatric Infect Dis* J 15: 1042–1044

20 Ferencz A (2000) Azithromycin in the therapy of ulceroglandular tularemia. In: SH Zinner, LS Young, JF Acar, C Ortiz-Neu (eds): *New considerations for macrolides, azalides, streptogramins, and ketolides.* Marcel Dekker, Inc., New York, 376–381.

21 Elewski BE (2000) Pulse azithromycin is effective in inflammatory acne vulgaris. In: SH Zinner, LS Young, JF Acar, C Ortiz-Neu (eds): *New considerations for macrolides, azalides, streptogramins, and ketolides.* Marcel Dekker, Inc., New York 362–366

22 Girgis NI, Brown FM, Tribble D, Butler T (2000) Randomized trial of azithromycin vs. ciprofloxacin for treatment of typhoid fever in Egypt. In: SH Zinner, LS Young, JF Acar, C Ortiz-Neu (eds): *New considerations for macrolides, azalides, streptogramins, and ketolides.* Marcel Dekker, Inc., New York, 336–340

23 Butler T, Sridhar CB, Daga MK, Pathak K, Pandit RB, Khakhria (2000) Treatment of typhoid fever in a randomized multicenter trial in India: a comparison of azithromycin and chloramphenicol. In: SH Zinner, LS Young, JF Acar, C Ortiz-Neu (eds): *New considerations for macrolides, azalides, streptogramins, and ketolides.*: Marcel Dekker, Inc., New York, 341–347

24 Markham A, Faulds D (1994) Roxithromycin, an update of its antimicrobial activity, pharmacokinetic properties and therapeutic use. *Drugs* 48: 297–326

25 Gurfinkel E, Bozovich G, Beck E, Testa E, Livellara B, Mautner B (1999) Treatment with the antibiotic roxithromycin in patients with acute non-Q-wave coronary syndromes. *Eur Heart* J 20: 121–127

26 Tanaka M, Tao T, Kaku K, Kaneko T (1995) Agranulocytosis induced by macrolide antibiotics. *Am J Hematol* 48: 133

27 Anonymous (1999) Hypertrophic pyloric stenosis in infants following pertussis prophylaxis with erythromycin-Knoxville Tennessee, MMWR 1999; 48: 1117–1120

28 Longo G, Valenti C, Gandini G, Ferrara L, Bertesi M, Emilia G (1997) Azithromycin-induced intrahepatic cholestasis. *Am J Med* 102: 217–218

29 Begue P, Astruc J (1995) The overall safety of oral roxithromycin in paediatric clinical studies. *Infection* 23(Suppl 1): S25–S27

30 Korzeniowski OM (2000) Macrolides, azalides, and streptogramins in patients with hepatic and renal failure. In: SH Zinner, LS Young, JF Acar, C Ortiz-Neu (eds): *New considerations for macrolides, azalides, streptogramins, and ketolides.* Marcel Dekker, Inc., New York, 45–52

31 Mole L (2000) Drug interactions with macrolides and related structures. In: SH Zinner, LS Young, JF Acar, C Ortiz-Neu (eds): *New considerations for macrolides, azalides, streptogramins, and ketolides.* Marcel Dekker, Inc., New York, 25–34

32 Wales D, Woodhead M (1998) The anti-inflammatory effects of macrolides. *Eur Respir J* 12: 57–63

33 Labro MT (1998) Anti-inflammatory activity of macrolides: a new therapeutic potential. *J Antimicrob Chemother* 41(Suppl B): 37–46

34 Shryock TR, Mortensen JE, Baumholtz M (1998) The effects of macrolides on the expression of bacterial virulence mechanisms. *J Antimicrob Chemother* 41: 505–512

35 Howe RA, Spencer RC (1997) Macrolides for the treatment of *Pseudomonas aeruginosa* infections. *J Antimicrob Chemother*; 40: 153–155

Macrolide Antibiotics
ed. by W. Schönfeld and H. A. Kirst

Pharmacokinetics/pharmacodynamics of macrolides

Holly M. Mattoes[1] and Charles H. Nightingale[1,2]

[1]Department of Pharmacy Research, [2]Office of Research Administration, Hartford Hospital, University of Connecticut, 80 Seymour Street, Hartford, CT 06102–5037, USA

Introduction

The macrolides are a class of antibiotics used to treat many different infections, and, in light of their excellent intracellular activity, they are especially important in the treatment of respiratory tract infections [1]. The pharmacokinetics and pharmacodynamics of macrolides differ dramatically from other antimicrobial agents [2]. Pharmacokinetics deals with the action of the drug in the body over a period of time, encompassing issues of absorption, distribution, metabolism, and elimination. Pharmacodynamics of antimicrobials is the study of the concentration of drug to which the bacteria is exposed as a function of time indexed to serum measurements of the drug's microbiological activity (minimum inhibitory concentration [MIC] or minimum bactericidal concentration [MBC]). The macrolide class began with erythromycin; however, its high side-effect profile, frequent dosing, and drug interactions make it a difficult drug to use clinically [1, 3, 4]. As a result, newer macrolides have been developed, and the newer macrolide/azalide drugs, azithromycin and clarithromycin, will be the focus of this chapter. Data on roxithromycin as well as the macrolides josamycin and spiramycin, which are more popular in Europe, also will be discussed.

Concentration-independent killing

Pharmacodynamically, a drug must achieve three goals before killing can occur. First, the antibiotic must bind to the specific binding site of the bacteria. Second, a certain number of binding sites must be occupied. Finally, the drug must remain at the binding site for a sufficient period of time [5]. For macrolides/azalides, killing seems to occur in a concentration-independent fashion, described by the pharmacodynamic parameter of time above the MIC (T > MIC). While there is some controversy about this point, most individuals from a clinical perspective consider, this class of agents to follow time-dependent killing [6].

Studies have shown that the time-dependent killing of macrolides relies on the amount of time that the bacteria are exposed to the antibiotic. This effect appears to be maximized when the serum drug concentration, measured as the area under the concentration *versus* time curve for plasma (AUC), approaches 2 to 4 times the

MIC value for the organism. Once this level is achieved, the rate of killing plateaus and the significance of any additional increase in serum drug concentration has a minimal effect, which generally can be ignored. Under these conditions, it is the time above the MIC that becomes the important component related to bacterial killing and optimal antibacterial activity in immunocompetent patients. Azithromycin's long post-antibiotic effect, lasting up to 4.7 hours for *Streptococcus pneumoniae*, and 8 hours for *Haemophilus influenzae*, provides for additional killing by extending the bactericidal effect when the serum concentrations of the drug fall below the MIC of the organism [7]. In studies utilizing *in vitro* and animal models, maximal killing for time-dependent antibacterials occurs when drug serum concentrations remain above the MIC for at least half of the dosing interval [8–11]. In neutropenic patients, the killing may require serum concentrations to exceed the MIC for 100% of the dosing interval [8, 9].

However, this theory of killing represents ideal situations. In some *in vivo* clinical situations, such as resistant strains of microorganisms whose MIC is increased, the extent of the serum concentration above the MIC (the AUC/MIC ratio) may become the more important determination of efficacy. The applicable pharmacodynamic parameters are a function of the drug's concentration-time profile (dose) and the susceptibility of the target microorganisms (MIC). Modifying doses or choosing particular microorganisms can result in pharmacodynamic parameters other than the T > MIC to predominate. For example, a study by Mazzei and colleagues found that in an *in vivo* thigh infection model in neutropenic mice and a mouse peritonitis model, erythromycin acted as a time-dependent killer, while clarithromycin demonstrated increased bacterial killing when given at doses that maximize the Peak/MIC or AUC/MIC [12]. These data suggest that when utilizing a similar dosing scheme (under the proper conditions), contrary to the widely held belief of concentration-independent killing by macrolides, the AUC/MIC may be the most important pharmacodynamic parameter for demonstrating efficacy.

Additionally, the pharmacodynamic model may hold true only for infections where serum concentrations of the drug mimic those seen at the site of infection. In infections such as pneumonia and meningitis, the drug concentrations at the site of infection (believed to be the cerebrospiral fluid (CSF) or epithelial lining fluid (ELF) in these examples) will most likely be different from the concentration achieved in the serum. It has been demonstrated already that the achievable ELF concentrations of clarithromycin and azithromycin are different from the concentration profile of these agents in the plasma [20, 22]. An effective antibiotic must be able to achieve high concentrations at the site of infection, and, therefore, the concentration of drug in serum or plasma may not be a good marker of success. In such a case, the concentration of drug at the site of infection would be a better predictor of *in vivo* success, but this concentration is often very difficult to assess. Usually, the concentration in serum is considered to be a good surrogate for the drug concentrations at the site of infection. While this relationship is generally true, it is not always true, and, in such a case, models that correlate microbiological activity to serum concentrations do not apply. Unfortunately, the usual pharmacodynamic models make exactly this assumption, since the AUC, plasma concentration, and time above the MIC all refer to the serum or plasma concentrations.

Pharmacokinetics

This section will concentrate on the differences in tissue distribution of the macrolides as well as their efficacy in treating both extracellular and intracellular respiratory pathogens. The pharmacokinetic profiles of these newer drugs differ in many aspects from each other, as well as from erythromycin, however, both are excellent at reaching high concentrations intracellularly. Azithromycin is unique because of 1) its long serum half-life, enabling it to function effectively in once-daily dosing, and 2) its extensive tissue distribution, reaching high concentrations in alveolar macrophages while low levels remain in the plasma [13–15]. Table 1 provides a summary of the pharmacokinetics of several macrolides.

Azithromycin has an extended half-life and high tissue penetration. A 500-mg oral dose has a maximum serum concentration (Cmax) of 0.4 mg/l, an apparent half-life ($t_{1/2}$) of 9.6 h, and an area under the curve (AUC) of 4.5 mg*h/l [16,17]. High concentrations in tissues reach sustained levels for 2.3 to 3.2 days, allowing for once-daily dosing and shorter treatment regimens [1]. Azithromycin concentrations in the lung, tonsil, and prostate tissues 7 days after a 1.5 g dose are projected to be 4.3, 6.2, and 3.5 mg/kg, respectively [18]. Because of azithromycin's long half-life, reaching as long as 68 h, clinically there is a concern that the prolonged subinhibitory serum/plasma concentrations may select resistant microorganisms from the populations of bacteria infecting the patient [19]. Because of low achievable serum concentrations, oral azithromycin is not recommended for use in the U.S. in the treatment of bacteremia and moderate to severe pneumonia in elderly or debilitated individuals or those patients with significant underlying health problems [1]. In these cases, treatment using parenteral azithromycin is more appropriate.

Contrary to azithromycin, clarithromycin has high concentrations in the ELF of the lungs and plasma, as well as in alveolar macrophages (AM) [15, 20]. Clarithromycin has greater acid stability, improved pharmacokinetics, better gastrointenstinal tolerance, and a broader spectrum of activity than erythromycin

Table 1. Pharmacokinetics of macrolides[a]

	Cmax (µg/ml)	**$t_{1/2}$** (hours)	**AUC 0–24** (mg*h/l)
Azithromycin (500 mg PO)	0.4	9.6	4.5
Clarithromycin (400 mg PO)	2.1	4.7	17
Erythromycin (500 mg PO)	3.0	2	4.4–14.3
Dirithromycin (500 mg PO)	0.29	23.3	3.2
Roxithromycin (150 mg PO)	6.61–7.9	8.4–15.5	72.6–81.0
Spiramycin (500 mg IV)	3.10	6.25	10.30

a) references [7, 16, 17, 39, 43, 44]

[13, 14]. Hepatic metabolism of an oral dose results in its principal metabolite, 14-hydroxyclarithromycin. Concentrations of clarithromycin and its metabolite, 14-hydroxyclarithromycin, that were measured following the last dose peaked at 4 h at 3.29 mg/l and 1.43 mg/l, respectively, while the azithromycin level peaked at 0.09 mg/l at 4 h post-dose. In this study, steady-state concentrations followed conventional dosing with clarithromycin 500 mg tablets BID and azithromycin 500 mg tablet on day one followed by 250 mg QD [20]. Additionally, the ELF concentration of azithromycin after multiple dosing was below the level of sensitivity (0.01 mg/l) for 15 out of 17 subjects, while the ELF concentration of clarithromycin following multiple dosing exceeded 20 mg/l for most subjects for up to 12 h [20]. Steady-state concentrations of clarithromycin in the lungs of patients scheduled to undergo elective lung resection achieved mean levels of 54.32 μg/g and 5.12 μg/g for the metabolite [21]. Additionally, corresponding mean plasma concentrations for clarithromycin and its metabolite, measured at the time of lung resection, were 54.3 and 5.12 μg/g, respectively [21]. Finally, a study of healthy human volunteers undergoing bronchoalveolar lavage (BAL) demonstrated that clarithromycin (at a dose of 500 mg every 12 hours for 5 days) achieved steady-state concentrations in the plasma, ELF, and AM equal to or higher than those of patients receiving 5 oral doses of azithromycin (500 mg on the first day, then 250 mg daily) (see Tab. 2) [22]. The mean concentration of clarithromycin was significantly higher than azithromycin in the intrapulmonary compartments for the first 12 h after receiving the last dose of drug [22].

Additionally, from an application perspective, one can develop a sustained release clarithromycin dosage form which optimizes the T > MIC or AUC/MIC

Table 2. Steady-state concentrations of azithromycin and clarithromycin in serum and lung pharmacokinetics[a]

	Mean concentrations (μg/ml)					
	Plasma		AM[b]		ELF[c]	
	Azi	Clari	Azi	Clari	Azi	Clari
4 hours post-dose	0.08	2.00	42.7	480	1.01	34.5
8 hours post-dose	0.09	1.55	57.2	220	2.18	26.1
12 hours post-dose	0.04	1.22	40.4	181	0.95	15.1

a) Compiled from [22]
b) AM = Alveolar macrophages
c) ELF = Epithelial lining fluid

Table 3. Pharmacokinetics of extended release (ER) and immediate release (IR) clarithromycin (CLA)[a]

	500 mg ER QD	250 mg IR BID
Cmax (mg/l)	1.45 ± 0.43	1.94 ± 0.68
Tmax (h)	5.6 ± 2.1	2.4 ± 1.4
AUC (mg*h/l)	20.4 ± 8.7	21.0 ± 6.9

a) Compiled from Reference 23

ratio such that once/day dosing with good effectiveness is obtained (see Tab. 3) [23–27]. Table 3 indicates that maximum serum concentration (Cmax) of the extended release clarithromycin demonstrated a statistically significantly lower value ($p = 0.0001$) than that observed in the immediate release compound. The AUC values for the extended release clarithromycin met the requirements for equivalence (90% confidence interval), and the Tmax was significantly longer ($p = 0.0001$) than that of the immediate release compound [23].

Roxithromycin appears to have different pharmacokinetics from clarithromycin and is characterized by high concentrations in serum and low levels in tissues, contrary to the high tissue concentrations observed with clarithromycin. A 150 mg oral dose of roxithromycin demonstrated a Cmax between 6.61 and 7.9 mg/l, a mean elimination $t_{1/2}$ between 8.4 and 15.5 h, and an AUC of 72.6 to 81.0 mg*h/l [28]. In lung tissue of patients undergoing lung surgery, mean concentrations of roxithromycin after a 150 mg oral dose reached 5.6 mg/l at 6 h post-dose [29]. A study evaluating roxithromycin's penetration into the nasal mucosa and tonsil found that peak tissue levels occurred 4–6 h post-dose in patients receiving 150 mg b.i.d. for three days. The mean peak concentration was found to be 1.78 mg/kg ± 0.73 in the nasal mucosa and 2.2 mg/kg ± 1.21 in tonsils [30].

The macrolides spiramycin and josamycin also exhibit intracellular accumulation and penetration into the bronchial secretions. An *in vivo* study of josamycin in patients receiving 1 g orally b.i.d. for three days demonstrated mean serum levels of 0.56 mg/l ± 0.47 at 3 h post-dose, which is lower than that observed with clarithromycin and roxithromycin but similar to the low serum levels observed with azithromycin [31]. This study also demonstrated AM and BAL supernatant concentrations in these healthy volunteers averaging 44.3 ± 61.4 mg/l and 0.185 ± 0.176 mg/l, respectively [31]. This high intrapulmonary concentration reflects findings observed with the other macrolides previously discussed. Spiramycin achieves high tissue to serum levels throughout the body, especially in the lungs. The pharmacokinetics of this drug on day six following repeated doses of 500 mg t.i.d. intravenously demonstrated a mean Cmax of 3.10 mg/l, an apparent half-life of 6.25 h, and an AUC of 10.30 mg*h/l [32]. An *in vivo* study of lung penetration of spiramycin demonstrated concentrations of bronchial secretions averaging 7.3 mg/l following a single 1.5 g oral dose [33]. Upper respiratory concentrations reached 21.5 to 40.0 mg/kg in the tonsils of adults after a 3 g loading dose [33].

Intracellular accumulation

Current theory proposes that there are at least two mechanisms that account for the high accumulation of macrolides by phagocytic cells [34]. First, there appears to be an energy-independent system mechanism, resulting in passive diffusion. Here the driving force is most likely pH and hydrophobicity. An acidic pH (6.0) appears to prevent the uptake of antibiotic by peritoneal macrophages, while an alkaline pH (8.4) did not appear to affect uptake [34]. A second mechanism is an energy-dependent pathway corresponding to a nucleoside transport system. The high intracellular concentrations of the macrolides are due to contributions of these two mechanisms.

Macrolides concentrate intracellularly, which results in the advantage of a targeted delivery system, bringing active drug to infection sites by the phagocytes [35]. While the uptake of erythromycin into polymorphonuclear cells and macrophages is completed within 30 minutes, the uptake of azithromycin into these cells continues for at least 24 hours [35]. Conversely, azithromycin is released slowly from macrophages after removing the drug extracellularly, resulting in the release of 19% of the antibiotic into the extracellular medium after 1 h and a relase of 93.3% after 24 h. For erythromycin, 85% of the intracellular antibiotic was released extracellularly within 1 h, and by 3 h essentially all the erythromycin had been eliminated [34, 35]. Phagocytosis by *Staphylococcus aureus* was also demonstrated to significantly enhance the release of azithromycin [35].

Azithromycin concentrations are 226 times greater intracellularly than extracellularly [35]. In alveolar macrophages of adult volunteers undergoing bronchoscopy and bronchoalveolar lavage, azithromycin after 24 hours achieved a concentration of 41.7 mg/l [22]. Clarithromycin and its primary metabolite also demonstrated increased intracellular concentrations in this study, with levels in alveolar macrophages remaining at 99.4 mg/l and 31.3 mg/l, respectively, after 24 hours. Extensive uptake of azithromycin by phagocytes followed by targeted delivery in tissues at the site of infections may enhance the antibacterial activity of azithromycin against both intracellular and extracellular pathogens [1]. Similar to the previously discussed macrolides, roxithromycin has extensive intracellular concentration. A study of volunteers who received roxithromycin 300 mg b.i.d. demonstrated that the steady-state concentration in BAL cells (21 ± 10 mg/l) was 2 and 10 times higher than the corresponding roxithromycin concentration in plasma (11.4 ± 5.7 mg/l) and epithelial lining fluid (2.0 ± 1.7 mg/l) [29]. Alveolar macrophage concentrations of josamycin reached approximately 44.3 mg/l after a 1 g oral dose, and spiramycin concentrations in alveolar macrophages reached 12.8 mg/l after receiving 500 mg t.i.d. [31, 36].

The magnitude of azithromycin's intracellular concentration exposes phagocytes and other cells to the drug for an extended period of time [35]. Azithromycin has two basic amine groups in its structure that may account for greater ionization and trapping than that observed with the classical macrolides, such as erythromycin, which only has one amine group. An *in vitro* study demonstrated the presence of a rapid release of azithromycin in response to bacteria, and results show the presence of a high concentration of active drug released into the extracellular medium [35]. The released drug may act with normal phagocytes to eradicate intracellular and extracellular infections. Additionally, the azithromycin level at the site of infection is possibly increased by degranulation of phagocytes containing the antimicrobial [18, 35].

Pharmacodynamics

The macrolides have effective activity against the major respiratory tract pathogens, *Moraxella cattarhalis* and *Streptococcus pneumoniae*; however, both erythromycin and roxithromycin do not adequately cover *Haemophilus influenzae*, while azithromycin and clarithromycin do. Clarithromycin's activity against this pathogen is due to the activity of the parent compound and its active metabolite 14-hydroxyclarithromycin [13, 37].

As previously discussed, for macrolides, it is the time above the MIC that is believed to be the major parameter in determining efficacy against an organism. To optimize activity against pathogens, the MIC of the organism must be exceeded for at least 50% of the dosing interval. However, in an immunocompromised host, the MIC of the organisms may be required to be exceeded for 100% of the dosing interval in order to be effective. For the common respiratory tract pathogens, typically, the macrolides achieve a time above the MIC that is greater than 50%, and they are therefore predicted to be a reasonable treatment option for these infections. The MICs for macrolides against common respiratory tract organisms are summarized in Table 4.

Much of clarithromycin's antimicrobial effect is believed to be due to its active metabolite, 14-hydroxyclarithromycin [13, 21, 37, 38]. The metabolite has demonstrated greater *in vitro* potency against *H. influenzae* than the parent compound alone and additive or synergistic properties when combined with the parent compound [13, 37]. In sera of human volunteers, the concentrations of clarithromycin and its metabolite were equally active *in vitro* against pathogens implicated in community acquired pneumonia, with the metabolite having two-fold more activity than clarithromycin against *H. influenzae* [37]. In an animal model, the *in vivo* combination of the two compounds was either synergistic or additive depending on the level of *H. influenzae* present at the time that treatment was initiated [37]. The combination of clarithromycin and its metabolite was most active when the MIC_{90} reached 2 mg/l. Additionally, the metabolite demonstrated more activity than the parent in reducing bacterial counts of *H. influenzae*. Individually, however, both the metabolite and parent were ineffective as single agents in decreasing colony counts or improving cure rates [37].

Table 4. MIC_{90} of common respiratory pathogens[a]

	Azi	Ery	Clari	Roxi
S. pneumoniae	0.12	0.02	0.06	0.25
H. influenzae	0.84	4.30	1.00[b]	12.39
M. cattarhalis	0.16	0.49	0.25	0.41
M. pneumoniae	0.0002	0.01	0.008	0.03
C. pneumoniae	0.125	0.125	0.03	0.25
Legionella spp.	0.50	0.50	0.06	0.30

a) references [7, 28, 38, 42, 43]
b) with 14-hydroxyclarithromycin

For azithromycin, the high and sustained tissue levels ensure that intracellular pathogens are continuously exposed to bactericidal levels [18]. Treatment efficacy depends on where the site of infection is located. When the bacteria are in intracellular fluid that is in equilibrium with serum, a high tissue level is not as beneficial because serum concentrations will be low. However, in the case where the intracellular fluid drug concentrations are not proportional to serum, there will be high levels of drug intracellularly, even when the serum drug concentration is low, resulting in enhanced killing. As previously noted, the levels of azithromycin in the lung, tonsils, and prostate at seven days after a 1.5 g dose were 4.3 mg/kg, 6.2 mg/kg, and 3.5 mg/kg, respectively, and the concentration of azithromycin in these tissues remained above 3 mg/kg during the standard dosing regimen [18, 39]. The concentrations achieved in these tissues are in excess of the MIC_{90} reported for the major targeted respiratory tract organisms, *H. influenzae, S. pneumoniae,* and *M. catarrhalis*, as well as for the atypical organisms *Legionella* spp., *Chlamydia pneumoniae*, and *Mycoplasma pneumonia* [18, 39]. Additionally, for clarithromycin, the observed steady-state concentrations in the plasma, ELF, and AM have been demonstrated to exceed the MIC at which 90% of the isolates are inhibited for the common extracellular and intracellular pathogens causing pulmonary infections [22]. Clarithromycin concentrations in the ELF reportedly exceeded the MIC at concentrations greater than 8 times for *H. influenzae* and 100 times for *S. pneumoniae,* while azithromycin concentrations surpassed the MIC at greater than 4 times for *H. influenzae* and 33 times the mean MIC for *S. pneumoniae* [13].

Kill rates between clarithromycin and azithromycin for the common respiratory tract pathogens *S. pneumoniae, S. aureus, H. influenzae,* and *M. catarrhalis* demonstrated similar efficacy. However, differences were present in their killing kinetics as measured by the serum concentration of drug, the Cmax achieved, and the relation to the MIC of the respective pathogen [40]. Azithromycin killed a lower proportion of the initial population as compared to clarithromycin, and the killing observed with azithromycin proceeded at a slower rate than that observed with clarithromycin. Azithromycin had a regrowth of cultures after a reduction in the initial inoculum, and additionally, there was an 8 to 16 fold increase in MIC for all species with an MIC below 1 mg/l after they were exposed to a concentration gradient. A similar increase was not observed with clarithromycin-treated species. It is important to remember that these data were obtained in static *in vitro* conditions and may not accurately predict *in vivo* conditions [40].

In *H. influenzae* infections, the serum concentrations of clarithromycin and azithromycin are often at levels below the MIC of the pathogen. It is important to keep in mind, however, that although poor serum concentrations are observed, the high tissue penetration is the more important predictor of success for macrolides in treating infections at sites where the serum is not in equilibrium with the intracellular fluid. Efficacy was measured against *H. influenzae* in one study by examining the reduction of pulmonary *H. influenzae* burden on days 3 and 7 post-inoculation [15]. Azithromycin was effective in reducing colony counts on day 7, although no effect was seen on day 3. Clarithromycin, however, was effective in decreasing the level of *H. influenzae* in the lungs on both days 3 and 7 of therapy. Both drugs demonstrated marked efficacy against all six strains of *H. influenzae* tested. The quicker efficacy rate of clarithromycin, seen by day 3, is probably due to the drug's ability to concentrate in both intracellular and extracellular locations of the lung, thus ensuring a rapid response to *H. influenzae* in all pulmonary locations. Also, the extracellular concentration of azithromycin is usually low, accounting for the delayed response observed due to a potential need for the drug to diffuse out of the cell and into the extracellular locations [15].

In treating pneumococcal infections, clarithromycin has a demonstrated MIC one or two dilutions lower than that seen with other macrolides. Erythromycin exhibited bactericidal activity at eight times the MIC while azithromycin and clarithromycin demonstrated similar activity at two times the MIC. Time kill data demonstrated 90% bactericidal efficacy for all three antimicrobial agents after 12 hours at 2 times the MIC [41].

Similarly, the macrolides exhibit efficacy in the treatment of atypical pneumonias. Against *C. pneumoniae*, clarithromycin was the most active compound tested with an MIC_{90} of 0.03 mg/l; the activity of azithromycin was similar to that of erythromycin, with an MIC of 0.125 mg/l, and roxithromycin demonstrated an MIC between 0.25 and 1.0 mg/l [29, 42]. *M. pneumoniae* is a major cause of pneumonia, accounting for up to 20% of all pneumonias, and *in vitro* MIC testing of this organism has demonstrated significantly increased activity with azithromycin compared with either erythromycin or clarithromycin [38].

Conclusion

In conclusion, in order to maximize the killing potential of the macrolides, the concentration of the drug must exceed the MIC for at least 50% of the dosing interval. The bactericidal effect is maximized when the AUC approaches two to four times the MIC value of the organism, but once this ratio is achieved, it is the time above the MIC that needs to be optimized to enhance killing. This concentration-independent killing is enhanced by the intracellular accumulation of drug, which is extensive for the macrolides and allows for very high concentrations intracellularly over a prolonged period of time, providing effective killing of common intracellular respiratory pathogens. Within the class of macrolides, these agents possess differing abilities to concentrate in the serum. However, even for those macrolides that achieve fairly low serum concentrations, it is the extended release of drug from the intracellular space into the extracellular fluid, along with a prolonged post-antibiotic effect such as that observed with azithromycin, that helps to ensure that extracellular organisms are effectively eradicated. The improved pharmacokinetic profile of these newer macrolides/azalides over erythromycin allows for less frequent dosing and improved patient adherence and, possibly, clinical cure rates.

References

1 Gunasekara NS, Barman Balfour JA (1999) Management of community-acquired pneumonia: defining the role of azithromycin. *Dis Manage Health Outcomes* 5: 41–54
2 Nightingale CH (1997) Pharmacokinetics and pharmacodynamics of newer macrolides. *Pediatr Infect Dis J* 16: 438–443
3 Ludden TM (1985) Pharmacokinetic interactions of the macrolide antibiotics. *Clin Pharmacokinet* 10: 63–79
4 Periti P, Mazzei T, Mini E, Novelli A (1992) Pharmacokinetic drug interactions of macrolides. *Clin Pharmacokinet* 23: 106–131
5 Quintiliani R, Nightingale CH, Freeman CD (1994) Pharmacokinetic and pharmacodynamic considerations in antibiotic selection, with particular attention to oral cephalosporins. *Infect Dis Clin Pract* 3: 1–7
6 Bauernfeind A, Jungwirth R, Eberlein E (1995) Comparative pharmacodynamics of clarithromycin and azithromycin against respiratory pathogens. *Infection* 23: 316–321
7 Dunn CJ, Barradell LB (1996) Azithromycin: A review of its pharmacological properties and use as 3-day therapy in respiratory tract infections. *Drugs* 51: 483–505
8 Owens RC, Nicolau DP, Quintiliani R, Nightingale CH (1997) Bactericidal activity of clarithromycin, azithromycin and cefuroxime against penicillin-susceptible, -intermediate, and -resistant pneumococci. In: Abstracts of 20th International Congress of Chemotherapy (Sydney, Australia), June 29-July 3
9 Den Hollander JG, Knudsen JD, Mouton JW, Fuursted F, Frimodt-Moller N, Verbrugh HA, Espersen F (1998) Comparison of pharmacodynamics of azithromycin and erythromycin *in vitro* and *in vivo*. *Antimicrob Agents Chemother* 42: 377–382
10 Craig WA (1995) Interrelationship between pharmacokinetics and pharmacodynamics in determining dosage regimens for broad-spectrum cephalosporins. *Diagn Microbial Infect Dis* 22: 89–96
11 Vogelman B, Gudmundson G, Leggett J, Turnidge J, Ebert S, Craig WA (1998) Correlation of antimicrobial pharmacokinetic parameters with therapeutic efficacy in animal model. *J Infect Dis* 158: 831–847
12 Mazzei T, Novelli A, Fallani S, Cassetta MI, Conti S. Bacterial killing by macrolides: concentration-dependent or time-dependent? In: Abstracts of 5th International Conference on the Macrolides, Azolides, Streptogramins, Ketolides and Oxazolidinones (Seville, Spain), January 26–28, 2000
13 Bergman KL, Olsen KM, Peddicord TE, Fey PD, Rupp ME (1999) Antimicrobial activities and postantibiotic effects of clarithromycin, 14-hydroxy-clarithromycin, and azithromycin in epithelial cell lining fluid against clinical isolates of *Haemophilus influenzae* and *Streptococcus pneumoniae*. *Antimicrob Agents Chemother* 43: 1291–1293
14 Girard AE, Girard D, English AR, Gootz TD, Cimochowski CR, Faiella JA, Haskell SL, Retsema JA (1987) Pharmacokinetic and *in vivo* studies with azithromycin (CP-62,993), a new macrolide with an extended half life and excellent tissue distribution. *Antimicrob Agents Chemother* 31: 1948–1954
15 Alder JD, Ewing PJ, Nilius AM, Mitten M, Tovcimak A, Oleksijew A, Jarvis K, Paige L, Tanaka SKT (1998) Dynamics of clarithromycin and azithromycin efficacies against experimental *Haemophilus influenzae* pulmonary infection. *Antimicrob Agents Chemother* 42: 2385–2390
16 Kirst HA, Sides GD (1989) New directions for macrolide antibiotics: pharmacokintics and clinical efficacy. *Antimicrob Agents Chemother* 33: 1419–1422
17 Cooper MA, Nye K, Andrews JM, Wise R (1990) The pharmacokinetics and inflammatory fluid penetration of orally administered azithromycin. *J Antimicrob Chemother* 26: 533–538
18 Retsema JA, Girard AE, Girard D, Milisen WB (1990) Relationship of high tissue concentrations of azithromycin to bactericidal activity and efficacy *in vivo*. *J Antimicrob Chemother* 25: 83–89
19 Data on file. Pfizer Inc, New York, NY.
20 Patel KB, Xuan D, Tessier PR, Russomanno JH, Quintiliani R, Nightingale CH (1996) Comparison of bronchopulmonary pharmacokinetics of clarithromycin and azithromycin. *Antimicrob Agents Chemother* 40: 2375–2379

21 Fish DN, Gotfried MH, Danziger LH, Rodvold KA (1994) Penetration of clarithromycin into lung tissues from patients undergoing lung resection. *Antimicrob Agents Chemother* 38: 876–878

22 Rodvold KA, Gotfried MH, Danziger LH, Servi RJ (1997) Intrapulmonary steady-state concentrations of clarithromycin and azithromycin in healthy adult volunteers. *Antimicrob Agents Chemother* 41: 1399–1402

23 Gustavson LE, Cao GX, Semia SJ, Palmer RN. Pharmacokinetics of a new extended release clarithromycin tablet at doses of 500 and 1000 mg daily. In: Abstracts of 39th Interscience Conference on Antimicrobial Agents and Chemotherapy (San Francisco, California), September 26–29, 1999

24 Shortridge D, Flamm RK. *In vitro* susceptibility testing of *Streptococcus pneumoniae* isolates from a Multi-Center European Clinical Treatment Trial: clarithromycin modified release treatment of the acute exacerbation of chronic bronchitis. In: Abstracts of 21st International Congress of Chemotherapy (Birmingham, England), July 5–9, 1999

25 Fraschini F, Scaglione F, Demartini G, Dugnani S. *In vitro* comparative dynamics of clarithromycin modified release and azithromycin. In: Abstracts of 21st International Congress of Chemotherapy (Birmingham, England), July 5–9, 1999

26 Hutton J, Ryan J, Conway D. Cost-effectiveness of once-daily clarithromycin compared to amoxycillin/clavulanic acid in the treatment of acute exacerbation of chronic bronchitis. In: Abstracts of 21st International Congress of Chemotherapy (Birmingham, England), July 5–9, 1999

27 Adam D. Short-course therapy of lower respiratory tract infection with a 500mg total daily dosage of clarithromycin: once daily vs. twice daily administration. In: Abstracts of 21st International Congress of Chemotherapy (Birmingham, England), July 5–9, 1999

28 Markham A, Faulds D (1994) Azithromycin: an update. *Drugs* 48: 297–321

29 Chastre J, Brun P, Fourtillan JB, Soler P, Basset G, Manuel C, Trouillet JL, Gibert C (1987) Pulmonary disposition of roxithromycin (RU 28965), a new macrolide antibiotic. *Antimicrob Agents Chemother* 31: 1312–1316

30 Fraschini F, Scaglione F, Pintucci G, Maccarinelli G, Dugnani S, Demartini G (1991) The diffusion of clarithromycin and roxithromycin into nasal mucosa, tonsil and lung in humans. *J Antimicrob Chemother* 27(Suppl A): 61–65

31 Panteix G, Harf R, de Montclos H, Verdier MF, Gaspar A, Leclercq M (1988) Josamycin pulmonary penetration determined by broncho-alveolar lavage in man. *J Antimicrob Chemother* 22: 917–921

32 Frydman AM, Le Roux Y, Desnottes JF, Kaplan, Debbar F, Cournot A, Duchier J, Gaillot J (1998) Pharmacokinetics of spiramycin in man. *J Antimicrob Chemother* 22(Suppl B): 93–103

33 Bergogne-Berezin E (1988) Spiramycin concentrations in the human respiratory tract: a review. *J Antimicrob Chemother* 22(Suppl B): 117–122

34 Bonnet M, Van der Auwera P (1992) *In vitro* and *in vivo* intraleukocyte accumulation of azithromycin (CP-62,993) and its influence on *ex vivo* leukocyte chemiluminescence. *Antimicrob Agents Chemother* 36: 1302–1309

35 Gladue RP, Bright GM, Isaacson RE, Newborg MF (1989) *In vitro* and *in* vivo uptake of azithromycin (CP-62,993) by phagocytic cells: possible mechanism of delivery and release at sites of infection. *Antimicrob Agents Chemother* 33: 277–282

36 Harf R, Panteix G, Desnottes JF, Diallo N, Leclercq M (1988) Spiramycin uptake by alveolar macrophages. *J Antimicrob Chemother* 22(Suppl B): 135–140

37 Hardy DJ, Swanson RN, Rode RA, Marsh K, Shipkowitz NL, Clement JJ (1990) Enhancement of the *in vitro* and *in vivo* activities of clarithromycin against *Haemophilus influenzae* by 14-hydroxy-clarithromycin, its major metabolite in humans. *Antimicrob Agents Chemother* 34: 1407–1413

38 Ishida K, Kaku M, Irifune K, Mizukane R, Takemura H, Yoshida R, Tanaka H, Usui T, Suyama N, Tomono K et al (1994) *In vitro* and *in vivo* activities of macrolides against *Mycoplasma pneumoniae*. *Antimicrob Agents Chemother* 38: 790–798

39 Foulds G, Shepard RM, Johnson RB (1990) The pharmacokinetics of azithromycin in human serum and tissues. *J Antimicrob Chemother* 25: 73–82

40 Bauernfeind A, Jungwirth R, Eberlein E (1995) Comparative pharmacodynamics of clarithromycin and azithromycin against respiratory pathogens. *Infection* 23: 316–321

41 Ednie LM, Visalli MA, Jacobs MR, Appelbaum PC (1996) Comparative activities of clarithromycin, erythromycin, and azithromycin against penicillin-susceptible and penicillin-resistant pneumococci. *Antimicrob Agents Chemother* 40: 1950–1952

42 Hammerschlag MR, Qumei KK, Roblin PM (1992) *In vitro* activities of azithromycin, clarithromycin, L-ofloxacin, and other antibiotics against *Chlamydia pneumoniae*. *Antimicrob Agents Chemother* 36: 1573–1574

43 Alvarez-Elcoro S, Enzler MJ (1999) The macrolides: erythromycin, clarithromycin and azithromycin. *Mayo Clin Proc* 74: 613–634

44 Mazzel TA, Surrenti C, Novelli A, Biagini MR, Fallani S, Cassetta MI, Conti S, Surrenti E (1999) Pharmacokinetics of dirithomycin in patients with mild or moderate cirrhosis. *Antimicrob Agents Chemother* 43: 1556–1559

Macrolide Antibiotics
ed. by W. Schönfeld and H. A. Kirst

Cellular accumulation of macrolide antibiotics. Intracellular bioactivity

Marie-Thérèse Labro

INSERM U479, CHU X. Bichat-Cl. Bernard, 46 rue Henri Huchard, 75018 Paris, France

Introduction

An extended classification of macrolides from the classical definition of Woodward presents a vast continuum of macrocyclic lactonic structures in which some molecules are mainly antibacterial (true macrolides) whereas others possess mainly immunosuppressant activity (FK 506, rapamycin) or antifungal activity with host cell inhibitory properties (bafilomycins, concannamycins). Traditional macrolide antibiotics are characterized by a 12- to 16-membered ring, macrocyclic lactone nucleus, with few double-bonds, and substituted by several amino and/or neutral sugars. Over the past few decades, there has been continuous research into the development of new macrolide antibiotics by chemical modifications of the existing natural derivatives [1, 2]. This dynamic research has provided modern therapeutic agents, particularly the semi-synthetic derivatives of erythromycin A, either by adding new substituents, or introducing a nitrogen atom into the lactone (azalides), or, more recently, by withdrawing the L-cladinose at position 3 of the lactone ring and replacing it by a 3-keto function (ketolides). All these compounds display a substantially homogeneous antimicrobial spectrum and the capability to concentrate within host cells (the subject of this review). This property has been one major reason behind the search for new compounds targeting intracellular pathogens. Other possible consequences of the cellular accumulation of these drugs, particularly the modulation of various cell functions, are a further incentive for research in this field. A simplified chemical approach to the macrolide continuum is presented in Figure 1 [2, 3].

This brief overview will deal with the main characteristics of the cellular uptake of macrolides as defined by *in vitro* analysis. Cellular concentrations obtained from *ex vivo* studies will then be discussed. Finally, the potential relevance of these results will be presented, particularly with reference to the antimicrobial activity of macrolides against intracellular pathogens *in vitro* and in some animal models. The therapeutic efficacy of these drugs in diseases caused by these latter organisms is outlined in other chapters of this book.

V-ATPase Inhibitors ---------- **"True Macrolides"** ------ **Immunosuppressants**

Bafilomycins(16) | (Therapeutic Uses) | FK506(23)

Concannamycins (18) | 12-**14**-**16**-17* | Rapamycin (31)

14 ---------------------------------- **16**

Natural	**Semisynthetic**	**Natural**	**Semisynthetic**
Oleandomycin		Leucomycins	Rokitamycin
Erythromycin A---------------- ↓		Spiramycins	Miokamycin
		Tylosins	

Modifications

Substituents	**Lactone**		**Sugars**	
(14)	**AZALIDES** (15)	Others	**KETOLIDES** (14)	Others
Roxithromycin	Azithromycin		HMR 3647	
Clarithromycin			HMR 3004	
Dirithromycin			HMR 3562	
Erythromycylamine			HMR 3787	
Flurithromycin			ABT 773	

Figure 1. Simplified classification of macrolides (adapted from references 2, 3).
True macrolides are those defined according to Woodward and which are used in infectious diseases (humans or animals).
The number of atoms in the lactone ring is given in parentheses.
17*: lankacidins are group of macrolide antibiotics which do not possess sugar substituents as the immunosuppressants FK506 and rapamycins..

In vitro analysis of the cellular uptake of macrolides

Various reviews have summarized the main data regarding cellular uptake [3–5]. However, parallel to the dynamic chemical evolution of the macrolide family, new data periodically appear in this area that require continuous updating. The techniques available to study macrolide uptake by host cells have not changed much in recent years. Roughly speaking, two types of methods are used: either the total amount of cell-associated drug is measured by HPLC (high performance liquid chromatography) or liquid scintillation counting (when radiolabeled drugs are available), or the antimicrobial activity of a cell-associated compound is determined with standard bacterial strains. The advantages, disadvantages, and pitfalls of these various techniques have been discussed elsewhere [4, 5] and must be kept in mind to avoid over- or understatement of the results. The cell subsets that have been preferentially analyzed in this context are the phagocytes, particularly polymorphonuclear neutrophils (PMN), owing to their large numbers and easy recovery from venous blood. Of practical importance are also various phagocytic/non-phagocytic cell lines, which overcome the inter-individual variability frequently observed with cells obtained from different donors. However, the ubiquity of the macrolide carrier (transport system) has not been demonstrated, which impedes extrapolation of the results obtained with one cell line to a wider range of host cells. Whatever the cell and technique used, two sets of data can be obtained:

1) the three classical parameters, namely the kinetics of accumulation and efflux, and the cellular location, which define the basic profile of the cellular pharmacokinetics of the drug in precise conditions; and

2) the influence of various factors (temperature, pH, inhibitors, phagocytosis, cytokines, etc.) on drug uptake and/or efflux, aiming to characterize the underlying mechanism(s).

The main parameter used to compare drugs is the ratio of accumulation (C/E), i. e., the ratio between the cellular (cell-associated) and extracellular concentrations.

Classical approach to macrolide cellular pharmacokinetics

Table 1 presents the results obtained with the cell type most extensively investigated, the PMN [3–10], and Table 2 summarizes the data obtained with other cell types (phagocytic/non-phagocytic cells and cell lines) [4, 5, 8, 11, 12].

Erythromycin A and its derivatives are the compounds most extensively analyzed in this context. A preliminary classification of these antibiotics has been proposed according to their classical parameters of uptake by PMN [3]. Two groups can be easily separated. Group I includes dibasic molecules whose uptake is not saturable over a three-hour incubation period. They are preferentially located within PMN granules and are moderately released from loaded cells; the activation energy of these drugs (a parameter linked to their transmembrane passage) is generally higher than 100 kj/mole.

Group II corresponds to erythromycin A and its monobasic derivatives, which are rapidly taken up by PMN but exhibit a saturation kinetics profile and plateau around 30 to 60 min of incubation. Conversely, they rapidly egress from loaded cells and are located to a similar extent in the cytosolic and granular compartments of PMN. Their activation energy is around 60 to 70 kj/mole. Interestingly, the ketolides, which have been assessed in this context [6–8] display characteristics intermediate between the two subgroups. HMR 3004 exhibits the most impressive accumulation profile among all the macrolides assessed up to now. The quinoline substituent is likely to be responsible for this phenomenon, since a similar uptake has been observed with chloroquine (a four-amino quinoline antimalarial) [13]. Interestingly, all erythromycin A derivatives, including the ketolides, exert important inter-individual variability in cellular pharmacokinetics, at least when PMN from different subjects are assessed [6, 7, 14]. Whether this phenomenon reflects the presence of a membrane carrier system that exhibits variable numbers, isotypes (?), or functions, as observed with other receptors on the PMN membrane, has not been studied. It is also intringuing to note that cells other

Table 1. Uptake of macrolides by human polymorphonuclear neutrophils

Macrolides	Uptake C/E [time min]	Efflux[a] 5 min	 60 min	Location (% in granules)
Erythromycin A and derivatives:		**Group I[b]**		
Dirithromycin	9[5], 60–80[180] ΔG: 109[c]	22	52	73
Erythromycylamine	5[5], 25 [180] ΔG: 119	36	63	45
Azithromycin	>30 [5],>300[180] 60[d] [5], 3–5[e][180] ΔG: 122	≤20	≤20	60
		Group II		
Erythromycin A	5 [5], 4–18 [30] ΔG: 61	70	80	35
Roxithromycin	29 [5], 40–100[f][60] 136[g] ΔG: 75	45	80	49
Clarithromycin	20[5], 9–100[30]	60	80	30
Flurithromycin	>10[5]			
		Ketolides		
HMR 3004	253 [5], 460 [180] ΔG: 63	27	27	70
HMR 3647	31 [5], 348 [180] ΔG: 128	30	45	56–75
HMR 3562	141[5],420[180] ΔG: 72	30	35	75
HMR 3787	117[5],296[180] ΔG: 76	32	45	75
16-membered-ring macrolides				
Josamycin	16[15], 21[45] ΔG: 114	> 70		13
Rokitamycin	30[15] plateau	> 70		

Results are those obtained by scintillation counting unless indicated
a: efflux=% of drug released in the extracellular medium.
b: Groups I and II have been defined in reference 3 (details are given in the text).
c: ΔG= activation energy in Kj/mole.
d: measured by HPLC.
e: measured by bioassay.
f: depends on the medium.
g: cells from smokers.

Table 2. Uptake of macrolides by phagocytic/non-phagocytic cell lines

Cell Types	C/E* [time min/h]
– Human cells	
Alveolar MP	ERY A: 18–38 (46)[a] [30]; ROX: 61 (190)[a] [30]; AZI: >300[b] ->600; SPI: 20–35[b, c] [120].
MP	ERY A: 1.5–7[d] [24 h]; ROX: 2–6[d] [24 h].
Mo	ERY A: 4 [30]; ROX: 14 [30]
Fibroblasts	ERY A 25 [60]-97 [72h]
– Phagocytic cell lines	
J774	ERY A: 4 [15]; ROX: 25 [15]; AZI: 29 [2h] -41 [24h]
HL-60[6]	ROX: 40 [30]; HMR3004: 90 [30]; HMR3647: 70 [30].
PLB-985[6]	ROX: 30 [30]; HMR3004: 80 [30]; HMR3647: 70 [30]
THP-1[6]	HMR3004: 160 [30]; HMR3647: 110 [30]
NB-4[6]	HMR3647: 20 [60]
– Non-phagocytic cell lines	
Jurkat, K562, Colo 205	HMR3647: 15 [5][e]
Mc Coy, Hep-2	ERY A 4–5 [20]
– Animal Cells	
Rabbit alveolar MP	ROK 120 [30]; JOS: 40 [15]
Guinea pig alveolar MP	SPI: 22 [45]
Mouse MP	DIR: 2.8 [24h]; AZI: 62 [2h] -100 [24h]
Rat hepatocytes	ROX: 31 [60]; ERY A/ 11 [60].

* Measured by scintillation counting unless indicated
abbreviations: MP: macrophages; Mo monocytes; ERY A: erythromycin A; ROX: roxithromycin; AZI: azithromycin; SPI: spiramycin; ROK rokitamycin; JOS josamycin; DIR dithromycin.
a: cells from smokers.
b: Concentration-dependent.
c: measured by HPLC.
d: measured by bioassay.
e: plateau

than PMN accumulate macrolides to an extent different from that observed with these latter cells (Tab. 2). In general, macrophages, another mature phagocytic lineage, concentrate macrolides to a larger extent than to PMN, and the accumulation ratio is even greater in the macrophages from smokers, which may reflect either a greater activation state or a larger granular (lysosomal) compartment. By contrast, non-phagocytic cells and phagocytic precursors (myelomonocytic cell lines) accumulate macrolides to a significantly lesser extent than to their mature counterparts [12, 8], with saturation kinetics and rapid egress from loaded cells.

Mechanism(s) of macrolide uptake

Despite abundant, mainly descriptive, information on the cellular accumulation of macrolides, the mechanisms underlying this phenomenon are still poorly understood. The physico-chemical properties of these drugs (lipophilicity, electronic environment, ionization state, etc.) certainly influence their transmembrane passage and could be the major factors participating in their uptake by non-phagocytic cells. However, many data argue for the existence of an active transport system, at least in PMN, and likely in other mature phagocytic cells. The high accumulation ratio (always greater than 10, and sometimes as high as 200- to 400-fold) cannot be explained by the sole trapping due to protonation mechanism often forwarded to sustain the granular location of these weak bases. Indeed, variations in the pH of the extracellular medium significantly modify the accumulation of dibasic macrolides (e. g. azithromycin or dirithromycin), whereas roxithromycin or ketolides were little influenced except at extreme non-physiological values [9, 7, 6]. Temperature- and viability-dependent uptake has been observed for all macrolides. A high activation energy (ΔG) has been proposed to reflect the existence of an active transport system, although this parameter also could be linked to granular trapping, which requires the crossing of two membranes, cytoplasmic and granular (or to the transmembrane passage of hydrophilic molecules, for instance erythromycylamine). A comparison of the results (Tab. 1) rather argues for this latter hypothesis, except for josamycin. Other discrepancies between ΔG and granular location could be explained by the hydrophilic (erythromycylamine) or lipophilic (HMR 3004) character of the molecules. A major argument supporting the existence of an active transmembrane transport system comes from the observation of a concentration-dependent saturable accumulation process characteristic of carrier-mediated transport [6, 7, 15]. The putative carrier seems to accept all macrolides, irrespective of their chemical structure [7]. Metabolic inhibitors (CN^-, NaN_3, 2,4-dinitrophenol) at concentrations that do not impair cell viability and do not modify extracellular pH seem to be poorly effective at impairing macrolide uptake, except for ouabain, a Na^+-K^+ ATPase inhibitor [9]. These data suggest that in resting PMN, the energy required for macrolide transport is not furnished by the classical pathways of anaerobic glycolysis or mitochondrial oxidative respiration but could be provided by transmembrane cation exchangers. In addition, we have observed that Ca^{2+} deprivation and the presence of various inorganic Ca^{2+} channel inhibitors (La^{3+}, Ni^{2+}) impaired the uptake in a concentration-dependent manner but did not affect the efflux of erythromycin A derivatives, including the ketolides [7, 8, 10]. Whether this is also the case for other macrolides has not been investigated. In PMN, these cations have been reported to impair the functioning of the Na^+-Ca^{2+}exchanger. Classical L-type Ca^{2+} channel blockers such as nifedipine do not interfere with macrolide uptake. Verapamil exerts different effects on the uptake of erythromycin A derivatives belonging to either group I (increase followed by decrease during incubation) or group II (decrease). However, verapamil rapidly and strongly increases the efflux of all macrolides, independent of their chemical nature [6, 7]. Similar effects on macrolide uptake and efflux are obtained with the protein kinase A inhibitor H89 [16]. These data also favour the existence of an active efflux system in PMN. Besides its effects on L-type Ca^{2+} channels, verapamil has many effects, including inhibition of various protein kinases. It also reverses the multiple drug resistance phenotype of some tumor cells by interfering with a membrane pump protein belonging to the P-glycoprotein (P-gP) family involved in the active efflux of various hydrophobic compounds [17, 18]. Some macrolides, as well the macrolidic immunosuppressants FK 506 and rapamycin, have been shown to interfere with P-gP activity in different cell lines [19–21]. FK 506 also has been shown to use the P-gP system to cross some cell membranes [22]. These arguments suggest a link between the P-gP family and the macrolide carrier. Whether a P-gP–like protein is involved in the active uptake or efflux of these drugs is under investigation. Other data, which are consistent with an active transport system for macrolides, have been provided: for instance, pentoxifylline, a methylxanthine, and two derivatives, have been reported to increase the uptake of roxithromycin and dirithromycin by PMN [23]. Pentoxifylline is a phosphodiesterase inhibitor, which could increase the intracellular cyclic adenosine monophosphate (cAMP) concentration, and potentially activate protein kinase A (PKA). PKA interferes with the activation (activity?) of the macrolide efflux system [16]; the effect of pentoxyfilline on macrolide efflux was not considered by the authors. The phosphorylation state of the macrolide carrier seems to be of major importance for its transport activity [24]. The activation pathway has not yet been clarified, but it does not appear to be expressed in phagocytic precursors [12]. It must be noted that various proinflammatory cytokines, which activate various kinase cascades in phagocytes (the basis for their priming action), have been shown to enhance the uptake of macrolides by macrophages [25], whereas they did not modify or even decrease their accumulation by PMN [24]. That the macrolide carrier or its activation pathway potentially differs between these two phagocytic lineages adds further complexity to macrolide transport. Among other possibilities that have been forwarded to explain macrolide accumulation was the use of the nucleoside transport system by josamycin, a hypothesis that has been excluded for erythromycin A derivatives [7, 8, 9, 15, 23].

In summary, many data are consistent with the existence of a common macrolide transport system on the PMN membrane. Whether the same carrier (depending on its phosphorylation state) is involved in both the entry and efflux of these molecules is under investigation. Other uncertainties concern macrolide transport across granular membranes and in cell types other than PMN.

Ex vivo analysis of the cellular uptake of macrolides

A major problem as to the clinical relevance of the cellular concentrations measured *in vitro* is linked to the protocol itself: the experimental medium is generally static with predetermined drug concentrations as well as other factors (pH, ions, etc.). In contrast, the extracellular conditions (cytokines, neurohormonal and inflammatory mediators, drug concentration, and metabolites, etc.) vary time-dependently *in vivo*. Theoretically, the analysis of drug uptake by host cells *ex vivo, i.e.*, after drug administration to volunteers, patients, or infected/non-infected animals, is a more clinically relevant approach. However, the possibility of drug efflux during cell recovery can lead to understatement of the results. Despite these difficulties, the majority of studies have confirmed the cellular concentration of macrolides, particularly those with moderate efflux [4, 26–32]. After a 3-day course of azithromycin (500 mg once a day), concentrations of the drug as high as 51.6 mg/l (24 h after the last dose) and 2.9 mg/l (30 days after) have been measured in alveolar macrophages of healthy volunteers [30]. After a 5-day course of azithromycin (500 mg followed by 250 mg once a day for 4 days), the drug was found highly associated with PMN (51 mg/l, 4 h after the first dose). The cells still retained 60 mg/l of azithromycin 7 days after the final dose, at a time when serum concentration fell below detection limits [27]. Similar data were obtained in human monocytes, with a peak concentration of 120 mg/l of azithromycin at 28 h of a 5-day course and concentrations remaining high (21 mg/l, 200 h after the last dose) [29]. In agreement with possible drug efflux during cell recovery, it was observed that erythromycylamine (the hydrolysis product of dirithromycin) was significantly more accumulated within PMN of volunteers (maximal concentration 13.4 mg/l, day 5) than was erythromycin (6.1mg/l, day 3) after a 5-day course of dirithromycin (500 mg once a day) or erythromycin (1 g b.i.d.) [26]. In animal models, intraphagocytic accumulation of azithromycin, erythromycin and spiramycin has been shown [4, 31, 32]. Intracellular concentrations of azithromycin and erythromycin in alveolar macrophages were significantly higher in *Legionella pneumophila*-infected animals compared with controls; intracellular concentrations of azithromycin were at least 5-fold higher than those obtained with erythromycin.

Consequences of macrolide uptake by host cells

General aspects

The intraphagocytic accumulation of macrolides is firmly established. Given the crucial importance of phagocytes in infectious/non-infectious diseases, a significant impact of drug concentrations on various pathophysiological processes is likely. In particular, three functional aspects of phagocytes deserve attention:

1) PMN are the most prominent defenders against microbial invaders, owing to their large number, rapid and oriented (infected tissue-targetted) mobilization, and potent oxygen-dependent/-independent bactericidal systems. In general, they do not permit the intracellular multiplication of pathogens (except for some *Ehrlichia* species), although they can serve as a reservoir for some *Staphylococcus aureus* strains.

2) PMN are also key cells in deleterious inflammatory reactions by uncontrolled production of reactive oxygen species and enzyme release.

3) In contrast, macrophages, which display a less potent bactericidal system are used as a safe habitat by many facultative/obligate intracellular pathogens. The interference of macrolides with these functional properties of phagocytes may occur in three ways: 1) specific and high accumulation within blood PMN that can, during infectious processes, specifically migrate toward the infected site where they can release the non-firmly-bound intracellular drug (tissue-directed pharmacokinetics); 2) modulation of phagocyte metabolism and/or functions, thus interfering with the pro-inflammatory potential of these cells; 3) accumulation in various cell compartments where the drug may act on resident pathogens.

The first point has been explored mainly with azithromycin *in vitro* and *in vivo* [4, 32–37]. Macrophage-mediated delivery into the peritoneal cavity of mice has been demonstrated in a model of caseinate-induced peritonitis [32], and other authors have shown that the delivery of biologically active azithromycin to infected tissues was enhanced by cellular inflammatory processes [35, 37]. Roxithromycin, clarithromycin, or erythromycin A (which are rapidly released from loaded cells *in vitro*) were not concentrated better in infected tissues compared with controls [35, 37].

The second possible consequence of macrolide accumulation within phagocytes concerns the modulation of the proinflammatory potential of these cells. Renewed interest in this field has come from the demonstrated therapeutic efficacy of various erythromycin A derivatives in non-infectious inflammatory diseases such as diffuse panbronchiolitis and cystic fibrosis. Updates in this area have been provided recently [38–40]. Down-modulation of pro-inflammatory cytokine and oxidant production by phagocytes seem to be the two key events supporting the anti-inflammatory activity of some macrolides. The cellular targets and transductional pathways modified by these drugs, as well as the chemical structures responsible for these effects, have been partially characterized [41].

The unambigous beneficial consequences of macrolide accumulation are explained by their activity against intracellular pathogens.

Intracellular bioactivity of macrolides

The host defence system can eradicate most invading pathogens. However, some microorganisms have evolved strategies to escape, inhibit, or even use to their benefit various defence mechanisms. Intracellular parasitism is the most common mechanism for evasion from host defence [42, 43], which was rapidly recognized as a key cause of failure of antibiotic therapy in infectious diseases caused by these obligate/facultative intracellular pathogens. Intracellular penetration and accumulation of antibacterial agents is crucial for effective treatment of infections caused by such microorganisms [44, 45]. It is widely acknowledged that cellular accumulation is only one factor explaining the intracellular activity of antibiotics. Discrepancies between high cellular uptake and intracellular antibacterial efficacy have been observed widely. Other factors that are crucial for intracellular activity have been reviewed elsewhere [46]. They can be classified into two groups: those

Table 3. Factors influencing the intracellular efficacy of antibiotics

1- Antibiotic-Pathogen encounter.	2- Antibiotic activity.
– Pharmacokinetics: tissue distribution; concentrations; metabolism. – Tissue-directed pharmacokinetics: phagocyte delivery; cell "reservoirs". – Cellular uptake (entry/efflux): ionization; lipophilicity; membrane transporter; activation mechanisms; cytokines, mediators. – Cellular location: drug/pathogen.	– MIC, MBC – Drug inactivation: pH, binding to cell constituents, intracellular metabolism. – Synergy/antagonism with natural bactericidal mechanisms. – Physiological state of the microorganism.

related to the encounter between the pathogen and the drug, and those related to the antibacterial activity of the drug (Tab. 3).

Macrolide antibiotics are strongly accumulated within phagocytic/non- phagocytic cells; they have a preferential granular/lysosomal location and, in general, retain their antibacterial activity inside the cells. Their intracellular activity has been investigated using various *in vitro* cellular models and some animal models.

The effect of macrolides on intracellular pathogens may be classified according to their main cellular localisation, such as phagolysosomes, phagosomes, or cytosol.

Pathogens that do not inhibit phagolysosomal fusion

Although *S. aureus* is not considered an intracellular pathogen, it may persist within phagocytes and has been chosen frequently as a test bacterium to explore a possible synergy between macrolides and PMN bactericidal mechanisms. Macrolides are active against susceptible *S. aureus* phagocytosed by PMN, monocytes, and the macrophage cell line J774. In some studies, similar activity was demonstrated when the drug was added before, during or after phagocytosis. The factor determining the intracellular antistaphylococcal activity of macrolides remains their intrinsic antibacterial activity, although synergy between these drugs and oxidative/non-oxidative bactericidal systems of phagocytes has been suggested in some studies [47–49]. The intracellular activity of ketolides against various macrolide-susceptible or -resistant *S. aureus* has recently been examined [50]: ketolide-susceptible organisms were killed to a similar extent in control broth supplemented with this drug or in the presence of PMN and the drug, added before, during, or after phagocytosis. An *in vitro* model has been proposed to reflect more closely what occurs during infection. It uses a mixture of various phagocytic and non-phagocytic cells to assess the intra/extracellular activity of antibacterial drugs [51]: azithromycin was primarily active against intracellular *S. aureus*, whereas clarithromycin exerted more balanced activity against intra/extracellular bacteria. Animal models have suggested a synergistic interaction between PMN and macrolides, for instance erythromycin [52].

Pathogens that inhibit phagolysosomal fusion

Most *in vitro* studies demonstrate good activity of macrolides against *Legionella* spp. [51–56]. In general, the newer macrolides display better activity than erythromycin A, likely due to their better cellular and tissue pharmacokinetics [54].

Chlamydia spp. are obligate intracellular pathogens of phagocytic/non-phagocytic cells. Growing cells (not inclusion bodies) are highly susceptible to the bactericidal action of macrolides [46, 57].

Mycobacterium avium survives and multiplies within macrophages. The bacteria inhibit phagolysosomal fusion and develop within non-mature phagosomes at neutral pH because of the lack of an ATPase-dependent proton pump on the phagosomal membrane. Macrolides, particularly clarithromycin, have shown intracellular activity against *M. avium* in various *in vitro* cellular models [58–63], and this effect correlated with therapeutic efficacy in animal models of infection. Potentiation of the bactericidal action of roxithromycin by tumor necrosis factor (TNF) *in vitro* [59] and of clarithromycin by granulocyte-colony stimulating factor (G-CSF) *in vivo* [64] has been observed.

Another pathogen that has been considered a target for macrolides is *Toxoplasma gondii. T. gondii* elaborates a complex membranous network within the phagosomal compartment, which may influence the diffusion and intracellular distribution of these drugs. It has been reported that azithromycin and erythromycin A accumulate and remain active inside *T. gondii*-infected macrophages and interfere with the growth of the parasite [65].

Pathogens that escape from the phagosome

Various microorganisms escape from the microbicidal environment of the phagocytic vacuole into the cytosol. Macrolides, which display a bimodal (cytoplasmic/granular) distribution, can exert their activity against these pathogens [46]. The few published data on the intracellular activity of macrolides for *Rickettsia* suggest that the older macrolides are marginally effective (erythromycin, josamycin) or ineffective (spiramycin). However, erythromycin A derivatives seem to exert interesting activities. Azithromycin has been reported to be effective against *Rickettsia tsutsugamushi* [66] and various erythromycin A derivatives are active against *Bartonella* spp. and *Rickettsia* spp. [67].

Macrolides are active against intracellular *Listeria monocytogenes,* and this activity is enhanced by gamma interferon [68, 69]. The listeriacidal activity of macrolides is related to their intracellular accumulation as demonstrated in cell lines that do not accumulate these drugs because of their MDR (multiple drug resistance) phenotype [68].

Lastly, the intracellular bioactivity of clarithromycin against *Mycobacterium leprae* has provided a basis for future development of macrolides [46].

Prospective targets

Enteric pathogens do not belong to the classical spectrum of macrolides; however, they display limited susceptibility to azithromycin. This property was used to demonstrate the potential intracellular activity of this drug against phagocytosed gram-negative bacilli [46, 70, 71]. In particular, azithromycin exerted intracellular bactericidal activity against *Shigella flexneri* [71] within J774 macrophages similar to that obtained with ciprofloxacin. Also, azithromycin and, to a lesser extent, erythromycin A were shown to kill various intracellular *Enterobacteriaceae* (*Salmonella enteritidis, S. typhi, S. sonnei, S. dysenteriae*, and enteroinvasive *Escherichia coli*) [70].

In summary, various studies have confirmed that the intracellular accumulation of macrolides largely supports their activity against susceptible intracellular pathogens. However, many questions remain unclarified:

How do the macrolides act synergistically with natural bactericidal mechanisms of host cells? How does intracellular activity persist despite differing cellular locations between macrolides and the pathogen (see for instance *Chlamydia* and *Legionella* spp.)? It has been shown that erythromycin A derivatives promote neutrophil degranulation into the extracellular medium [72, 41]. Whether a similar mechanism operates within cells infected by such pathogens has not been investigated. However, this does not seem to be true for *M. avium*. Frehel and colleagues [73] have explored why macrolides exert bacteriostatic activity against this bacterial species despite high intracellular accumulation. The authors used transparent and opaque variants of *M. avium*, which respectively inhibit and do not prevent phagolysosomal fusion. They demonstrated that the inability of clarithromycin to completely destroy the bacteria resulted from limited accessibility of the drug, which was due to prevention of fusion between the compartments where the pathogen and the drug were located.

In vitro cellular models and experimental animal infections provide practical and fundamental approaches to assess the potential efficacy of macrolides in infections caused by intracellular pathogens. Clinical experience remains essential to define appropriate uses of these agents. Classical recommendations for intracellular pathogens have been summarized recently [44]. In adults and children, macrolides are first-choice antibiotics for chlamydial infections and legionellosis; erythromycin A combined with gentamicin is recommended in bacillary angiomatosis and *Bartonella* endocarditis. It is likely that other indications will be developed with the newest macrolides/ketolides, although cost-effectiveness is still an issue.

Conclusions

Intracellular accumulation of antibiotics has become a major consideration with respect to their antibacterial spectrum. In the future, this property will be recognized as important for other aspects of antibiotic interference with various pathophysiological processes. This phenomenon is well acknowledged in the case of some macrolides that display interesting immunomodulatory properties linked to their cellular (phagocytic) accumulation.

Progress in the understanding of transmembrane transport of these molecules should rapidly clarify the underlying mechanism(s), and the chemical structures involved at the site of the cell membrane and on the macrolidic backbone. Elucidation of these fundamental aspects may direct, in the future, chemical modifications of macrolide structure to propose new compounds with improved clinical efficacy in infections and/or inflammation.

References

1 Kirst HA (1991) New macrolides: expanded horizons for an old class of antibiotics. *J Antimicrob Chemother* 28: 787–790

2 Bryskier A (1999) New research in macrolides and ketolides since 1997. *Exp Opin Invest Drugs* 8: 1171–1194

3 Labro MT (1997) Effects of macrolides on leukocytes and inflammation. In: SH Zinner, LS Young, JF Acar, HC Neu (eds): *Expanding indications for the new macrolides, azalides and streptogramins* Marcel Dekker, New York, 101–116

4 Labro MT (1993) Intraphagocytic penetration of macrolide antibiotics. In: AJ Bryskier, J-P Butzler, HC Neu, PM Tulkens (eds): *Macrolides: Chemistry, pharmacology and clinical uses* Arnette-Blackwell, Paris, 379–388

5 Labro MT (1997) Pénétration intracellulaire des macrolides. *Presse Med* 26 (Suppl.11): 11–15

6 Vazifeh D, Abdelghaffar H, Labro MT (1997) Cellular accumulation of the new ketolide RU 64004 by human neutrophils: comparison with that of azithromycin and roxithromycin. *Antimicrob Agents Chemother* 41: 2099–2107

7 Vazifeh D, Preira A, Bryskier A, Labro MT (1998) Interactions between HMR 3647, a new ketolide, and human polymorphonuclear neutrophils. *Antimicrob Agents Chemother* 42: 1944–1951

8 Miossec-Bartoli C, Pilatre L, Peyron P, N'Diaye E-N, Collart-Dutilleul V, Maridonneau-Parini I, Diu-Hercend A (1999) The new ketolide HMR 3647 accumulates in the azurophilic granules of human polymorphonuclear cells.*Antimicrob Agents Chemother* 43: 2457–2462

9 Mtairag E M, Abdelghaffar H, Labro MT (1994) Investigation of dirithromycin and erythromycylamine uptake by human neutrophils in vitro. *J Antimicrob Chemother* 33: 523–536

10 Mtairag E.M, Abdelghaffar H, Douhet C, Labro MT (1995) Role of extracellular calcium in *in vitro* uptake and intraphagocytic location of macrolides. *Antimicrob Agents Chemother* 39: 1676–1682

11 Wildfeuer A, Reisert I, Laufen H (1993) Uptake and subcellular distribution of azithromycin in human phagocytic cells. *Arzneim Forsch* 43: 484–486

12 Vazifeh D, Labro MT (1999) Investigation of the uptake of HMR 3647, HMR 3004 and roxithromycin by myelomonocytic cell lines. Abstr 1929 In *Program and abstracts of the 39th Intersci Conf Antimicrob Agents Chemother* ASM Washington DC, p. 48

13 Raghoebar M, Van den Berg WB, Van Ginneken CAM (1987) Alteration of chloroquine accumulation in human polymorphonuclearleucocytes under inflammatory conditions. *Int J Tissue React* 9: 255–261

14 Laufen H, Wildfeuer A, Lach P (1990) Mechanism of azithromycin uptake in human polymorphonuclear leucocytes *Arzneim Forsch* 40: 686–689

15 Hand WL, King-Thompson N, Holman JW (1987) Entry of roxithromycin (RU 965), imipenem, cefotaxime, trimethoprim, and metronidazole into human polymorphonuclear leukocytes. *Antimicrob Agents Chemother* 31: 1553–1557

16 Labro MT, Abdelghaffar H, Vazifeh D, Bryskier A (1996) Roxithromycin uptake by human neutrophils is mediated by a protein kinase A-dependent mechanism. Abstr 110–018 In *Program and abstracts of the 7 h Intern Congr Infect Dis.* p. 278

17 Endicott JA, Ling V (1989) The biochemistry of P-glycoprotein-mediated multidrug resistance. *Ann Rev Biochem* 58: 137–171

18 Fardel O, Lecureur V, Guillouzo A (1996) The P-glycoprotein multidrug transporter. *Gen Pharmac* 27: 1283–1291
19 Wakasugi H, Yano I, Ito T, Hashida T, Futami T, Nohara R, Sasayama S, Inui K (1998) Effect of clarithromycin on renal excretion of digoxin: interaction with P-glycoprotein. *Clin Pharmacol Ther* 64: 123–128
20 Arceci RJ, Stieglitz K, Bierer BE (1992) Immunosuppressant FK506 and rapamycin function as reversal agents of the multidrug-resistance phenotype. *Blood.* 80: 1528–36
21 Crosta L, Candiloro V, Meli M, Tolomeo M, Rausa L, Dusonchet (1994) Lacidipine and josamycin: two new multidrug resistance modulators. *Anticancer Res* 14: 2685–2690
22 Saeki T, Ueda K, Tanigawara Y, Hori R, Komano T (1993) Human P-glycoprotein transports cyclosporin A and FK506. *J BiolChem* 268: 6077–6080
23 Hand WL, Hand DL (1995) Influence of pentoxifylline and its derivatives on antibiotic uptake and superoxide generation by human phagocytic cells. *Antimicrob Agents Chemother* 39:1574–1579
24 Vazifeh D, Bryskier A, Labro MT (2000) Effect of proinflammatory cytokines on the interplay between roxithromycin, HMR 3647, or HMR 3004 and human polymorphonuclear neutrophils. *Antimicrob Agents Chemother* 44: 511–21
25 Bermudez LE, Inderlied C, Young LS (1991) Stimulation with cytokines enhances penetration of azithromycin into human macrophages. *Antimicrob Agents Chemother* 35: 2625–2629
26 Geerdes-Fenge HF, Goetschi B, Rau M, Borner K, Koeppe P, Wettich K, Lode H (1997) Comparative pharmacokinetics of dirithromycin and erythromycin in normal volunteers with special regard to accumulation in polymorphonuclear leukocytes and in saliva. *Eur J Clin Pharmacol* 53: 127–133
27 Ballow CH, Amsden GW, Highet VS, Forrest A (1998) Pharmacokinetics of oral azithromycin in serum, urine, polymorphonuclear leucocytes and inflammatory vs non-inflammatory skin blisters in healthy volunteers. *Clin Drug Invest* 15: 159–67
28 Baldwin DR, Wise R, Andrew JM, Ashby JP, Honeybourne D (1990) Azithromycin concentrations at the site of pulmonary infections. *Eur Resp J* 3: 886–90
29 Olsen KM, San Pedro GS, Gann LP, Gubbins PO, Halinski DM , Campbell GD jr (1996) Intrapulmonary pharmacokinetics of azithromycin in healthy volunteers given five oral doses. *Antimicrob Agents Chemother* 40: 2382–2385
30 Aubert J-D, Juillerat-Jeanneret L, Fioroni P, Dayer P, Plan P-A, Leuenberger P (1998) Function of alveolar macrophages after a 3-day course of azithromycin in healthy volunteers. *Pulm Pharmacol Therapeut* 11: 263–269
31 Stamler DA, Edelstein MAC, Edelstein PH (1994) Azithromycin pharmacokinetics and intracellular concentrations in *Legionella pneumophila* -infected and uninfected guinea pigs and their alveolar macrophages. *Antimicrob Agents Chemother* 38: 217–222
32 Gladue RP, Bright GM, Isaacson RE, Newborg MF (1985) *In vitro* and *in vivo* uptake of azithromycin (CP-52,993) by phagocytic cells: possible mechanism of delivery and release at sites of infection. *Antimicrob Agents Chemother* 33: 277–282
33 Frank MO, Sullivan GW, Carper HT, Mandell GL (1992) In vitro demonstration of transport and delivery of antibiotics by polymorphonuclear leukocytes. *Antimicrob Agents Chemother* 36: 2584–2588
34 Paul TR, Knight ST, Raulston JE, Wryck PB (1997) Delivery of azithromycin to *Chlamydia trachomatis*-infected polarized human endometrial epithelial cells by polymorphonuclear leucocytes. *J Antimicrob Chemother* 39: 623–630
35 Milisen WB, Girard AE (1993) Preferential concentrations of azithromycin in an infected mouse thigh model. *J Antimicrob Chemother* 31 (Suppl. E): 5–16
36 Fontan PA, Buzzola FR, Spinedi EG, Sordelli DO (1996) *Haemophilus influenzae* type b exoproducts induce chemotaxis and macrolide antibiotic release by human polymorphonuclear leukocytes. *Chemother* 42: 71–77.
37 Girard D, Bergeron JM, Milisen WB, Retsema JH (1993) Comparison of azithromycin, roxithromycin and cephalexin penetration kinetics in early and mature abscesses. *J Antimicrob Chemother* 31 (Suppl. E): 17–28

38 Labro MT (1993) Effects of macrolides on host natural defenses. In: AJ Bryskier, J-P Butzler, HC Neu, PM Tulkens (eds): *Macrolides: Chemistry, pharmacology and clinical uses* Arnette-Blackwell, Paris, 389–408
39 Labro MT (1998) Antiinflammatory activity of macrolides: a new therapeutic potential? *J Antimicrob Chemother* 41 (Suppl.B): 37–46
40 Labro MT (1998) Immunological effects of macrolides. *Curr Opin Infect Dis* 11: 681–688.
41 Abdelghaffar H, Vazifeh D, Labro MT (1997) Erythromycin A-derived macrolides modify the functional activities of human neutrophils by altering the phospholipase D-phosphatidate phosphohydrolase transduction pathway. *J Immunol* 159: 3995
4005
42 Hackstadt T (1998) The diverse habitats of obligate intracellular parasites. *Curr Opin Microbiol* 1: 82–87
43 Moulder JW (1985) Comparative biology of intracellular parasitism. *Microbiol Rev* 49: 298–337
44 Maurin M, Raoult D (1996) Optimum treatment of intracellular infections. *Drugs.* 52: 45–59
45 Butts JD (1994) Intracellular concentrations of antibacterial agents and related clinical implications. *Clin Pharmacokinet* 27: 63–84
46 Labro MT (1996) Intracellular bioactivity of macrolides. *Clin Microbiol Infect* 1 (Suppl.1): S24–S30
47 Anderson R, Van Rensburg CEJ, Jooné G, Lukey PT (1987) An *in vitro* comparison of the intraphagocytic bioactivity of erythromycin and roxithromycin. *J Antimicrob Chemother* 20 (Suppl.B): 57–68
48 Labro MT, Amit C, Babin-Chevaye C, Hakim J (1986) Synergy between RU 28965 (roxithromycin) and human neutrophils for bactericidal activity in vitro. *Antimicrob Agents Chemother* 30: 137–142
49 Torigoe R (1993) The intracellular activity of ofloxacin and roxithromycin against *Staphylococcus aureus* phagocytosed in human neutrophils. *Chemother* 41: 955–62
50 Labro MT, Vazifeh D, Bryskier A (1999) Bactericidal activity of the ketolide HMR 3647 and roxithromycin in combination with human neutrophils. Abstr 1246 In *Program and abstracts of the 39th Intersci Conf Antimicrob Agents Chemother* ASM Washington DC, p. 258
51 Scaglione F, Demartini G, Dugnani S, Fraschini F (1993) A new model examining intracellular and extracellular activity of amoxicillin, azithromycin and clarithromycin in infected cells. *Chemother* 39: 416–423
52 Hoogeterp JJ, Mattie H, Van Furth R (1993) Activity of erythromycin and clindamycin in an experimental *Staphylococcus aureus* infection in normal and granulocytopenic mice. *Scand J Infect Dis* 25: 123–132
53 Stout JE, Arnold B, Yu VL (1998) Activity of azithromycin, clarithromycin, roxithromycin, dirithromycin, quinupristin/dalfopristin and erythromycin against *Legionella* species by intracellular susceptibility testing in HL-60 cells. *J Antimicrob Chemother* 41: 289–291
54 Donowitz GR, Earnhardt KI (1993) Azithromycin inhibition of intracellular *Legionella micdadei* .*Antimicrob Agents Chemother* 37: 2261–2264
55 Baltch AL, Smith RP, Franke MA, Michelsen PB (1998) Antibacterial effects of levofloxacin, erythromycin, and rifampin in a human monocyte system against *Legionella pneumophila. Antimicrob Agents Chemother* 42: 3153–3156
56 Ramirez JA (1993) Comparative study of the bactericidal activity of ampicillin/sulbactam and erythromycin against intracellular *Legionella pneumophila. J Antimicrob Chemother* 32: 93–99
57 Hammerschlag MR, Qumel KK, Roblin PM (1992) *In vitro* activities of azithromycin, clarithromycin, L-ofloxacin, and other antibiotics against *Chlamydia pneumoniae. Antimicrob Agents Chemother* 36: 1573–1574
58 Rastogi N, Labrousse V, Bryskier A (1995) Intracellular activities of roxithromycin used alone and in association with other drugs against *Mycobacterium avium* complex in human macrophages. *Antimicrob Agents Chemother* 39: 976–978
59 Bermudez LEM, Young LS (1988) Activities of amikacin, roxithromycin, and azithromycin alone or in combination with Tumor necrosis factor against *Mycobacterium avium* complex. *Antimicrob Agents Chemother* 32: 1149–1153

60 Skinner PS, Furney SK, Jacobs MR, Klopman G, Ellner JJ, Orme IM (1994) A bone marrow-derived murine macrophage model for evaluating efficacy of antimycobacterial drugs under relevant physiologic conditions. *Antimicrob Agents Chemother* 38: 2557–2563.

61 Yajko DM , Sanders CA, Mady JJ, Cawthon VL, Hadley WK (1996) *In vitro* activities of rifabutin, azithromycin, ciprofloxacin, clarithromycin, clofazimine, ethambutol, and amikacin in combinations of two, three, and four drugs. *Antimicrob Agents Chemother* 40: 743–749.

62 Mor N, Heifets L (1993) MICs and MBCs of clarithromycin against *Mycobacterium avium* within human macrophages. *Antimicrob Agents Chemother* 37: 111–114.

63 Baradelli IE, Plosker GL, Metavish D (1993) Clarithromycin. A review of its pharmacologic properties and therapeutic use in *mycobacterium avium* intracellulare complex infection in patients with acquired immune deficiency syndrome. *Drugs* 46: 289–312

64 Lazard T, Perronne C, Cohen Y, Grosset J, Vildé JL, Pocidalo JJ (1993) Efficacy of granulocyte colony-stimulating factor and RU-40555 in combination with clarithromycin against *Mycobacterium avium* complex infection on C57 BL/6 mice.*Antimicrob.Agents Chemother* 37: 692–695.

65 Blais J, Beauchamp D, Chamberland S (1994) Azithromycin uptake and intracellular accumulation by *Toxoplasma gondii*-infected macrophages. *J Antimicrob Chemother.*34: 371–382

66 Strickman D, Sheer T, Salata K, Hershey J, Dasch G, Kelly D, Kuschner R (1995) *In vitro* effectiveness of azithromycin against doxycycline-resistant and -susceptible *Rickettsia tsutsugamushi,* etiologic agent of scrub typhus. *Antimicrob Agents Chemother* 39: 2406–2410

67 Ives TJ, Manzewitsch P, Regnery RL, Butts JD. Kebede M (1997) *In vitro* susceptibilities of *Bartonella henselae, B. quintana, B. elisabethae, Rickettsia rickettsii, R. conorii, R. akari,* and *R. prowazekii* to macrolide antibiotics as determined by immunofluorescent-antibody analysis of infected vero cells monolayers *Antimicrob Agents Chemother* 41: 578–582

68 Nichterlein T, Kretschman M, Schadt A, Meyer A, Wildfeuer A, Laufen H, Hof H (1998) Reduced intracellular activity of antibiotics against *Listeria monocytogenes* in multidrug resistant cells. *Int J Antimicrob Agents* 10: 119–125

69 Ouadrhiri Y, Scorneaux B, Sibille Y, Tulkens PM (1999) Mechanism of the intracellular killing and modulation of antibiotic susceptibility of *Listeria monocytogenes* in THP-1 macrophages activated by gamma interferon. *Antimicrob Agents Chemother* 43: 1242–1251

70 Rakita RM, Jacques-Palaz K, Murray BE (1994) Intracellular activity of azithromycin against bacterial enteric pathogens. *Antimicrob Agents Chemother* 38: 1915–1921

71 Willot I, Scorneaux B, Tulkens PM (1993) Comparative intracellular activity of antibiotics against virulent *L. monocytogenes* and *S. flexneri* and their non-virulent mutants in a model of J774 macrophages. Abstr 769 In *Program and abstracts of the 33rd Intersci Conf Antimicrob Agents Chemother*

72 Abdelghaffar H, Mtairag EM, Labro MT (1994) Effect of dirithromycin and erythromycylamine on human neutrophil degranulation. *Antimicrob Agents Chemother* 38: 1548–1554

73 Fréhel C, Offredo C, de Chastelier C (1997) The phagosomal environment protects virulent *Mycobacterium* from killing and destruction by clarithromycin. *Infect Immun* 65: 2792–2802

Macrolide Antibiotics
ed. by W. Schönfeld and H. A. Kirst

Clarithromycin and new derivatives of erythromycin

Takashi Adachi and Shigeo Morimoto

Medicinal Research Laboratories, Taisho Pharmaceutical Co., Ltd., 403 Yoshino-cho 1-chome, Saitama-shi, Saitama 330–8530, Japan

Introduction

Since erythromycin's the discovery in 1952 [1], it has been one of the most useful macrolide antibiotics, having the highest antibacterial activity and low toxicity. In order to achieve high antibacterial activities against a wide variety of pathogens and favorable pharmacokinetic properties, tremendous efforts have been made related to chemical modification [2, 3]. In the 1970s and 1980s, dirithromycin, flurithromycin, and davercin were synthesized and evaluated. Erythromycin itself is quite unstable under acidic conditions, so esters, salts, and various formulations also have been developed.

At Taisho Pharmaceutical Co. Ltd., we were interested in the role of the hydroxyl groups of erythromycin (**2**), and a series of *O*-alkylated derivatives was synthesized [4–8]. Among them, clarithromycin (6-*O*-methylerythromycin A, **1**) exhibited antibacterial activities against aerobic gram-positive bacteria, some gram-negative bacteria, anaerobic bacteria, *Mycoplasma,* and *Chlamydia.* The antibacterial activities of clarithromycin were equal to or two-fold better than erythromycin A (**2**) *in vitro*. However, clarithromycin is fairly stable in acidic conditions due to 6-*O*-methylation, which brought about excellent biological properties, especially *in vivo* antibacterial activities, pharmacokinetic properties, and metabolism. The structural difference between clarithromycin and erythromycin is only the 6-*O*-methyl group, but the biological properties of clarithromycin were improved considerably.

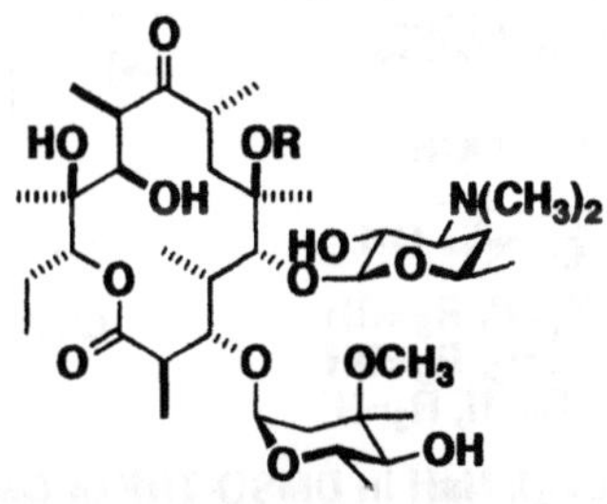

Clarithromycin (1) R=CH_3
Erythromycin A (2) R=H

Figure 1. Structures of clarithromycin (1) and erythromycin A (2).

Clarithromycin was developed by Taisho Pharmaceutical Co., Ltd. and Abbott Laboratories and has been used for infectious diseases throughout the world.

From the viewpoint of the chemistry of macrolide antibiotics, structure-activity relationships of erythromycin derivatives, the selective synthesis of clarithromycin for industrial production, biological properties, and also our recent research activities on macrolide antibiotics will be described.

Synthesis of erythromycin derivatives and structure-activity relationships

The synthesis of *O*-alkylerythromycins is shown in Scheme 1 [4, 5]. According to Flynn's method [9], 2'-*O*,3'-*N*-bis-carbobenzoxy-*N*-demethylerythromycin (**3**) was obtained. Methylation of **3** with MeI/KOH in a mixture of dimethylsulfoxide (DMSO) and 1, 2-dimethoxyethane (DME) gave the mixture of 6-*O*-methylated (**4**) and 11-*O*-methylated compounds (**5**). Hydrogenation to remove the carbobenzoxy groups and hydrogenation with formaldehyde to regenerate the dimethylamino group (DME) gave clarithromycin (**1**) and 11-*O*-methylerythromycin A (**6**). Minor by-products, 6,11-di-*O*-methyl (**7**) and 6,12-di-*O*-methylerythromycins A (**8**), were obtained by methylation by using a slight excess of KOH, successive

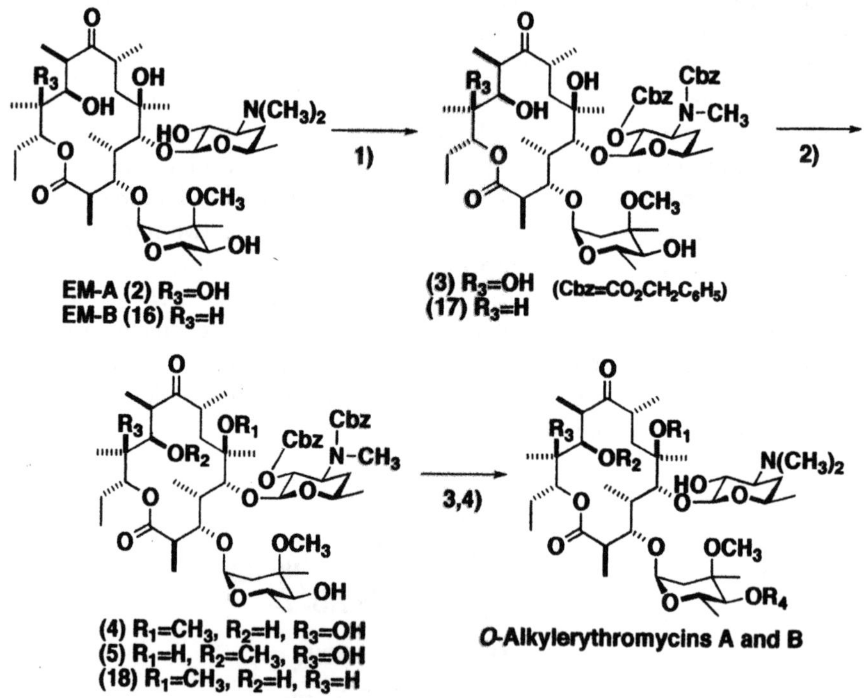

1) CbzCl, $NaHCO_3$ 2) CH_3I, NaH in DMSO-THF or DMSO-DME(1:1) or DMF
3) H_2 / Pd-C in EtOH-Acetate buffer 4) HCHO, H_2 / Pd-C in EtOH-Acetate buffer

Scheme 1. Synthesis of *O*-alkylerythromycins A and B.

hydrogenation, and *N*-methylation. Methylation of **3** with dimethylsulfate/NaH in DMF gave 11-*O*-methyl (**6**) and 11,4"-di-*O*-methyl derivatives (**9**). Methylation of **3** with excess MeI and NaH gave 11,12,4"-tri-*O*-methyl (**11**) and 6,11,12,4"-tetra-*O*-methyl derivatives (**12**). Methylation of **4** with excess KOH gave the 6,11,4"-tri-*O*-methyl derivative (**10**). By alkylation similar to that of **3** using the corresponding alkyl halide, 6-*O*-ethyl (**13**), 11-*O*-ethylerythromycin A (**14**) and 11-*O*-propylerythromycin A (**15**) were obtained [5]. By similar methods, *O*-alkylerythromycins B (**19–23**) were obtained from erythromycin B (**16**) [6].

In vitro antibacterial activities are shown in Table 1 [8]. Against *Staphylococcus aureus* and *Bacillus subtilis*, clarithromycin (**1**) was equal to or two-fold more active than erythromycin (**2**). 6,12-di-*O*-Methylerythromycin A (**8**) and 6-*O*-methylerythromycin B (**19**) showed activity equal to **2**. 11-*O*-Methylerythromycin A (**6**) was slightly less active than **2**. 6-*O*-Ethyl (**13**) and 11-*O*-ethylerythromycins A (**14**) were slightly less active than the corresponding *O*-methylerythromycins. Tri- and tetra-*O*-methylerythromycins showed weak activities. The activities of *O*-alkyl derivatives decreased with the number of methyl groups and with increasing alkyl chain length. Although clarithromycin was the most active compound, the effect of 6-*O*-methylation was not so remarkable *in vitro*.

Table 2 shows the *in vivo* antibacterial activities against systemic infections in mice induced by *S. aureus* [5, 6, 8]. 11-*O*-Methylerythromycin A (**6**) was slightly more active than erythromycin (**2**). On the other hand, 6-*O*-methylerythromycins (**1, 7, 8, 19**) were more active than erythromycin. Clarithromycin (**1**) was 3.6 to 7.6 times more active than **2**.

Table 1. *In vitro* antibacterial activities of *O*-alkylerythromycins A and B.

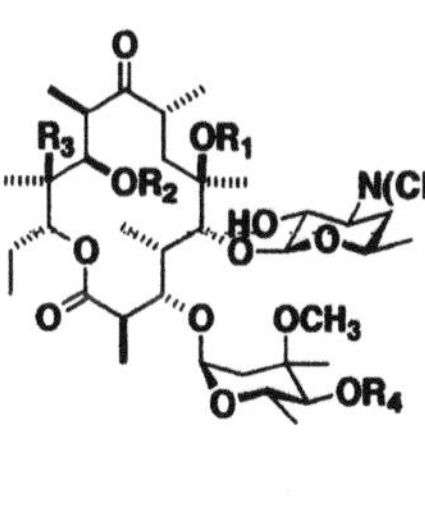

Compound	R_1	R_2	R_3	R_4	MIC(μg/ml) Staphylococcus aureus Smith 4	Bacillus subtilis ATCC 6633
1	CH_3	H	OH	H	0.10	0.05
2	H	H	OH	H	0.20	0.10
6	H	CH_3	OH	H	0.39	0.39
7	CH_3	CH_3	OH	H	0.39	0.20
8	CH_3	H	OCH_3	H	0.20	0.05
9	H	CH_3	OH	CH_3	1.56	0.78
10	CH_3	CH_3	OH	CH_3	1.56	1.56
11	H	CH_3	OCH_3	CH_3	12.5	3.13
12	CH_3	CH_3	OCH_3	CH_3	6.25	1.56
13	C_2H_5	H	OH	H	0.39	0.10
14	H	C_2H_5	OH	H	0.78	0.39
15	H	C_3H_7	OH	H	1.56	0.78
16	H	H	H	H	0.20	0.10
19	CH_3	H	H	H	0.20	0.10
20	H	CH_3	H	H	0.39	0.10
21	CH_3	H	H	CH_3	3.13	0.78
22	CH_3	CH_3	H	CH_3	3.13	1.56
23	C_2H_5	H	H	H	0.78	0.10

Table 2. *In vivo* antibacterial activities of *O*-methylerythromycins against systemic infections in mice induced by *Staphylococcus aureus* Smith 4.

Compound[a)]	ED_{50} (mg/mouse)	
	Test-1 (n=20)	Test-2 (n=15)
Erythromycin A (2)	0.977 (0.760-1.22)	0.652 (0.519-0.851)
Clarithromycin (1)	0.273 (0.222-0.333)	0.086 (0.058-0.111)
6,11-*di-O*-Methylerythromycin A (7)	0.446 (0.370-0.534)	
6,12-*di-O*-Methylerythromycin A (8)		0.216 (0.161-0.285)
11-*O*-Methylerythromycin A (6)	0.738 (0.554-0.914)	
6-*O*-Methylerythromycin B (19)		0.358 (0.253-0.458)

a) : Compounds were administered orally to ICR mouse (4 week, male) 1 h after infection

Kurath reported the mechanism of the acid-catalyzed decomposition of erythromycin [10]. The 6-hydroxyl group and the 9-carbonyl group form erythromycin enol ether by dehydration, and then the 12-hydroxyl group attacks the 9-position to give a spiroketal. The 6-hydroxyl group is protected by the methyl group in 6-*O*-alkylerythromycins, which gives stability to the molecule. 6-*O*-alkylerythromycins showed higher acid stabilities than erythromycin A. The half-lives ($t_{1/2}$) of clarithromycin and erythromycin A were 25.1 hours and 0.03 hours, respectively [8].

The pharmacokinetic properties of 6-*O*-methylerythromycins were then compared. After oral administration of clarithromycin (**1**), 6,11-di-*O*-methylerythromycin A (**7**), 6-*O*-methylerythromycin B (**19**), and erythromycin (**2**) at a dose of 50 mg/kg to rats, peak plasma concentrations (C_{max}) were 2.40, 2.53, 1.70, and 0.64 µg/ml, respectively. The areas under the plasma concentration-time curves (AUCs) of these derivatives were 11.17, 15.07, 15.2, and 2.37 µg·h/ml, respectively [5, 6]. A favorable distribution of 6-*O*-methylerythromycins in the lung tissue and cells was observed in rats [11]. Taking into account the antibacterial activities, clarithromycin had the highest potency in the lung. Clarithromycin was selected as being the most promising candidate for a new antibiotic.

Selective synthesis of clarithromycin

The original synthetic process (Scheme 1) for clarithromycin using the intermediate, **3**, was not selective, and the reactivity of the 11-hydroxyl group was higher than that of the 6-hydroxyl group [4, 5]. In spite of an exhaustive examination of reaction conditions, selective 6-*O*-methylation was not achieved. The 11-hydroxyl group was protected by acetyl, methoxyethoxymethyl, and 11,12-carbonate groups (Scheme 2). But the protected compounds existed as

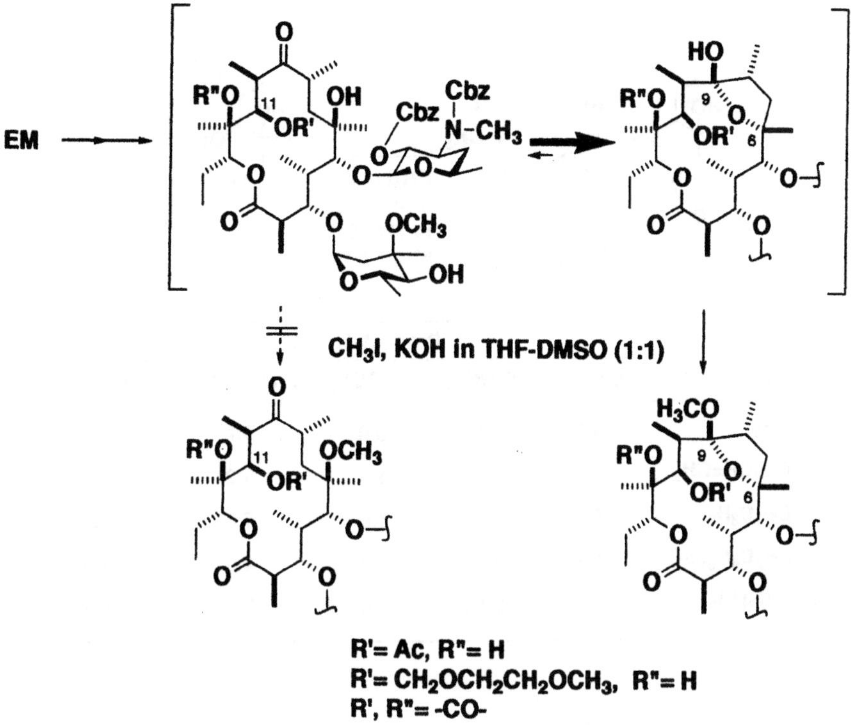

Scheme 2. Protection of 11-hydroxyl group.

the 6,9-hemiketal form, and the 9-*O*-methyl-6,9-hemiketal compound was obtained.

However, selectivity was greatly different between erythromycins A (**2**) and B (**16**). Erythromycin B is a minor component of the fermentation of erythromycin A and lacks the 12-hydroxyl group (Scheme 1). Methylation of 2'-*O*,3'-*N*-bis-carbobenzoxyerythromycin B (**17**) by MeI and KOH (1.3 equivalent) in a mixture of DMSO-DME gave the 6-*O*-methylated compound (**18**) as a major product [6]. Small amounts of the 11-*O*-methylated and 6,4"-di-*O*-methylated compounds were obtained. It was thought that a lack of the 12-hydroxyl group influenced the conformation of the aglycone and selectivity of methylation was greatly improved.

To change the conformation of the aglycone in erythromycin A, the 9-carbonyl group was converted to oximes, hydrazones, amines, and alcohol. From these studies, regioselective methylation was achieved by using 9-oxime derivatives [12]. Protective groups on the oxime influenced the selectivity, and allyl, benzyl, substituted benzyl, and trityl groups were examined (Tab. 3). *o*-Chlorobenzyl oxime gave the highest selectivity.

Scheme 3 shows the synthesis of clarithromycin. Oximation of **3** with hydroxylamine, and protection of the oxime with *o*-chlorobenzyl chloride afforded the bis-carbobenzoxy 9-oxime derivative **24**. Compound **24** was then methylated with MeI/KOH in DMSO-tetrahydrofuran (THF) to give the

Table 3. Methylation of erythromycin 9-oxime derivatives (1).

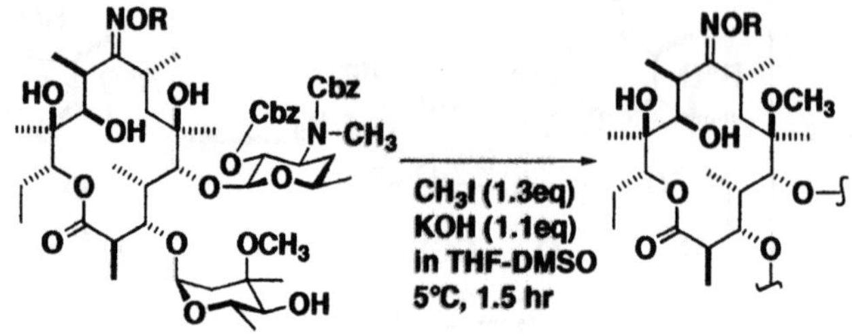

R	Product, % yield				
	6-OH	6-OCH$_3$	11-OCH$_3$	6,11-di-OCH$_3$	6,4"-di-OCH$_3$
-CH$_3$	9.1	79.9	0.9	6.7	1.6
-CH$_2$CH=CH$_2$	8.6	84.5	1.4	5.2	1.5
-CH$_2$C$_6$H$_5$	7.1	84.1	1.6	5.6	1.2
-CH$_2$C$_6$H$_5$(2-Cl)	4.6	86.2	1.2	4.0	1.3
-C(C$_6$H$_5$)$_3$	18.2	78.4	1.4	0.4	0.9

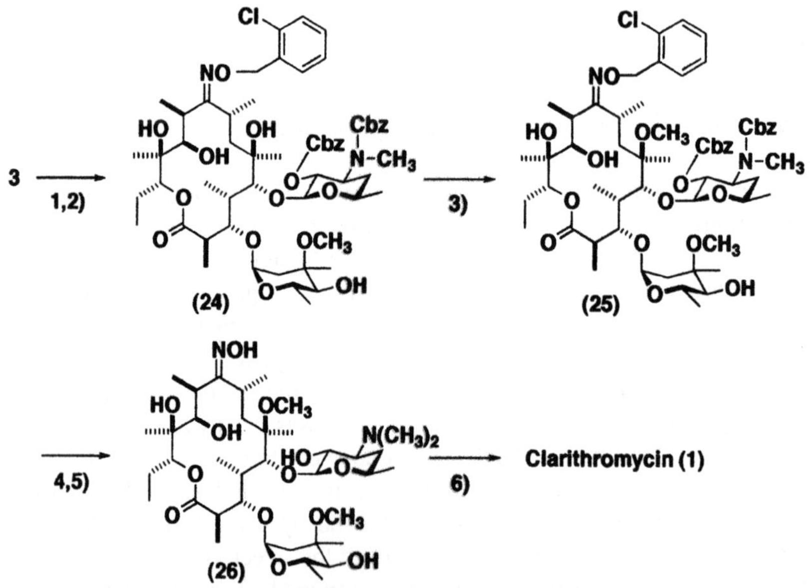

1) NH_2OH-HCl, AcONa in MeOH 2) (2-Cl)$C_6H_4CH_2Cl$, KOH in DMF
3) CH_3I, KOH in THF-DMSO 4) H_2 / Pd-Black in MeOH-AcOH-H_2O
5) HCHO, HCO_2H in EtOH 6) $NaHSO_3$ in EtOH-H_2O

Scheme 3. Synthesis of clarithromycin *via* regioselective methylation (1).

6-*O*-methyl derivative (**25**) as a major product. Hydrogenation to remove the carbobenzoxy groups and *N*-methylation by the Eschweiler-Clarke reaction gave 6-*O*-methylerythromycin A 9-oxime (**26**). Deoximation of **26** was achieved under mild conditions by using sodium bisulfite to give clarithromycin (**1**).

The above method had several problems as an industrial production process. A large amount of carbobenzoxy chloride is used. Hydrogenation could not be carried out at times because of contamination by an unknown catalyst poison. More efficient protective groups were investigated, and it was found that the bulky trimethylsilyl (TMS) group on the 2'-hydroxyl group prevents the formation of 3'-*N*-trimethylammonium salt with MeI due to steric hindrance [13]. Then we investigated the protective group of the oxime, which could be removed together with the TMS groups under acidic conditions, and ketals were found to be efficient for the protection of the oxime. Table 4 shows the selectivity of 6-*O*-methylation of various ketal oximes. Among these protective groups, the 1-isopropoxycyclohexyl group gave the best selectivity, which was superior to the previous *o*-chlorobenzyl group. Bulky protecting groups were favorable for 6-*O*-methylation.

Scheme 4 shows the whole synthetic route. Oximation of erythromycin A (**2**) with hydroxylamine gave the oxime (**27**). Trimethylsilylation of **27** with 1,1,1,3,3,3-hexamethyldisilazane (HMDS)/pyridine hydrochloride and successive ketalization with cyclohexanone diisopropyl ketal gave bis-TMS ketal (**28**), which

Table 4. Methylation of erythromycin 9-oxime derivatives (2).

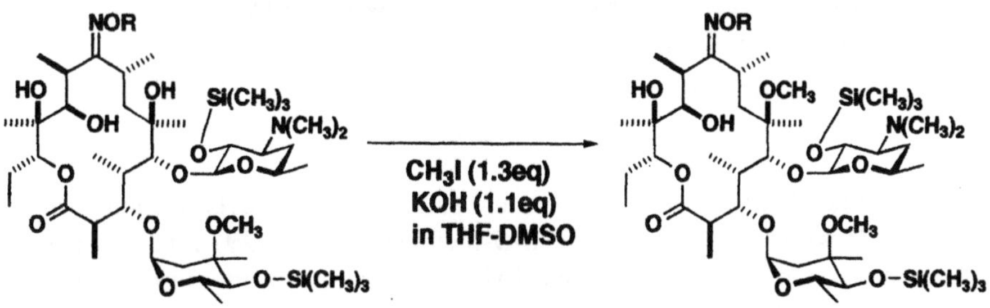

R	Product, % yield 6-OH	6-OCH$_3$	6,11-di-OCH$_3$
-CH$_2$CH=CH$_2$	11.6	77.4	5.5
-CH$_2$C$_6$H$_5$(2-Cl)	7.0	84.8	4.8
-CH(OC$_2$H$_5$)$_2$	11.7	71.4	14.1
-C(CH$_3$)$_2$-O-i-Pr	4.9	87.0	2.6
-C(CH$_3$)$_2$-O-n-Bt	4.0	87.2	2.3
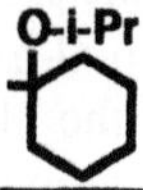 O-i-Pr	5.5	90.0	1.0

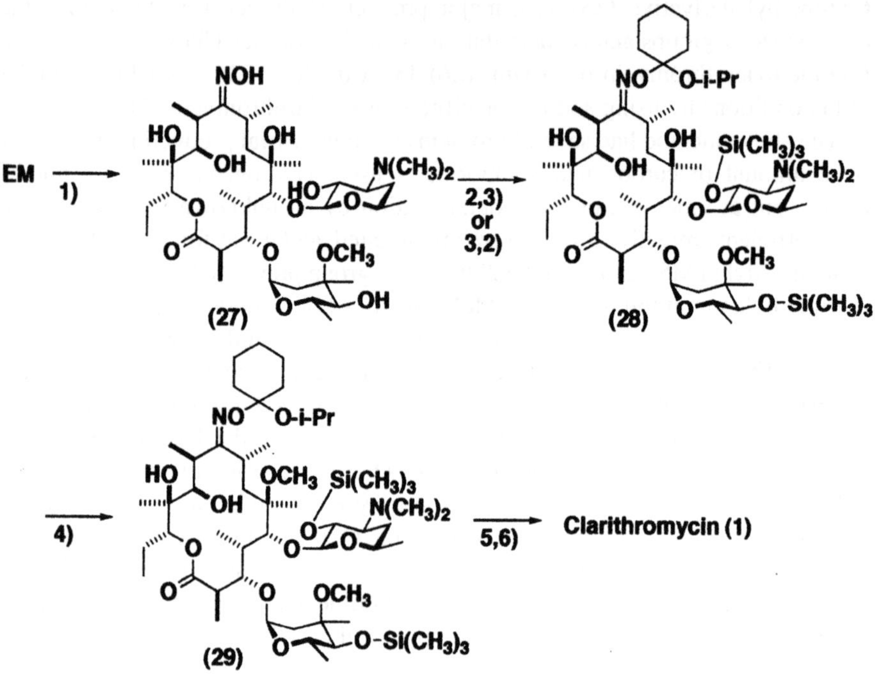

1) NH_2OH, HCO_2H in MeOH 2) HMDS, Pyr·HCl in MeCN 3) Cyclohexanone diisopropyl ketal, Pyr·HCl in MeCN 4) CH_3I, KOH in THF-DMSO 5) HCO_2H in EtOH-H_2O 6) $NaHSO_3$ in EtOH-H_2O

Scheme 4. Synthesis of clarithromycin *via* regio-selective methylation (2).

also could be obtained by ketalization and successive trimethylsilylation. Methylation of **28** with MeI/KOH gave the 6-*O*-methyl derivative (**29**). Finally, removal of all protective groups (ketal and TMS) by treatment with formic acid and deoximation with sodium bisulfite gave clarithromycin [14]. The advantages of this process are as follows: 1) excellent selectivity of 6-*O*-methylation; 2) catalytic hydrogenation is avoided; 3) protection and deprotection can be done under mild conditions; 4) *N*-Methylation is unnecessary; and 5) protection of 4"-hydroxyl groups by TMS decreases the 4"-*O*-methylated by-products.

The selectivities of 6-*O*-methylation were completely different between erythromycin A, erythromycin A oxime, and erythromycin B, which were investigated using a conformation search program, CONFLEX, coupled with MM2 geometry optimization [15, 16]. Two stable clusters A and B were generated mainly for erythronolide A. In cluster A, the 11-hydroxyl group was stabilized more than the 6-hydroxyl group by hydrogen bonding. On the other hand, the 6-hydroxyl group was stabilized in cluster B. In erythronolide A, the proportion of clusters A and B was 78% and 21%, respectively, suggesting that 6-*O*-methylation proceeds more than 11-*O*-methylation. But it was calculated that the 11-hydroxyl anion in cluster B was considerably more stable than the 6-hydroxy anion in cluster A. As a result, 11-*O*-methylation from cluster B proceeds more than 6-*O*-methylation from cluster A in erythromycin A. On the other hand, erythronolide A oxime and erythronolide B take cluster A and cluster D, respectively. Neither compound takes cluster B. In clusters A and D, the 11-hydroxyl groups were masked from methylation. Thus, 6-*O*-methylation proceeds regio-selectively in erythromycin A oxime and erythromycin B derivatives.

Biological properties of clarithromycin

Clarithromycin showed a broad antibacterial spectrum similar to that of erythromycin [8, 17–20]. *In vitro* antibacterial activities of clarithromycin are shown in Table 5 [8]. Clarithromycin showed strong activities against gram-positive bacteria (*Staphylococcus aureus*, *Staphylococcus epidermidis*, *Streptococcus pneumoniae*, *Streptococcus pyogenes*: MIC_{50} ≤ 0.025 to 0.20 μg/ml), some gram-negative bacteria (*Branhamella catarrhalis*, *Neisseria gonorrhoeae*, *Hae-*

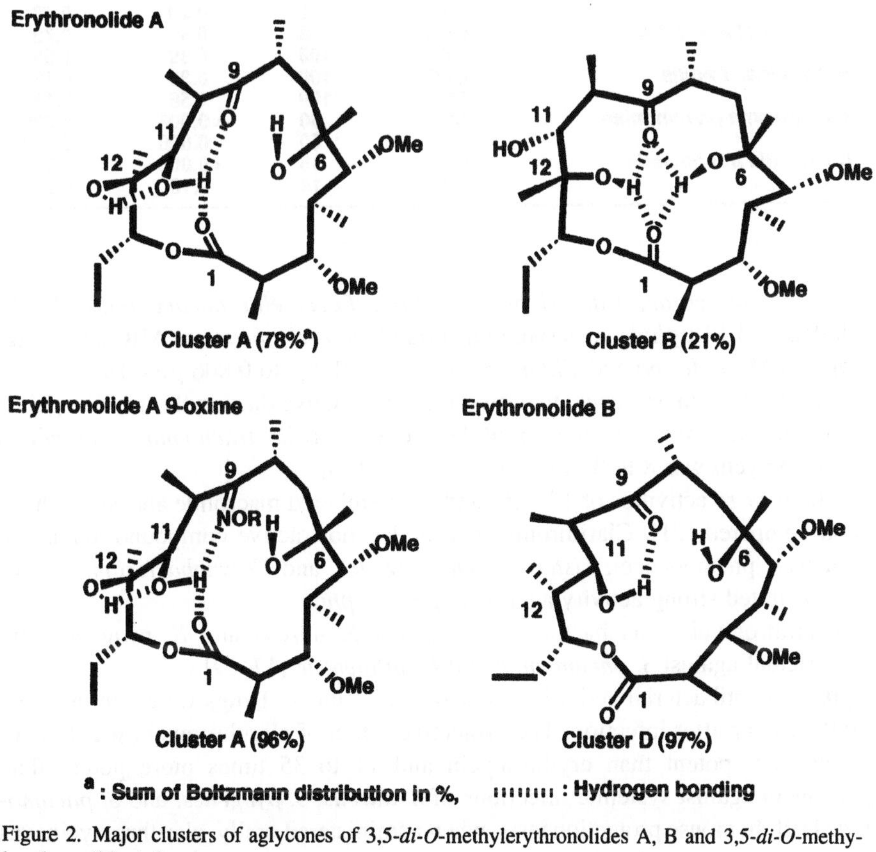

Figure 2. Major clusters of aglycones of 3,5-*di-O*-methylerythronolides A, B and 3,5-*di-O*-methylerythronolide A 9-oxime.

Table 5. *In vitro* antibacterial activity of clarithromycin (CLR) and erythromycin (EM) against clinical isolates.

Strain	Drug	No. of strain	MIC_{50} (μg/ml)	MIC_{80} (μg/ml)
Staphylococcus aureus	CLR	765	0.20	>100
	EM	765	0.39	>100
Staphylococcus epidermidis	CLR	262	0.10	>100
	EM	262	0.20	>100
Streptococcus pyogenes	CLR	274	0.05	>100
	EM	274	0.05	>100
Streptococcus pneumoniae	CLR	166	≤0.025	0.05
	EM	166	0.05	0.05
Enterococcus faecalis	CLR	300	0.78	>100
	EM	300	1.56	>100
Branhamella catarrhalis	CLR	110	0.10	1.56
	EM	110	0.10	0.20
Neisseria gonorrhoeae	CLR	63	0.20	0.78
	EM	63	0.20	1.56
Bordetella pertussis	CLR	22	≤0.012	0.025
	EM	22	0.025	0.05
Haemophilus influenzae	CLR	345	3.13	6.25
	EM	345	3.13	3.13
Campylobacter jejuni	CLR	83	0.39	1.56
	EM	83	0.78	1.56
Legionella pneumophila	CLR	8	≤0.025	0.05
	EM	8	0.20	0.78
Peptostreptococcus sp.	CLR	108	0.39	0.78
	EM	108	0.39	1.56
Bacteroides fragilis	CLR	100	0.39	0.78
	EM	100	1.56	3.13
Mycoplasma pneumoniae	CLR	50	≤0.003	0.006
	EM	50	0.006	0.012
Chlamydia trachomatis	CLR	15	≤0.006	≤0.006
	EM	14	0.10	0.20

mophilus influenzae, *Campylobacter jejuni*, *Legionella pneumophila*: MIC_{50} ≤ 0.012 to 3.13 μg/ml), anaerobic bacteria (*Peptostreptococcus*: MIC_{50} 0.39 μg/ml), and *Mycoplasma* and *Chlamydia* (MIC_{50} ≤ 0.003 to 0.006 μg/ml).

Clarithromycin was equal to or two-fold more active than erythromycin against all organisms except *L. pneumophila* and *Chlamydia trachomatis*, for which clarithromycin was 8 to 30 times more potent [20].

The *in vitro* activities of 14-, 15- and 16-membered macrolide antibiotics have been compared [21]. Clarithromycin was the most active compound against *S. pyogenes*, pneumococci, *Listeria monocytogenes,* and *Corynebacterium* species and exhibited strong activity against *L. pneumophila*.

Clarithromycin was bacteriostatic against *S. aureus* and *S. pyogenes*, but bactericidal against *S. pneumoniae* and *H. influenzae* [17–19].

In vivo antibacterial activities are shown in Table 6. Drugs were administered orally 1 hour after infection. The protective effect of clarithromycin was 6 to 15 times more potent than erythromycin and 11 to 35 times more potent than josamycin against systemic infections of *S. aureus*, *S. pyogenes,* and *S. pneumoniae* [19]. In mouse protection tests, when administered orally, clarithromycin was more potent than erythromycin against *H. influenzae*, *S. pyogenes*, *S. pneumoniae,*

Table 6. Protective effect of clarithromycin, erythromycin and josamycin on systemic infection in mice (ICR mouse, 4 week, male, n=10).

Strain	Challenge dose (cfu/mouse)	Drug[a)]	ED_{50} (mg/mouse)	MIC (μg/ml)
Staphylococcus aureus Smith 4	2.0×10^7 (5% Mucin)	Clarithromycin	0.212	0.10
		Erythromycin	1.23	0.20
		Josamycin	3.01	0.78
Staphylococcus aureus BB	2.0×10^7 (5% Mucin)	Clarithromycin	0.340	0.10
		Erythromycin	3.32	0.10
		Josamycin	11.9	0.39
Streptococcus pyogenes J-1	3.9×10^7 (5% Mucin)	Clarithromycin	0.055	0.05
		Erythromycin	0.837	0.05
		Josamycin	1.92	0.20
Streptococcus pneumoniae IID553	3.3×10^6	Clarithromycin	0.332	0.025
		Erythromycin	3.31	0.05
		Josamycin	3.74	0.10

[a)]: Drugs were administered orally to ICR mouse 1 h after infection

and *S. aureus* [20]. Clarithromycin was more potent than erythromycin against *Legionella* infection in guinea pigs [20].

The strong *in vivo* activities of clarithromycin may be due to its excellent pharmacokinetic properties. After oral administration to mice, C_{max}, AUC, and $t_{1/2}$ of clarithromycin were approximately 3, 6 to 7 and 1.3 to 1.6 times higher than those of erythromycin, respectively [22]. Tissue concentrations of clarithromycin were generally higher than in plasma, especially in the lung of rats and mice [22]. The peak level in lung and the AUC value for clarithromycin were 36 and 69 times higher than those of erythromycin in rats, respectively [22]. Urinary excretions (1 to 24 h) of clarithromycin and erythromycin were 23.2% and 3.3%, respectively, after oral administration to rats [22].

The pharmacokinetic properties of clarithromycin were compared by using [*N*-methyl-^{14}C]clarithromycin and [*N*-methyl-^{14}C]erythromycin in rats [23]. Plasma and tissues levels of clarithromycin were significantly higher than those of erythromycin. Among the tissues, the peak level of [^{14}C]clarithromycin in the lung was especially high. Levels of radioactivity and bioactivity amounted to 15 and 73 times the corresponding levels of [^{14}C]erythromycin, respectively. A high distribution of clarithromycin, especially in lung, was observed by whole-body autoradiograms of rats after intravenous administration of [^{14}C]clarithromycin. Excretions of the total radioactivity of [^{14}C]clarithromycin and [^{14}C]erythromycin were 60% and 20%, respectively [23]. Microautoradiography revealed that radioactivity in the lung was confined almost entirely to the alveolar wall but was rather low in the vascular system [24]. Concerning the affinity of clarithromycin for lung tissue, it is suggested that clarithromycin is transported *via* a carrier-mediated system [25].

In order to evaluate antibiotics, whole-body autobacteriography was established [26]. By combination with autoradiography, antibiotic activity in the whole-body and distribution of the antibiotic could be compared visually. By these techniques, it was found that clarithromycin distributed in high concentration to the tissues, particularly in the lung, and exhibited strong antibacterial activities.

Favorable pharmacokinetic properties were observed in humans, too [27]. Clarithromycin and erythromycin were administered orally at a dose of 200 mg to adult male volunteers in Phase 1 clinical studies. The peak serum concentrations were reached 2 h after administration, showing values of 1.07 μg/ml for clarithromycin and 0.38 μg/ml for erythromycin. The AUC values of clarithromycin and erythromycin were 7.18 μg·h/ml and 1.37 μg·h/ml, respectively. The urinary concentration of clarithromycin was considerably higher than that of erythromycin, and the cumulative recovery rate at 8 h was 31.2% for clarithromycin and only 1.5% for erythromycin.

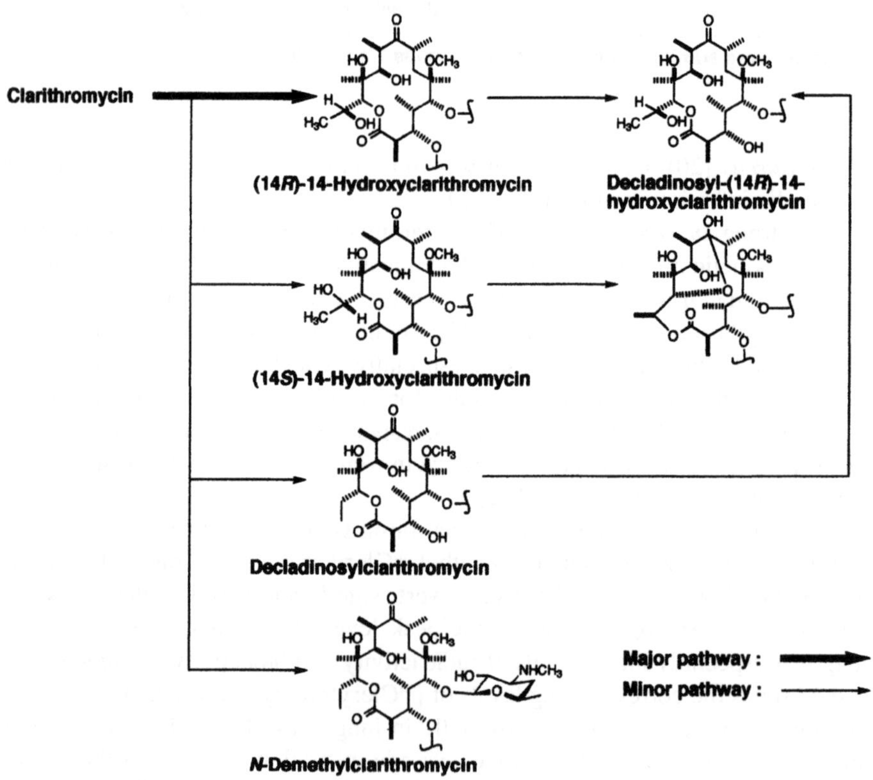

Figure 3. Structures of metabolites of clarithromycin and proposed metabolic pathway in humans.

A unique metabolic pathway in clarithromycin was discovered. Six metabolites were isolated from human urine obtained in Phase 1 clinical studies [28–31]. The proposed metabolic pathway is shown in Figure 3. (14*R*)-14-Hydroxyclarithromycin is the major active metabolite in human. The (14*S*)-epimer was obtained as a minor metabolite. 14-Hydroxylation has never been reported in roxithromycin, azithromycin, or erythromycin. In the metabolism of erythromycin, *N*-demethylation and hydrolysis of cladinose have been well known, whereas *N*-demethylation was a minor metabolic pathway in clarithromycin. 6-*O*-Methylation of erythromycin greatly changed the metabolism of the drug, too.

The metabolism of clarithromycin was considerably different between that in humans and that in animals. *N*-Demethylation is preferential to 14-hydroxylation in rats and dogs [32]. It is noteworthy that hydroxylations have been reported in the metabolism of 16-membered macrolide antibiotics [33–35].

(14*R*)-14-Hydroxyclarithromycin showed *in vitro* activities comparable to clarithromycin [29, 36]. When administered orally, (14*R*)-14-hydroxyclarithromycin was 1.5-fold and 3-fold more active than clarithromycin *in vivo* against systemic infections of *S. aureus* and *S. pneumonaie,* respectively, as is shown in Table 7 [36].

(14*R*)-14-Hydroxyclarithromycin exists in significant quantity in serum and urine [37]. The synergistic effects of 14-hydroxyclarithromycin with clarithromycin were reported against *H. influenzae* [38–40]. It is thought that (14*R*)-14-hydroxyclarithromycin contributes to the clinical efficacy of clarithromycin.

(14*R*)-14-Hydroxyclarithromycin was prepared by microbial conversion of clarithromycin using *Mucor circinelloides* for further biological studies. Microbial conversion is a useful method for preparing metabolites of medicinal substance [41, 42].

Table 7. Protective effect of (14*R*)-14-hydroxyclarithromycin, clarithromycin and erythromycin on systemic infection in mice (ICR mouse, 4 week, male, n=10).

Strain	Challenge dose (cfu/mouse)	Drug[a)]	ED_{50} (mg/mouse)	MIC (μg/ml)
Staphylococcus aureus BB	5.0×10^7 (5% Mucin)	(14*R*)-14-Hydroxyclarithromycin	0.232	0.20
		Clarithromycin	0.370	0.10
		Erythromycin	2.27	0.20
Streptococcus pneumoniae IID553	3.3×10^6	(14*R*)-14-Hydroxyclarithromycin	0.076	0.025
		Clarithromycin	0.222	≥ 0.012
		Erythromycin	1.41	≥ 0.012

a): Drugs were administered orally to ICR mouse 1 h after infection

New clinical uses

Clarithromycin has been used for the treatment of upper and lower respiratory infections, skin and soft tissue infections, and urogenital infections [43, 44].

Additional clinical applications of clarithromycin for the treatment of mycobacterial infections and *Helicobacter pylori*-associated gastroduodenal disease have been approved. Disseminated *Mycobacterium avium* complex (MAC) infection is a common opportunistic disease in AIDS patients and is associated with significant morbidity and mortality. Clarithromycin, having strong antibacterial activities against this pathogen, is useful for the treatment and prevention of MAC infections [45–47]. Clarithromycin has been used for treatment and prevention of the recurrence of gastroduodenal ulcers caused by *H. pylori* by combination therapy with β-lactam antibiotics and proton pump inhibitors. The strong antibacterial activity of clarithromycin against *H. pylori* and high acid stability are thought to contribute to the efficacy [48–51].

Long-term administration of erythromycin as well as clarithromycin is useful for the treatment of diffuse panbronchiolitis (DPB). DPB is a disease characterized by chronic inflammation of the respiratory bronchioles and the infiltration of chronic inflammatory cells. The disease results in respiratory failure due to infection by *Pseudomonas aeruginosa* or *H. influenzae* and was previously difficult to treat. The efficacy of erythromycin for this disease was reported in 1987 [52]. Erythromycin and clarithromycin do not show antibacterial activity against *P. aeruginosa*, but they do improve pulmonary functions [53]. Efficacy of 16-membered macrolides has not been reported.

The mechanism of 14-membered macrolides in DPB has been investigated, and new biological properties of macrolides have been revealed. For example, erythromycin inhibited respiratory glycoconjugate secretion [54] and chloride secretion across canine tracheal cells [55]. The number of neutrophils and the neutrophil-derived elastolytic-like activity in bronchoalveolar lavage fluid decreased after treatment with erythromycin along with a significant improvement in pulmonary function [56]. Erythromycin inhibited intrapulmonary influx of neutrophils in mice with intratrachial injection of recombinant IL-8 [57]. Erythromycin suppressed the proliferation of lymphocytes [58] and promoted differentiation of monocytes to macrophages [59]. Many pathogens produce glycocalyx and form biofilm. Erythromycin and clarithromycin degraded the biofilm, which may be related to the efficacy in the treatment of DPB [60].

Recent chemical modification of erythromycin

In the early 1990s, three new macrolides, clarithromycin, roxithromycin, and azithromycin, were developed, and they have expanded the indications of this class of drug into new therapeutic areas. For further improvement of erythromycin derivatives, macrolide resistant *S. pneumoniae* and *H. influenzae* have been regarded as key pathogens.

At Taisho Pharmaceutical Co., Ltd., chemical modification has been continued and a new class of macrolides has been synthesized (Fig. 4).

TE-802 (**32**), a 9,11,12-tricyclic ketolide, exhibited strong *in vitro* antibacterial activities against both erythromycin-susceptible bacteria and erythromycin-resis-

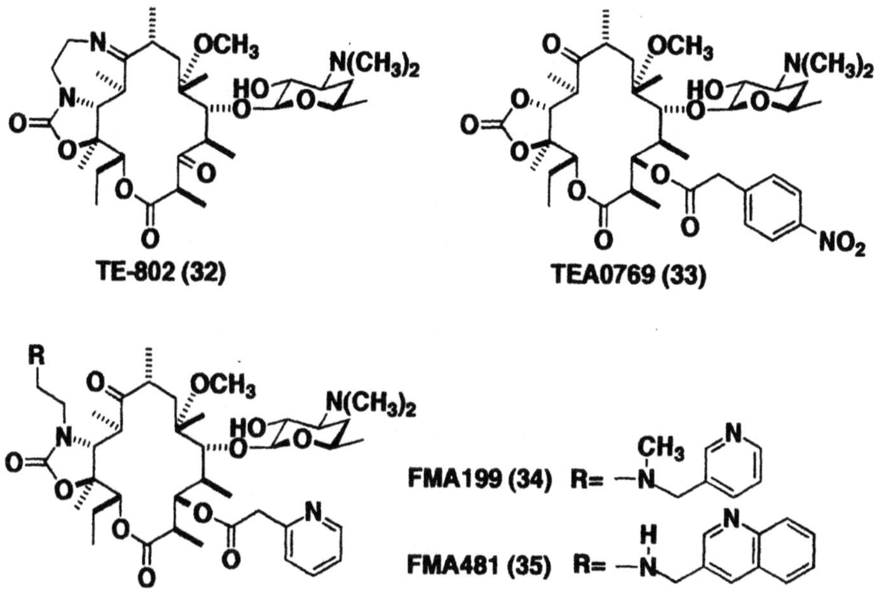

Figure 4. Structures of newly synthesized ketolide and acylides.

Table 8. *In vitro* antibacterial activity of TE-802, clarithromycin and azithromycin.

Strain	MIC(μg/ml)		
	TE-802	Clarithromycin	Azithromycin
S. aureus 209P-JC	0.10	0.10	0.39
S. aureus B1	0.20	>100	>100
S. pyogenes IID689	0.05	0.05	0.10
E. faecalis ATCC 29212	0.20	0.78	12.5
E. faecalis ATCC 19434	0.025	0.78	3.13
S. pneumoniae BM210	0.10	0.78	0.78
S. pneumoniae BM225	6.25	>100	>100
H. influenzae ATCC43095	6.25	6.25	1.56

tant *S. aureus* and *S. pneumoniae* [61]. Against clarithromycin-resistant strains of *S. aureus* B1 and *S. pneumoniae* 225, TE-802 was significantly more active than clarithromycin and azithromycin (Tab. 8). TE-802 was 1.5 to 12 times more active than clarithromycin and azithromycin *in vivo* against systemic infections in mice (Tab. 9). The strong *in vivo* activities of TE-802 could be explained by its significantly high acid stability and good pharmacokinetic properties [61].

A series of 3-*O*-acyl derivatives of erythromycin, named acylides, were synthesized and their biological properties were evaluated. Among them, TEA0769 (**33**), a 3-*O*-(*p*-nitrophenylacetyl)-11,12-carbonate, showed strong activity against erythromycin-susceptible strains. It was found that cladinose could be substituted by acyl groups without any decrease of activity [62]. FMA199 (**34**)

Table 9. Protective effect of TE-802, clarithromycin and azithromycin on systemic infection in mice (ICR mouse, 4 week, male, n=10).

Strain	Challenge dose (cfu/mouse)	Drug[a)]	ED_{50} (mg/mouse)	MIC (μg/ml)
Staphylococcus aureus Smith 4	4.8×10^7	TE-802	0.22	0.20
		Clarithromycin	0.33	0.20
		Azithromycin	0.47	0.78
Streptococcus pneumoniae IID553	1.1×10^3	TE-802	0.047	0.05
		Clarithromycin	0.58	0.05
		Azithromycin	0.45	0.20

[a)]: Drugs were administered orally to ICR mouse 1 h after infection

Table 10. *In vitro* antibacterial activity of acylides and erythromycin.

	MIC(μg/ml)		
Strain	FMA199	FMA481	EM
S. pneumoniae IID553	0.10	0.05	0.10
S. pneumoniae BM210	0.39	0.10	1.56
S. pneumoniae BM205	0.39	0.10	>100
S. pneumoniae BM211	1.56	0.39	>100
H. influenzae ATCC43095	3.13	3.13	6.25

and FMA481 (**35**), 3-*O*-(2-pyridylacetyl)-11,12-carbamates, showed strong activities against erythromycin-susceptible and -resistant *S. pneumoniae* (Tab. 10) [63]. The combination of 3-*O*-acyl groups and 11,12-carbamates is thought to be important for the activity against erythromycin-resistant strains.

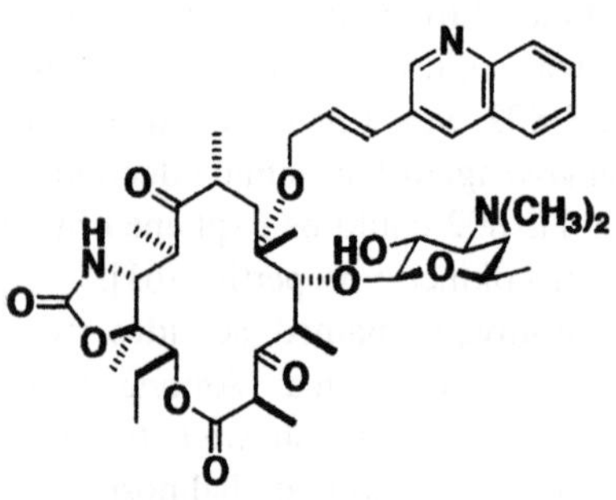

ABT-773 (36)

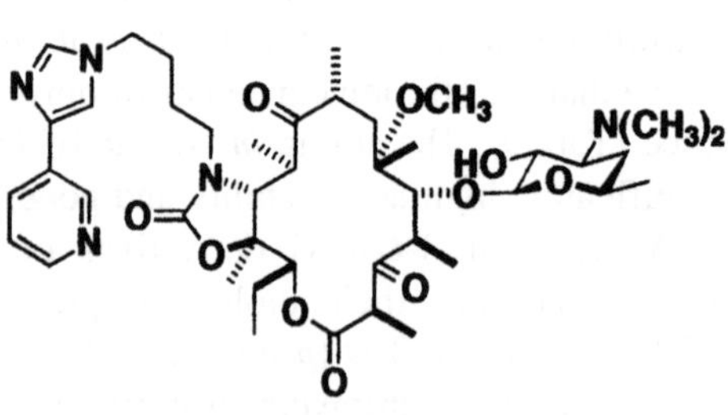

HMR3647 (37)

Figure 5. Structures of ABT-773 and HMR3647 (telithromycin).

Recently, two ketolides , ABT-773 (**36**) and HMR3647 (telithromycin, **37**) were reported (Fig. 5) [64, 65]. These compounds exhibit strong activities against erythromycin-resistant *S. pneumoniae*. It had been thought that cladinose was essential for antibacterial activities, but these derivatives lack cladinose. These recent studies show that there is still room for the discovery of new semi-synthetic macrolide antibiotics.

References

1 McGuire JM, Bunch PL, Anderson RC, Boaz HE, Flynn EH, Powell EH, Smith JW (1952) Ilotycin, a new antibiotic. *Antibiot Chemother* 2: 281–283

2 Ōmura S (ed) (1984) *Macrolide antibiotics – chemistry, biology and practice*. Academic Press, Orlando, FL

3 Bryskier AJ, Butsler J-P, Neu HC, Tulkens PM (eds) (1993) *Macrolides – chemistry, pharmacology and clinical uses*. Arnette Blackwell, Paris

4 Morimoto S, Takahashi Y, Watanabe Y, Omura S (1984) Chemical modification of erythromycins I. Synthesis and antibacterial activity of 6-*O*-methylerythromycins A. *J Antibiot* 37: 187–189

5 Morimoto S, Misawa Y, Adachi T, Nagate T, Watanabe Y, Omura S (1990) Chemical modification of erythromycins II. Synthesis and antibacterial activity of *O*-alkyl derivatives of erythromycin A. *J Antibiot* 43: 286–294

6 Morimoto S, Adachi T, Misawa Y, Nagate T, Watanabe Y, Omura S (1990) Chemical modification of erythromycins IV. Synthesis and biological properties of 6-*O*-methylerythromycin B. *J Antibiot* 43: 544–549

7 Iwasaki H, Sugawara Y, Adachi T, Morimoto S, Watanabe Y (1993) Structure of 6-*O*-methylerythromycin A (clarithromycin). *Acta Cryst* C49: 1227–1230

8 Ōmura S, Morimoto S, Nagate T, Adachi T, Kohno Y (1992) Research and development of clarithromycin. *Yakugaku zasshi* 112: 593–614

9 Flynn EH, Murphy HW, McMahon RE (1955) Erythromycin. II. Des-*N*-methylerythromycin and *N*-methyl-C^{14}-erythromycin. *J Am Chem Soc* 77: 3104–3106

10 Kurath P, Jones PH, Egan RS, Perun TJ (1971) Acid-degradation of erythromycin A and erythromycin B. *Experientia* 21: 362

11 Suwa T, Kohno Y, Yoshida H, Morimoto S, Suga T (1989) Uptake of *O*-alkylerythromycin derivatives in the lung tissue and cell of rats. *J Pharm Sci* 79: 783–784

12 Watanabe Y, Morimoto S, Adachi T, Kashimura M, Asaka T (1993) Chemical modification of erythromycins IX. Selective methylation at the C-6 hydroxyl group of erythromycin A oxime derivatives and preparation of clarithromycin. *J Antibiot* 46: 647–660

13 Watanabe Y, Adachi T, Asaka T, Kashimura M, Matsunaga T, Morimoto S (1993) Chemical modification of erythromycins XII. A facile synthesis of clarithromycin (6-*O*-methylerythromycin A) *via* 2'-silylethers of erythromycin A derivatives. *J Antibiot* 46: 1163–1167

14 Morimoto S, Adachi T, Matsunaga T, Kashimura M, Asaka T, Watanabe Y, Sota K, Sekiuchi K (1991) Erythromycin A derivatives. *US Patent* 4990602 [*Chem Abstr* (1990)113: 1326941]

15 Kawashima Y, Morimoto S, Matsunaga T, Kashimura M, Adachi T, Watanabe Y, Hatayama K, Hirono S, Moriguchi I (1990) Studies on selectivity of *O*-methylation of erythromycin derivatives based on molecular mechanics and molecular orbital methods. *Chem Pharm Bull* 38: 1485–1489

16 Gotō H, Kawashima Y, Kashimura M, Morimoto S, Osawa E (1993) Origin of regioselectivity in the *O*-methylation of erythromycin as elucidated with the aid of computational conformational space search. *J Chem Soc Perkin Trans* 2: 1647–1654

17 Morimoto S, Nagate T, Sugita K, Ono T, Numata K, Miyachi J, Misawa Y, Yamada K, Omura S (1990) Chemical modification of erythromycins III. *In vitro* and *in vivo* antibacterial activities of new semisynthetic 6-*O*-methylerythromycins A, TE 031 (clarithromycin) and TE-032. *J Antibiot* 43: 295–305

18 Ono T, Numata K, Inoue M, Mitsuhashi S (1988) Bacteriological evaluation of TE-031 (A-56268), a new macrolide antibiotic: *in vitro* and *in vivo* antibacterial activity. *Chemother* 36 (Suppl. 3): 1–34
19 Nagate T, Sugita K, Numata K, Ono T, Miyachi J, Morikawa E, Omura S (1988) Antibacterial activities of TE-031 (A-56268), a new macrolide antibiotic. *Chemother* 36 (Suppl. 3): 129–155
20 Fernandes PB, Bailer R, Swanson R, Hanson CW, McDonald E, Ramer N, Hardy D, Shipkowitz N, Bower RR, Gade E (1986) *In vitro* and *in vivo* evaluation of A-56268 (TE-031), a new macrolide. *Antimicrob Agents Chemother* 30: 865–873
21 Hardy DJ, Hensey DM , Beyer JM, Vojtko C, McDonald EJ, Fernandes PB (1988) Comparative *in vitro* activities of new 14-, 15- and 16 membered macrolides. *Antimicrob Agents Chemother* 32: 1710–1719
22 Suwa T, Yoshida H, Fukushima K, Nagate T (1989) Comparative pharmacokinetics of TE-031 and erythromycin stearate in rats and mice. *Chemother* 36 (Suppl. 3): 198–204
23 Kohno Y, Yoshida H, Suwa T, Suga T (1989) Comparative pharmacokinetics of clarithromycin (TE-031), a new macrolide antibiotic, and erythromycin in rats. *Antimicrob Agents Chemother* 33: 751–756
24 Kohno Y, Yoshida H, Yoshitomi S, Suwa T (1989) Metabolic fate of TE-031 (A-56268)(VII) uptake into the lung. *Chemother* 36 (Suppl. 3): 257–263
25 Kohno Y, Yoshida H, Suwa T, Suga T (1990) Uptake of clarithromycin by rat lung cells. *J Antimicrob Chemother* 26: 503–513
26 Kohno Y, Ohta K, Suwa T, Suga T (1990) Autobacteriographic studies of clarithromycin and erythromycin in mice. *Antimicrob Agents Chemother* 34: 562–567
27 Saito A, Ishikawa K, Shinohara M, Fukuhara I, Nakayama I, Tomizawa M, Sato K (1988) Preclinical and clinical studies on TE-031 (A-56268). *Chemother* 36 (Suppl. 3): 521–537
28 Adachi T, Morimoto S, Watanabe Y, Sota K (1988) Isolation and identification of metabolites of TE-031 (A-56268) in human. *Chemother* 36 (Suppl. 3): 264–273
29 Adachi T, Morimoto S, Kondoh H, Nagate T, Watanabe Y, Sota K (1988) 14-Hydroxy-6-*O*-methylerythromycins A, active metabolites of 6-*O*-methylerythromycin A in human. *J Antibiot* 41: 966–975
30 Adachi T, Morimoto S, Watanabe Y, Kamiya N, Iwasaki H (1989) Crystal and molecular structure of (14*R*)-14-hydroxy-6-*O*-methylerythromycin A. *J Antibiot* 42: 1012–1014
31 Adachi T (1989) 15-Membered macrolides *via* translactonization in 14-hydroxy-6-*O*-methylerythromycin A. *J Org Chem* 54: 3507–3510
32 Suwa T, Yoshida H, Kohno Y, Yoshitomi S, Kamei K (1988) Metabolic fate of TE-031 (A-56268) (IV) Metabolism of ^{14}C-TE-031 in rats and dogs. *Chemother* 36 (Suppl. 3): 227–237
33 Inouye S, Shomura T, Tsuruoka T, Omoto S, Niida T, Umemura K (1972) Isolation and structure of two metabolites of macrolide antibiotic, SF-837 substance. *Chem Pharm Bull* 20: 2366–2371
34 Shomura T, Someya S, Murata S, Umemura K, Nishio M (1981) Metabolism of 9,3"-diacetylmidecamycin. II. The structures of several metabolites of 9,3"-diacetylmidecamycin. *Chem Pharm Bull* 29: 2413–2419
35 Morishita M, Ohno M, Serizawa K, Fujiwara T, Sakakibara H (1984) Isolation and identification of metabolites of TMS-19-Q. *Chemother* 32 (Suppl. 6): 85–92
36 Nagate T, Ono T, Sugita K, Akashi T, Morikawa E, Miyazaki M, Takeichi C, Omura S (1988) Antibacterial activities of M-5, the most active metabolite of TE-031 (A-56268) in man. *Chemother* 36 (Suppl. 3): 156–169
37 Suwa T, Ohtake T, Urano H, Kodama T, Nakamura M, Iwatate C, Watanabe T (1988) Metabolic fate of TE-031 (A-56268) (IX), Absorption and excretion in humans (HPLC method). *Chemother* 36: 933–940
38 Hardy DJ, Swanson RN, Rode RA, Marsh K, Shipkowitz NL, Clement JJ (1990) Enhancement of the *in vitro* and *in vivo* activities of clarithromycin against *Haemophilus influenzae* by 14-hydroxy-clarithromycin, its major metabolite in humans. *Antimicrob Agents Chemother* 34: 1407–1413
39 Powel M, Chen HY, Weinhardt B, Williams JD (1991) *In-vitro* cidal activity of clarithromycin and its 14-hydroxy metabolite (A-62671) against *Haemophilus influenzae*. *J Antimicrob Chemother* 27: 694–696

40 Olsson-Liljequist B, Hoffman BM (1991) *In-vitro* activity of clarithromycin combined with its 14-hydroxy metabolite A-62671 against *Haemophilus influenzae. J Antimicrob Chemother* 27(Suppl. A): 11–17

41 Sasaki J, Mizoue K, Morimoto S, Adachi T (1988) Microbial transformation of 6-*O*-methylerythromycin derivatives. *J Antibiot* 41: 908–915

42 Adachi T, Sasaki J, Omura S (1989) Hydroxylation and *N*-demethylation of clarithromycin (6-*O*-methylerythromycin A) by *Mucor circinelloides. J. Antibiot* 42: 1433–1437

43 Finch RG (1997) Overview of the clinical use of macrolides and streptogramins. *Infect Dis Ther* 1997: 3–26

44 Langtry HD, Brogden RN (1997) Clarithromycin. A review of its efficacy in the treatment of respiratory tract infections in immunocompetent patients. *Drugs* 53: 973–1004

45 Tartaglione TA (1996) Therapeutic options for the management and prevention of *Mycobacterium avium* complex infection in patients with the acquired immunodeficiency syndrome. *Pharmacother* 16: 171–182

46 Mertl SL (1996) The role of clarithromycin in the prophylaxis of disseminated *Mycobacterium avium-intracellulare* infection in patients with AIDS. *Pharmacother* 16: 393–400

47 Wright J (1998) Current strategies for the prevention and treatment of disseminated *Mycobacterium avium* complex infection in patients with AIDS. *Pharmacother* 18: 738–747

48 Markham A, McTavish D (1996) Clarithromycin and omeprazole, as *Helicobacter pylori* eradication therapy in patients with *H. pylori*-associated gastric disorders. *Drugs* 51: 161–178

49 NIH consensus development panel on *Helicobacter pylori* in peptic ulcer disease (1994) *Helicobacter pylori* in peptic ulcer disease. *JAMA* 272: 65–69

50 Soll AH (1996) Medical treatment of peptic ulcer disease: Practical guidelines. *JAMA* 275: 622–629

51 The European *Helicobacter pylori* study group (1997) Current European concepts in the management of *Helicobacter pylori* infection. The Maastricht Consensus Report. *Gut* 41: 8–13

52 Kudoh S, Uetake T, Hagiwara K, Hirayama M, Hus L, Kimura H, Sugiyama Y (1987) Clinical effect of low-dose long-term erythromycin chemotherapy on diffuse panbronchiolitis. *Jpn J Thorac Dis* 25: 632–642

53 Sawaki M, Mikasa K, Konishi M, Maeda K, Narita N (1998) Clinical study of long-term treatment using erythromycin in chronic lower respiratory tract infection *Jpn J Chemother* 46: 239–247

54 Goswami SK, Kivity S, Marom Z (1990) Erythromycin inhibits respiratory glycoconjugate secretion from human airways *in vitro. Am Rev Respir Dis* 141: 72–78

55 Tamaoki J, Isono K, Sakai N, Kanemura T, Konno K (1992) Erythromycin inhibits Cl secretion across canine tracheal epithelial cells. *Eur Respir J* 5: 234–238

56 Ichikawa Y, Ninomiya H, Koga H, Tanaka M, Kinoshita M, Tokunaga N, Yano T, Oizumi K (1992) Erythromycin reduces neutrophils and neutrophil-derived elastolytic-like activity in the lower respiratory tract of bronchiolitis patients. *Am Rev Respir Dis* 146: 196–203

57 Kadota J, Sakito O, Kohno S, Sawa H, Mukae H, Oda H, Kawakami K, Fukushima K, Hiratani K, Hara K (1993) A mechanism of erythromycin treatment in patients with diffuse panbronchiolitis. *Am Rev Respir Dis* 147: 153–159

58 Keicho N, Kudoh S, Yotsumoto H, Akagawa KS (1993) Antilymphocytic activity of erythromycin distinct from that of FK506 or cyclosporin. *J Antibiot* 46: 1406–1413

59 Keicho N, Kudoh S, Yotsumoto H, Akagawa KS (1993) Erythromycin promotes monocyte to macrophage differentiation. *J Antibiot* 47: 80–89

60 Takeda H, Ohotami H, Ohgaki N (1994) Basic action of macrolide to diffuse panbronchiolitis *Antibiot Chemother* 10: 1305–1312

61 Kashimura M, Asaka T, Misawa Y, Matsumoto K, Morimoto S (2001) Synthesis and antibacterial activity of the tricyclic ketolides TE-802 and its analogs. *J Antibiot* 54:664–678

62 Asaka T, Kashimura M, Ishii T, Matsuura A, Suzuki K, Ohyauchi R, Matsumoto K, Numata K, T, Akashi T, Adachi T, Morimoto S (1997) New macrolide antibiotics, acylides (3-*O*-acyl-5-*O*-desosaminylerythronolides); Synthesis and biological properties. *37th ICAAC*, Toronto, Canada, Abstract F-262

63 Asaka T, Kashimura M, Manaka A, Tanikawa T, Ishii T, Sugimoto T, Suzuki K, Sugiyama H, Akashi T, Saito H, Adachi T, Morimoto S (1999) Structure activity studies leading potent

acylides: 3-*O*-acyl-5-*O*-desosaminylerythronolide 11,12–carbamates. *39th ICAAC*, San Francisco, California, Abstract F-2159
64 Or Y, Clak RF, Wang S, Chu DTW, Nilius AM, Flamm RK, Mitten M, Ewing P, Alder J, Ma Z (2000) Design, synthesis and antimicrobial activity of 6-*O*-substituted ketolides active against resistant respiratory tract pathogens. *J Med Chem* 43: 1045–1049
65 Denis A, Agourideas C, Auger JM, Benedetti Y, Bonnefoy A, Bretin F, Chantot JF, Dussarat A, Fromentin C, D'Ambrieres SG et al (1999) Synthesis and antibacterial activity of HMR3647. A new ketolide highly potent against erythromycin-resistant and susceptible pathogens. *Bioorg Med Chem Lett* 9: 3075–3080

Macrolide Antibiotics
ed. by W. Schönfeld and H. A. Kirst

Azithromycin and novel azalides

Wolfgang Schönfeld and Stjepan Mutak

PLIVA Research, Antiinfective Research, Prilaz Baruna Filipovića 25, 10000 Zagreb, Croatia

Introduction

Macrolides represent a well-known family of oral antibiotics. Their spectrum of activity covers most relevant bacterial species responsible for upper and lower respiratory tract infections. In 1952 the first macrolide, erythromycin, was introduced into the market. Erythromycin is active against gram-positive and certain gram-negative microorganisms and is still used to treat infections of the respiratory tract, skin and soft tissues, and genital tract. Macrolides express their antibiotic activity by inhibition of protein synthesis by binding to a 50S ribosome subunit. The precise mode of action is reported elsewhere in this monograph.

After confirmation of the precise structure of the fermentation products, world-wide efforts in medicinal chemistry were undertaken to improve the biological profile (better activity, higher stability, and improved bioavailability). This effort yielded various new chemical entities, reviewed in [1, 2, 3] and in other chapters of this monograph. Erythromycin A is the most important starting point for preparation of 14-membered semi-synthetic macrolide antibiotics. The key intermediate for this group of new derivatives was erythromycin A oxime (**2**), which is prepared from erythromycin A (**1**) and hydroxylamine hydrochloride in the presence of weak base or buffer (Scheme 1). All important semi-synthetic macrolides from this generation are derived from erythromycin oxime. Its O-alkoxyalkyl derivative is roxithromycin [4]. Catalytic reduction of the oxime yielded 9(S)-erythromycylamine, which was subsequently converted to dirithromycin [5]. Another approach described by Taisho Pharmaceutical Company was the successful synthesis of 6-O-methylerythromycin (clarithromycin). The key steps were the use of protected erythromycin oxime [6] to achieve selective O-methylation at position 6. PLIVA has a long tradition in chemical synthesis of various antibacterials. At the beginning of the 1960s, chemical transformation programs were started using erythromycin A as a starting material.

This chapter describes the chemical synthesis of azithromycin [7] based on its key reaction of Beckmann rearrangement and gives an outlook on further derivatisation of various nitrogen bearing compounds. This will include synthesis of a new group of macrolides named ketolides, of which two 14-membered representatives [8, 9] are in clinical development as a third generation of macrolides active against inducible resistant *Streptococcus pneumoniae* and *Staphylococcus aureus*.

Synthesis of azithromycin and 9a-azalides

Azithromycin is the first and presently the only 15-membered macrolide antibiotic on the market with a basic nitrogen atom inserted into the macrocyclic ring. The starting compound for the synthesis of azithromycin was erythromycin oxime (**2**), which was synthesised in the research laboratories at PLIVA [10].

First efforts concentrated on the carbonyl group at position 9. Reaction conditions to oximate the hindered 9-keto group were identified, and to prove the structure, the oxime was subsequently transformed into an amine by catalytic reduction [10]. At the same time, the 9-amine was synthesised at Eli Lilly [1b]. Initial antimicrobial testing demonstrated that the oxime and amine showed activity against gram-positive bacteria similar to erythromycin, but they showed significantly better activity against some gram-negative bacteria. It was decided to start a derivatisation program on these scaffolds [11]. Using erythromycin oxime and amine, various substituted derivatives were prepared. One of the ideas was to combine erythromycin and sulphonamide properties [12].

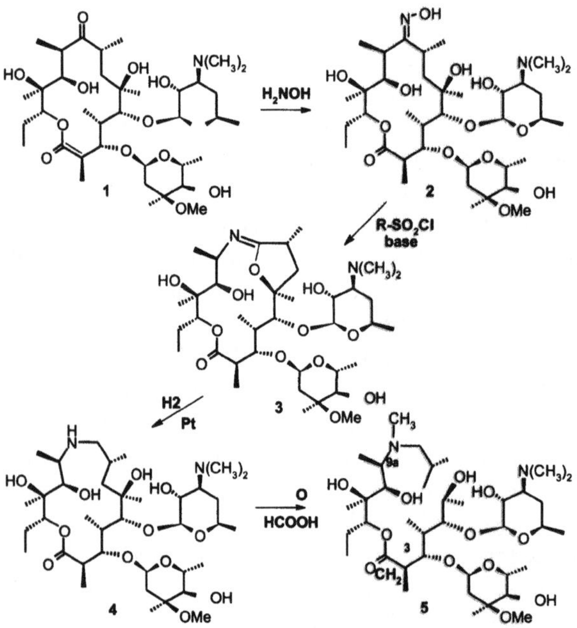

Scheme 1. Synthesis of azithromycin.

The key reaction was established during the synthesis of O-sulfonyl derivatives of oxime **2** [13–15]. It is well known that sulfonyl chlorides are catalysts for the Beckmann rearrangement to transform oximes to amides. However, this chemical derivatisation step was not experienced before on macrolactone scaffolds [16]. Treatment of oxime **2** with benzenesulfonyl chloride in an acetone-water mixture with sodium bicarbonate yielded a degradation product. Physico-chemical analysis indicated that in the assumed structure, one water molecule was missing and that the compound exhibited a bicyclic structure. The presumed structure therefore was erythromycin-6,9-imino-ether **3**, which was later confirmed by x-ray structural analysis [17]. The product had no antibacterial activity and was further derivatised in various subsequent reactions. Catalytic hydrogenation in the presence of PtO_2 or Pt/C gave the cyclic amine **4** named 9-dihydro-9-deoxo-9a-aza-9a-homoerythromycin A, which was cited earlier as 10-dihydro-10-deoxo-11-azaerythromycin A according to the older nomenclature. The structures of the imino-ether **3** and the 15-membered amine **4** were determined by mass spectral and ^1H or ^{13}C NMR data. Finally, the structures were confirmed by x-ray of the respective aglycone derivatives prepared by removal of both sugars [16].

The antibacterial activity of this new cyclic 15-membered amino-lactone **4** was close to that of the oxime **2**: similar activity against gram-positive bacteria and better activity against gram-negative bacteria than erythromycin (Tab. 1). Starting from the cyclic amine **4**, a number of derivatives were produced. The best activity was achieved with 9a(N)-methyl derivative **5**, which was prepared by reductive methylation with formaldehyde and formic acid [17]. The new product 9-dihydro-9-deoxo-9a-methyl-9a-aza-9a-homoerythromycin (**5**), named azithromycin, showed broad antibacterial activity (Tab. 1) and strongly improved acid stability.

Table 1. Antibacterial *in vitro* activity of azithromycin and its precursors (MIC in µg/ml) [7] N.D. = not determined

Microorganism	**Compound**			
	1	**2**	**4**	**5**
Streptococcus faecalis ATTC 8043	0.50	0.50	0.25	0.25
Staphylococcus aureus ATTC 6538-P	0.50	0.50	0.50	0.50
Micrococcus flavus ATTC 10240	0.05	0.05	0.05	0.01
Sarcina lutea ATTC 9341	0.12	0.12	0.05	0.06
Escherichia coli ATTC 10536	25.0	25.0	10.0	2.00
Pseudomonas aeruginosa NTTC 1049	128.0	N.D.	N.D.	32.0
Klebsiella pneumoniae ATTC 10031	4.00	N.D.	N.D.	1.00

Soon after the publication of the Belgian patent and initial biological data, negotiations with various pharmaceutical companies were started to develop this compound for worldwide markets. At a similar time to PLIVA, chemists at Pfizer identified azithromycin as a result of its own derivatisation programs [18, 19]. Pfizer and PLIVA signed an option agreement in 1985, and preclinical and clinical development started. Both parties shared the data, and in October 1987 a Licence and Supply Agreement was signed between both companies.

During the process development, azithromycin was first isolated as the anhydrous substance [16] then was crystallised from ethanol-water as the monohydrate [18] and finally as the more stable dihydrate [17]. Azithromycin dihydrate was crystallised from a mixture with THF-hexane [20] or acetone-water, the method currently used in production. The crystal structure was confirmed by x-ray crystallographic parameters [17,21] of a sample obtained from diethyl ether. For intravenous application, water-soluble salts were prepared [17,22], and some stable divalent metal ion complexes were formed [23] as possible oral dosage forms for treatment of stomach ulcers. Further investigation of the biological properties of azithromycin (**5**) revealed evidence for its high activity against some important gram-negative microorganisms [24] such as *H. influenzae, Neisseria gonorrheae*, and *M. catarrhalis*. Preclinical investigations very soon revealed evidence for its promising and favourable profile, such as stability in acid environment [25], high oral bioavailability as compared with erythromycin [26], longer half-life, and high tissue concentrations [27]. This profile allowed a short-time dosing regimen, one of the key advantages of azithromycin compared with other antibacterials and macrolides [28]. The pharmacokinetic properties of azithromycin in relation to other macrolides are described in detail in other chapters of this monograph.

Macrolide antibiotics are metabolised mainly through demethylation by the cytochrome P450 microsomal enzyme system. Azithromycin is mainly excreted *via* the bile either as the parent substance or as up to as 10 inactive metabolites [29, 30].

The conformation of azithromycin (**5**) in solution was determined by nuclear magnetic resonance (NMR) spectroscopy and molecular modelling and was compared with its crystal structure and with some erythromycin derivatives [31]. In $CDCl_3$ solution **5** exists predominantly in a "folded-in" conformation in the C-3 to C-5 region, whereas its dihydrate crystal state conformation is "folded-out". The "folded-out" conformation increases with solvent polarity [31] and dominates in water [32]. In 1988 Azithromycin was introduced to the Yugoslavian market in its dihydrate form by PLIVA under its brand name "Sumamed". Pfizer achieved market approval in its first markets in 1990 under the name "Zithromax".

Further investigations showed evidence that imino-ether **3**, the main product of the first successful Beckmann rearrangement, was formed from readily available 9(E)-erythromycin oxime (**2**) [33]. When the Beckmann rearrangement is performed in ether in the presence of pyridine at –45 °C, the mixture of 6,9-iminoether **3** and 9,11-iminoether **6** was formed [34].

The same condition and temperature (0 to 5 °C) yielded the lactam **7** [34], which did not show antibacterial activity and could not be reduced to cyclic amine **4** [16].

The introduction of the Beckmann rearrangement opened a completely new derivatisation line, and various attempts were undertaken to improve the proper-

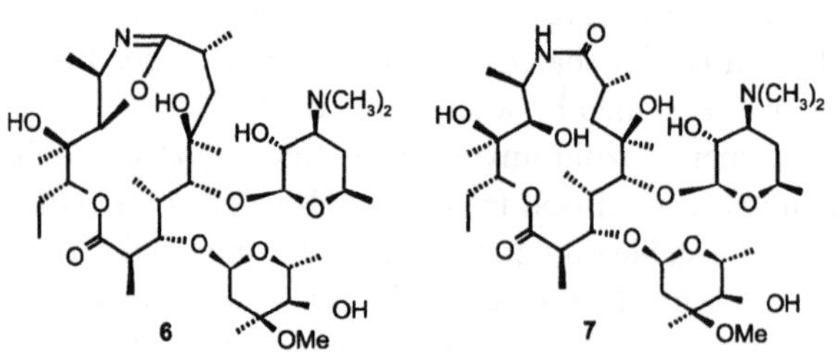

6

7

Figure 1. Structures of 9a-aza-homoerythromycin-9,11-iminoether and 9a-aza-homoerythromycin.

ties of azithromycin. The following sections describe the derivatisation of erythromycin to its 8a-azalides, N-and O-substituted azalides.

Synthesis of 8a-azalides

As mentioned above, 9(E)-oxime **2** [33] is the main product of oximation of erythromycin A (**1**). After isolation of 9(Z)-erythromycin oxime (**8**) [35] and basic isomerisation of the E isomer into the Z isomer, researchers at Merck applied the Beckmann rearrangement and synthesised isomeric 8a-homoerythromycin-6,9-iminoether (**9**), 8a-homoerythromycin-9,12-iminoether (**10**), and isomeric 8a-lactam (**11**) [36]. Under aqueous conditions imino-ether **9** and lactam **11** were formed.

When anhydrous conditions were used, imino-ethers **9** and **10** were isolated. The imino-ether **10** was in equilibrium with its 10-methyl epimer. Conformational analysis and molecular modelling techniques of imino-ether **3** and its corresponding 8a-isomer **9** were used to establish the predominant solution-state conformation [35] and to explain chemical reactivity. Imino-ethers **9** and **10** were further reduced with hydrogen and PtO_2 or $NaBH_4$ to the corresponding 9-dihydro-9-deoxo-8a-aza-8a-homoerythromycin (**12**) and methylated to 9-dihydro-9-deoxo-8a-methyl-8a-aza-homoerythromycin (**13**). The reduction rate of 9a-aza- and 8a-aza- 6,9-imino-ethers **3** and **9,** as well as 9a-aza-9,11-imino-ether **6**, have been studied using molecular modelling techniques [37]. The various positions varied with their susceptibility to reduction. Accessibility of the C-9 carbon atom explains the order of susceptibility of compounds as **6 > 3 > 9**.

The lactam **11** was N-alkylated at position 8a with alkyl halides and NaH with prior protection of the hydroxyl groups by trimethylsilyl (TMS) [36]. Another method for preparation of N-substituted lactams **11a** was based on the primary oxidation of imino-ethers **9** or **10** to the N-oxide of the sugar's dimethylamino

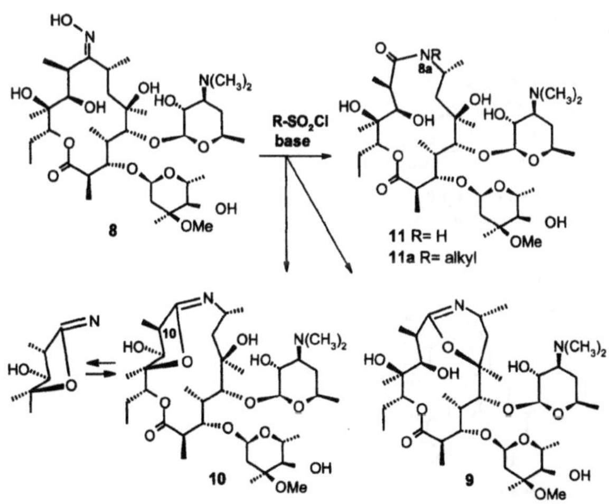

Scheme 2. Synthesis of 8a-azalides.

group, followed by reaction with alkyl halides [36] and finally by hydrolysis to yield the lactam and deoxygenation of the N-oxide.

Antibacterial activities of 8a-azalide **12** and its N-methyl derivative **13** were similar to those of 9a-azalide **4** and azithromycin (**5**), respectively.

Synthesis of other N-substituted azalide derivatives

The generation of the first azalide 9-dihydro-9-deoxo-9a-aza-9a-homoerythromycin (**4**) opened the derivatisation line at the 9a-nitrogen. Using reductive alkylation with formaldehyde or acetaldehyde, 9-dihydro-9-deoxo-9a-methyl-9a-aza-9a-homoerythromycin (**5**) (azithromycin) or its 9a-ethyl analogue were prepared. To avoid the formation of the quaternary ammonium salt, some N-alkyl substituted derivatives were prepared by reaction of the corresponding halides, and the N-hydroxy derivative **14** was generated from amine **4** [19].

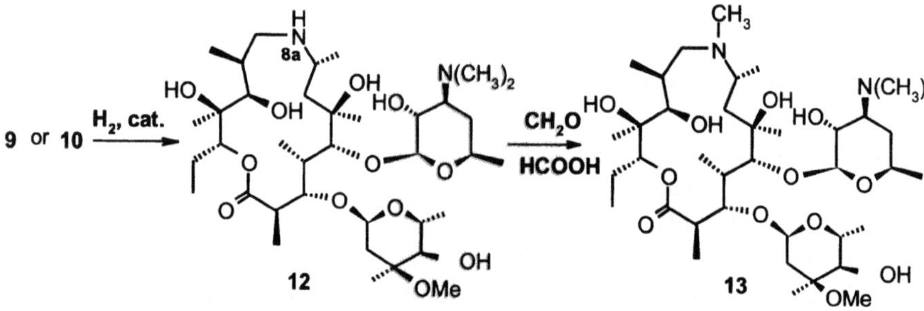

Scheme 3. Synthesis of 8a(N)-methyl-9-dihydro-8a-aza-8a-homoerythromycin.

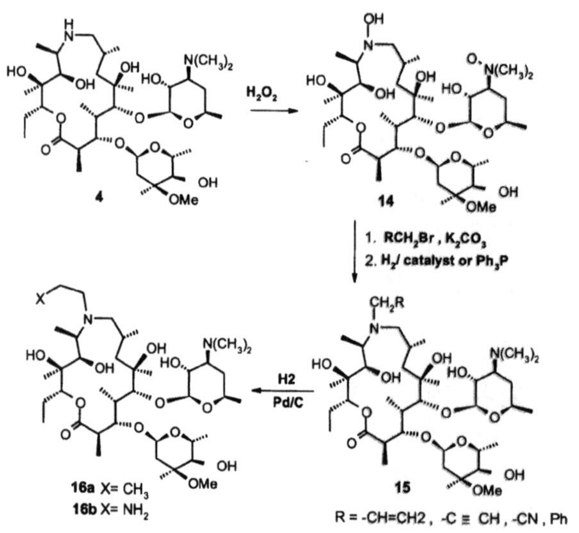

Scheme 4. Synthesis of 9a(N)-substituted-9-dihydro-9a-aza-9a-homoerythromycins.

These new derivatives, *e. g.*, **15,** were transformed further into their N-allyl derivatives, subsequently transformed by hydrogen and Pd catalyst to the N-propyl derivative **16,** and confirmed by X-ray analysis of its aglycone backbone [38]. New cyano-alkyl derivatives were reduced with hydrogen and Raney Ni to corresponding amino-alkyl compounds, but none of these derivatives showed better biological activity than azithromycin **5**.

Starting from 9-dihydro-9-deoxo-9a-aza-9a-homoerythromycin (**4**), various 9a-N-carbamoyl and thiocarbamoyl derivatives were prepared by reaction with corresponding isocyanates or isothiocyanates [39]. Reactions were usually conducted in toluene to achieve easily crystallisable N'-alkyl or N'-aryl substituted ureas. The structures of the N'-isopropyl and N'-(4-pyridyl) derivatives were confirmed by x-ray structural analysis [40].

Representatives of various ureas included isopropyl- (**17a**), 4-methyl-5-oxazolyl- (**17b**), 2-furyl- (**17 c**), 4-pyridyl- (**17 d**), phenyl- (**17e**), benzyl- (**17f**), and 1-naphthyl- (**17g**) ureas and N'-benzyl-thiourea (**17 h**). In biological testing, only a few derivatives showed moderate antibacterial activity (Table 2).

Table 2. Antibacterial *in vitro* activity of N-carbamoyl and thiocarbamoyl derivatives of 9-deoxo-9-dihydro-9a-aza-9a-homoerythromycins (MIC in μg/ml) [39]

Microorganism	**Compound**						
	5	**17a**	**17b**	**17d**	**17e**	**17f**	**17h**
S. epidermidis ATCC 12228	0.78	6.25	6.25	25.0	3.12	6.25	6.25
S. aureus ATCC 6538P	1.56	1.56	12.5	12.5	6.25	3.12	3.12
M. flavus ATCC 10240	–	3.12	12.5	12.5	6.25	3.12	1.56
S. faecalis ATCC 8043	0.78	3.12	6.25	6.25	3.12	3.12	1.56
B. subtilis NCTC 8236	0.19	1.56	12.5	25.0	6.25	3.12	1.56
E. coli ATCC 10536	1.56	12.5	25.0	12.5	12.5	25.0	12.5
S. pyogenes -J-21	1.56	–	6.25	12.5	3.12	–	–

As a further line of derivatisation of 9a-azalides [19], another amino group was introduced on the cladinose sugar starting from azithromycin **5.** After protection of the 2'-hydroxyl group by acetyl (**18**), the 4"-hydroxyl group was oxidised using Moffat-Pfitzer conditions to get the respective 4"-oxo derivative (**19**), which was oximated to (**20**) and then reduced to 4"-amine (**21**).

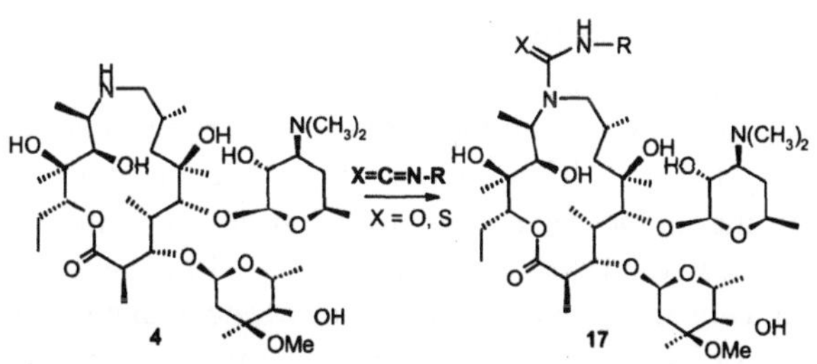

Scheme 5. Synthesis of 9a(N)-carbamoyl- and thiocarbamoyl-9-dihydro-9a-aza-9a-homoerythromycins.

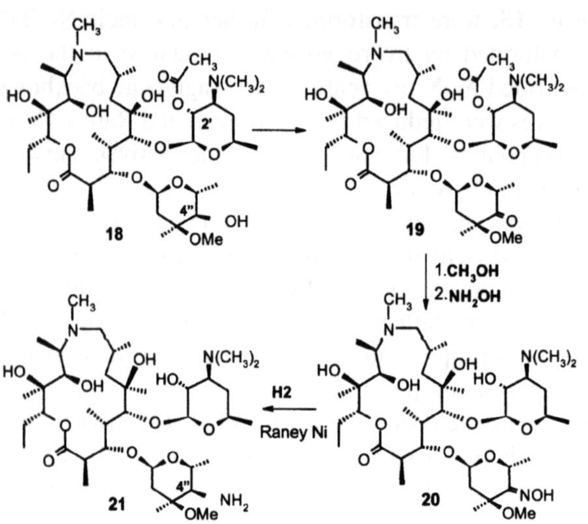

Scheme 6. Synthesis of 4"-oximino- and 4"-amino-9a(N)-methyl-9-dihydro-9a-aza-9a-homoerythromycins.

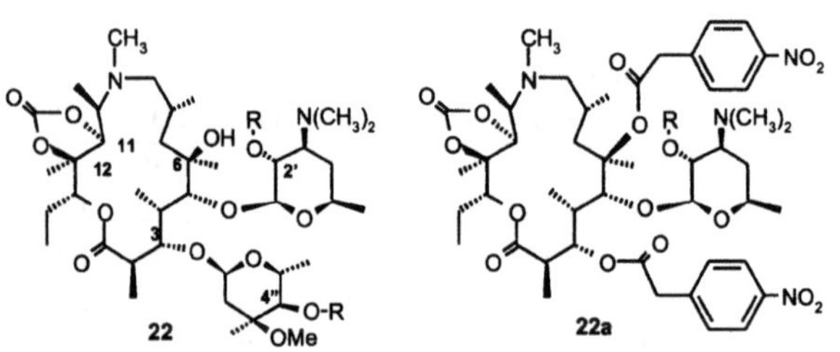

Figure 2. Structures of acyl derivatives of azithromycin 11,12-carbonates.

In vitro and *in vivo* activity of the amine **21** were better that of erythromycin and equalled that of azithromycin, especially against gram-negative microorganisms.

Synthesis of O-substituted azalide derivatives

Azithromycin and its 8a-aza isomer possess five hydroxyl groups, two of them are secondary hydroxyl groups on sugar moieties, while one secondary and two tertiary hydroxyl groups are located on the aglycone ring itself. Their presence explains the difficulties in targeted derivatisation. The most reactive hydroxyl group is at the 2'-position on the amino sugar. Initial derivatives targeting the hydroxyl groups were esters: mono-, di-, or tri-acetyl on the 2'-O- (**18**), 4"-O-, and 11-O- hydroxyl groups, which were prepared using acetic anhydride with pyridine [22]. Reaction of azithromycin or its diacetyl derivative with ethylene carbonate and potassium carbonate yielded the corresponding 11,12-carbonates (**22**) or its diacetyl derivatives. Acetyl groups could be easily removed by hydrolysis in methanol.

All esters and carbonates of free hydroxyl groups failed to show any improvement over erythromycin in antibacterial activity against gram-positive bacteria, but they were found to exhibit higher activity against gram-negative strains.

The synthesis of various esters was described by Taisho. Especially 3-decladinosyl-arylacetyl macrolides demonstrated activity against inducible resistant strains. The 14-membered macrolides included 3-decladinosyl-3,6-di(*p*-nitrophenyl)acetyl-azithromycin and its 11,12-carbonate **22a** [41]. However, biological activity of aza-acylides was not mentioned.

Since esters most often are cleaved in biological fluids, formation of ether bonds could be more appropriate to generate stable O-substituted derivatives. The first focus was on the synthesis of the 6-O-methyl derivative of azithromycin, similar to the synthesis of clarithromycin. Using benzyloxycarbonyl chloride in the presence of sodium bicarbonate, azithromycin (**5**) was protected at the 2'-O- and 3'-N- positions to get di-benzyloxycarbonyl derivative (**23**), which was methylated with methyl iodide and sodium hydride in dimethylsulfoxide tetrahydrofurane (DMSO-THF) or dimethylformamide (DMF) [42]. Unfortunately, only mixtures of 11-O- and 12-O-methyl derivatives with small amounts of di- or tri-methylated products (**24**) were generated. These products were hydrogenated using palladium on carbon and then remethylated on position 3'-N- with formaldehyde and formic acid. The mixture of mono- and some di- or tri-methylated azithromycins (**25**) was separated by column chromatography.

In the first publication, the structure of 12-O-methyl derivative **25a** was wrongly interpreted as 6-O-methyl azithromycin [42]. This error was corrected later by a publication from Merck [43] and was confirmed by PLIVA using x-ray structural analysis of the trimethylated compound **25 d** [44]. Finally, structure-reactivity studies using quantum mechanics of azithromycin, revealed evidence that alkylation of the 6-hydroxyl group is practically impossible to achieve.

Antibacterial testing of 12-O-methyl derivative **25a** indicated weaker activity than azithromycin **5**, while 11-O-methyl **25b** was equally or slightly more active.

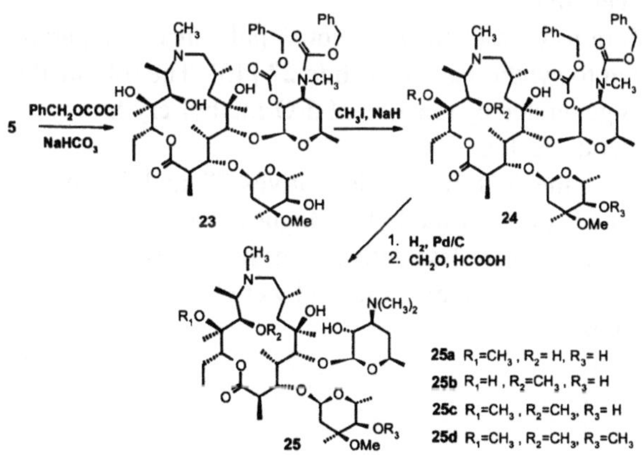

Scheme 7. Synthesis of O-methyl derivatives of azithromycin.

The antibacterial activities (Tab. 3) decreased with increasing degree of methylation [42,44].

Table 3. Antibacterial activity of azithromycin (**5**) and its O-methyl derivatives (MIC in μg/ml) [42,43]

Microorganism	Compound					
	5	**25a**	**25b**	**25c**	**25d**	**27**
S. pneumoniae MB 3957	< 0.06	0.03	0.03	1.0	2.0	0.5
S. pyogenes MB 2874	0.03	0.03	0.03	0.12	0,25	0.12
S. aureus MB 2865	0.5	1.0	1.0	8.0	8.0	2.0
E. faecalis MB 5407	4.0	4.0	8.0	16.0	16.0	8.0
E. faecium MB 516	0.25	0.25	0.5	0.25	2.0	1.0
B. subtilis MB 5586	1.0		1.0	4.0	8.0	1.0

Merck published the synthesis of mono-, di-, and trimethyl derivatives of 9-dihydro-9-deoxo-8a-methyl-8a-aza-homoerythromycin (**26**), and the authors established rates of O-methylation from 8a-aza- and 9a-aza-homoerythromycins: 11-OH(9a) ≥ 12-OH(9a) > 4"-OH(9a) ≡ 4"-OH(8a) > 12-OH(8a) > 11-OH(8a). To methylate the 6-hydroxyl group, they started with the 11,12-carbonate of 8a-azalide **13** and obtained the 2-methylated 3,6-ether accompanied by removal of cladinose. Direct methylation of the 6-hydroxyl group of 8a-azalide was achieved only after removal of cladinose, which yielded the 3,6,11,12-tetra-O-methyl derivative. Furthermore, the 6-O-methyl-9a-azalide **27** and 6-O-methyl-8a-azalide **28** starting from clarithromycin (6-O-methyl-erythromycin A) have been described [45]. The E- and Z-oximes were prepared, and then converted using the reaction with TsCl in ether/pyridine to the corresponding 9a-aza-9,11-iminoether or 8a-aza-9,12-iminoether. Beckmann reaction of E-oxime in aqueous acetone resulted in the 6-O-methyl derivative of 9a-lactam **7**. After reduction of iminoethers and reductive methylation of 9a-and 8a-amines, the desired 6-O-methyl compounds **27** and **28** were generated.

Authors from Hoechst-Marion-Roussel (now Aventis) published comparable results using the same reaction to synthesise the azalide **27** [46]. The 6-O-methyl derivative of 9a-lactam **7** was generated by reaction of 6-O-methyl-erythromycin-9(E)-oxime with TsCl in aqueous acetone [46].

Antibacterial examination of the 6-O-methyl derivatives **27** and **28** showed lower activity compared to its 11- or 12-O-methyl analogues (Tab. 4). Generally O-methyl derivatives of 8a-azalides were less active than the corresponding 9a-azalides [45]. 6-O-methyl derivatives of lactams **7** and **11** were less active than the corresponding amines **27** and **28**.

Table 4. Antibacterial activity of azithromycin (**5**) 8a-azalide **13** and its O-methyl derivatives (MIC in µg/l) [45].

Microorganism	**Compound**					
	13	**26a**	**26b**	**26c**	**26d**	**28**
S. pneumoniae MB 3957	< 0.06	0.5	2.0	1.0	4.0	0.5
S. pyogenes MB 2874	< 0.06	0.03	0.5	0.25	0.5	0.06
S. aureus MB 2865	0.3	8.0	32.0	8.0	32.0	2.0
E. faecalis MB 5407	2.0	8.0	32.0	16.0	32.0	16.0
E. faecium MB 516	0.125	2.0	16.0	4.0	8.0	1.0
B. subtilis MB 5586	0.3	4.0	16.0	4.0	2.0	1.0

In an effort to synthesise O-methyl azalides before introducing the 9a-N-methyl group, 9-dihydro-9-deoxo-9a-aza-9a-homoerythromycin A (**4**) was protected as its tris-carbobenzoxy derivative **29** and treated with methyl iodide in the presence of NaH in DMF [47]. The reaction resulted in a mixture of 2'-O,3'-N-bis-carbobenzoxy-9-dihydro-9-deoxo-9a-aza-9a-homoerythromycin-9a,11-cyclic carbamate and its 12-O-methyl derivative. The cyclic carbamates were deprotected using catalytic reduction and 3'-N-methylated with formaldehyde and formic acid to reintroduce the dimethylamino group. Finally 9-dihydro-9-deoxo-9a-aza-9a-homoerythromycin-9a,11-cyclic carbamate (**30a**) and its 12-O-methyl derivative (**30b**) were isolated by column chromatography.

In comparison to azithromycin, these novel bicyclic azalides **30a** and **30b** exhibited substantially decreased antibacterial activities *in vitro*.

Pfizer described the derivatisation of macrolides at the 4"-position and prepared novel 4"-O-(aryl-methyl-amino)-alkyl carbamates of 9-erythromycylamine. These compounds showed activity against resistant strains comparable to

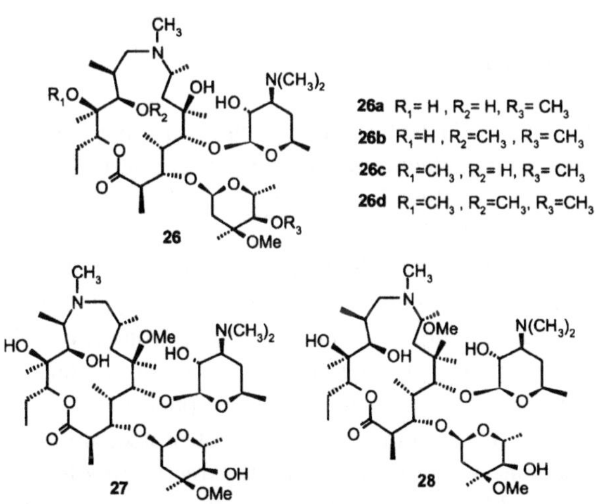

Figure 3. Synthesis of O-methyl derivatives of azithromycin and its 8a-aza- analog.

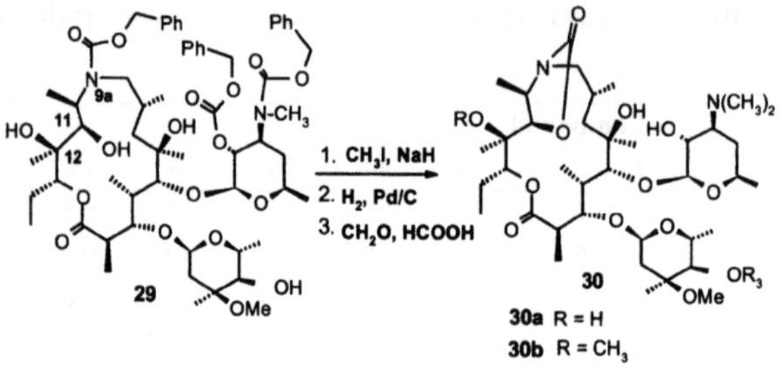

Scheme 8. Synthesis of azithromycin-9a(N),11(O)-cyclic carbamates.

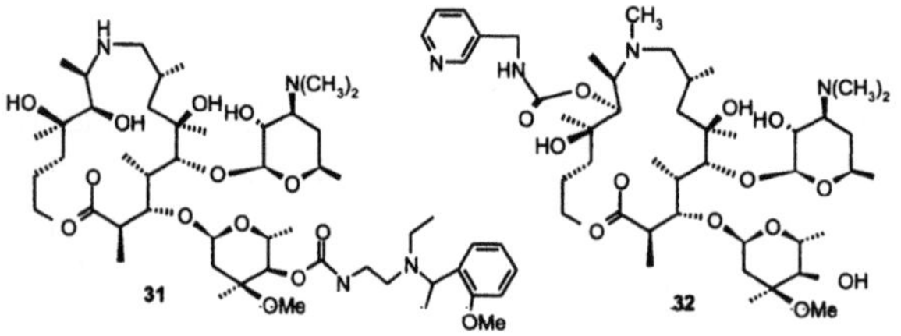

Figure 4. Structures of O-carbamoyl derivatives of 9a-aza-9-dihydro-homoerythromycin and azithromycin.

the ketolide telithromycin (HMR 3647, Ketek). The corresponding azalide derivative **31** was less active than the 14-membered compounds [48].

Subsequently a number of carbamate derivatives of the 11-hydroxyl group of 9a azalides (**32**) or 8a-azalides were prepared [49]. Mainly the family comprised carbamoyl substituents with various isomers of pyridyl or dimethoxybenzyl side chains.

Intramolecular rearrangement of azalides

In recent years several reports have evidenced a growing interest in ring opening reactions of macrolide antibiotics, which led to the synthesis of chimeric 9a- and 8a-azalides [50]. Two different types of base-catalysed ring-opening reactions of erythromycin A have been reported [51, 52].

Compounds containing carbon-nitrogen double bonds are easily hydrolysed to the corresponding aldehydes or ketones. The key intermediate in synthesis of azithromycin 6,9-iminoether **3** has a C-9/9a -C=N (or carbon-nitrogen) double bond, which in acid catalysed hydrolysis (AcOH) yielded the amino-lactone **33** [53]. The amino group was acylated or methylated to its corresponding N-acetyl or N,N-dimethylamino derivative. If the amino group was not protected during this reaction, amine **33** in acetone-water solution reacted by intermolecular transacylation to yield the amide **34**, which was further reduced to its amido-alcohol **35**. Various O-acetyl derivatives have been prepared. Compounds **33–35**

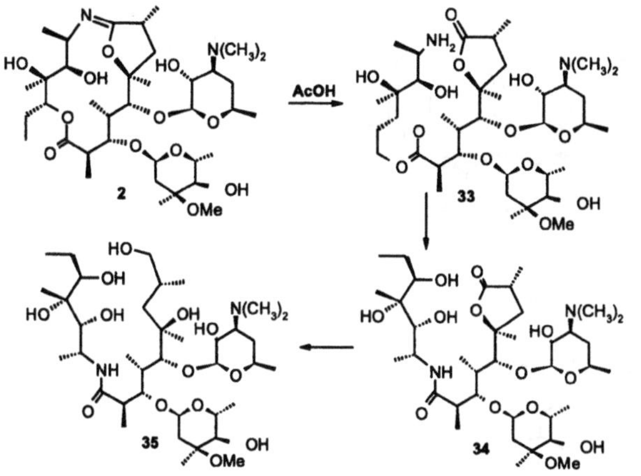

Scheme 9. Acid induced degradation of 9a-aza-9a-homoerythromycin-6,9-imino-ethers and formation of secomacrolides and secoazalides.

and their acetyl derivatives, named secomacrolides or secoazalides, did not show any antibacterial activity, but they are useful as intermediates for novel macrolides or azalides. Another ring-opening reaction was observed if the imino-ether **3** was treated with hydroxylamine hydrochloride [54]. During preparation of the lactam oxime, a simultaneous cleavage of the double bond led to formation of the seco-oxime **36**. The amino-oxime **36** was acetylated to N- and O-acetyl derivatives, or trans-acylated to seco-amide **37**. Catalytic reduction of the imino-ether group of amide **37** yielded the amine **38**, which was converted to the corresponding N,N-dimethylamine.

Compounds **36–38** and their acetyl or N,N-dimethyl derivatives did not show any antibacterial activity.

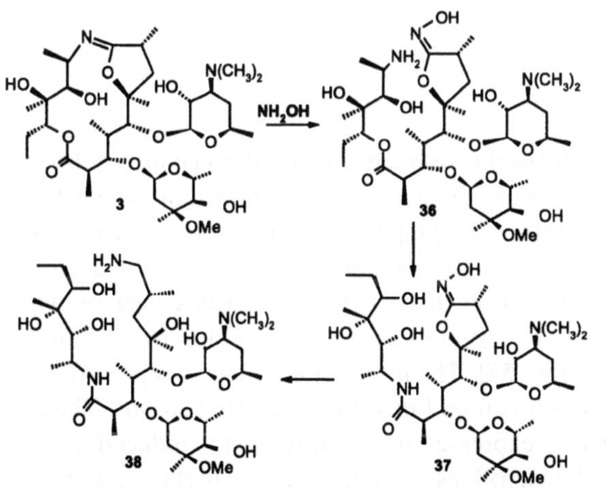

Scheme 10. Reaction of 9a-aza-9a-homoerythromycin-6,9-imino-ether with hydroxylamine and formation of secomacrolides and secoazalides.

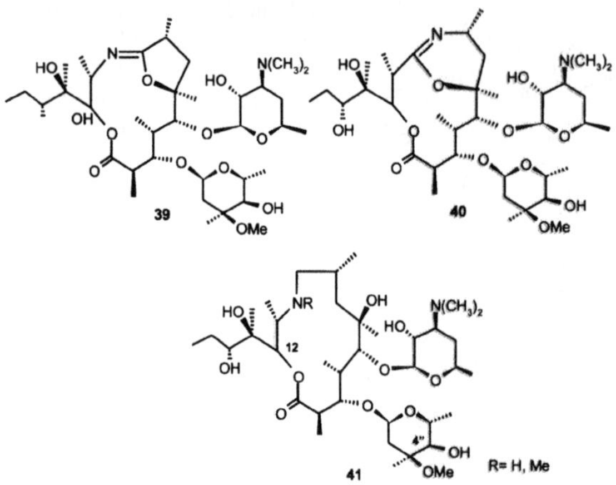

Figure 5. Structures of 13-membered azalides.

Other rearrangements of azalide imino-ethers were described by Merck [36]. The trans-annular reactions between the aglycone hydroxyl groups and imino-ether and lactone groups of the 9a- (**3**) and 8a-azalide (**9**) were investigated. Translactonisation of **3** and **9**, which included the 11-hydroxyl group, resulted in 13-membered imino-ethers **39** and **40**.

The thermal rearrangement of 9a-aza-6,9-imino-ether **3** produced an isomeric mixture of 9a-aza-9,11-imino-ether **6** and 8a-aza-9,11-imino-ether **10**, which were further transformed to azithromycin and its 8a-methyl isomer. Starting from imino-ether **6** in reaction with acetic acid, a dilactone was formed, which was then transformed by warming in methanol to 9a-aza-lactam **7**.

13-membered azalides **41** were prepared at Pfizer by intramolecular translactonisation of 9-dihydro-9-deoxo-9a-aza-9a-homoerythromycin (**4**). Various azalides were described by derivatisation on positions 10 and 4", but without any biological data given [55].

Ketoazalides

During the last few years an increased resistance to macrolides could be observed worldwide. The different mechanisms of resistance are described in more detail by Sutcliffe and Leclerq within this monograph. One of the most wide-spread mechanisms of macrolide resistance in pathogenic bacteria resulted from a base-specific mono- and dimethylation of 23S ribosomal RNA near or within the macrolide binding site, so that antibiotics such as macrolides, lincosamide, or streptogramin now fail to bind [56, 57]. The responsible reaction is performed by the enzyme erm-methylase, which is found in various bacterial strains. The erm-methylase is either constitutively expressed or its expression is induced, *e. g.*, by macrolides. The capability of macrolides to induce the methylase differs substantially. Early reports on the 3-keto macrolides narbomycin [58] and picromycin

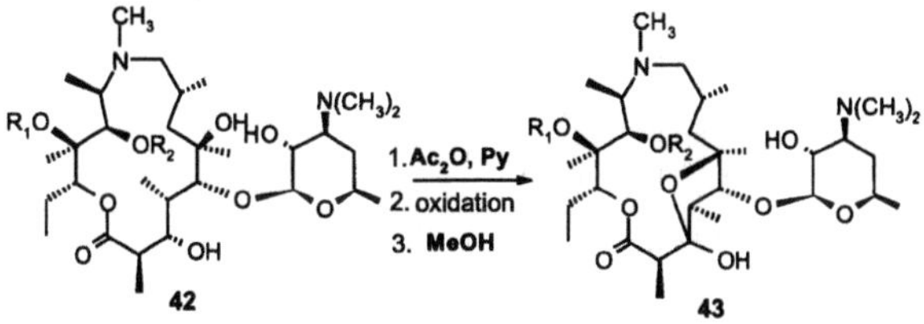

Scheme 11. Oxidation of azithromycin derivatives and formation of 3,6-hemiketals.

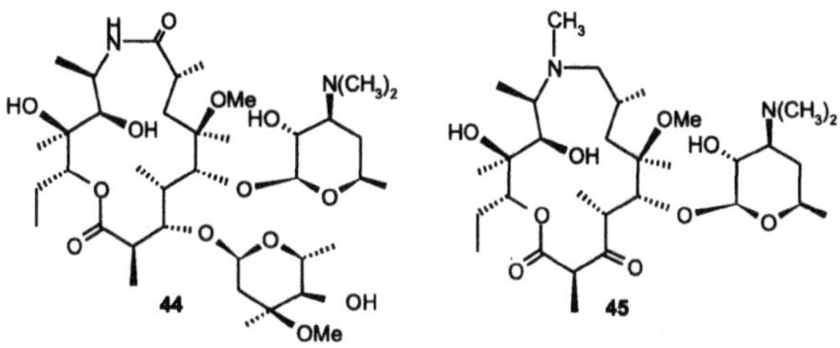

Figure 6. Structures of 6-O-methyl-9a-aza-homoerythromycin and 3-decladinosyl-3-oxo-6-O-methyl-azithromycin.

[59] described that these compounds, themselves showing only weak antibacterial activity, were not able to induce resistance [59]. This observation was the rationale for transformation of 3-decladinosyl-erythromycin-oxime derivatives to 3-oxo compounds [8]. However, the reaction resulted in the formation of 3,6-hemiketals, if the hydroxyl group at position 6 was not protected, *e. g.*, by prior methylation. A comparable hemiketal formation is observed if azalides are used [61].

Azithromycin (**5**) and its 11- or 12-O-methyl derivatives (**25b** or **25a**) yielded by acid hydrolysis the corresponding 3-decladinosyl derivatives **42**, which were protected by acylation of the 2'-hydroxyl group, oxidized and deprotected to 3-decladinosyl-3-oxo-9a-methyl-9-dihydro-9a-aza-9a-homoerythromycin-3,6-hemiketals (**43**). All hemiketals failed to show any antibacterial activity.

In contrast, 3-keto-9a-azalide was prepared starting from 6-O-methyl-erythromycin-9(E)-oxime, which was converted to the 6-O-methyl derivative of 9,11-imino-ether (**6**) or, under aqueous conditions, to the corresponding lactam 6-O-methyl-9a-aza-9a-homoerythromycin (**44**) [46]. The imino-ether **6** was transformed to 6-O-methyl-azithromycin **27**, which after hydrolysis of cladinose, subsequent protection, oxidation and deprotection yielded the ketoazalide **45**.

Unfortunately, the antibacterial activities of azalides compared with azithromycin and ketolide HMR-3647 (Ketek, telithromycin) [62] decreased, while the ketoazalide **45** was significantly less active (Tab. 5).

Table 5. Antibacterial *in vitro* activity of ketoazalide **45,** 9a-azalide **27** and lactam **44** compared with azithromycin (**5**) and ketolide HMR 3647 , (MIC in µg/ml) [46].

Microorganism	**Compound**				
	5	**3647**	**45**	**27**	**44**
S. aureus	0.3	0.04	40.0	1.2	1.2
S. pneumoniae Ery_{Rcon}	40.0	0.02	40.0	40.0	40.0
S. pneumoniae Ery_{Rind}	40.0	0.02	40.0	40.0	10.0
S. pneumonia	0.15	0.02	40.0	0.15	1.2
S. pyogenes	0.6	0.02	40.0	0.15	0.6
H. influenzae	1.2	1.2	40.0	2.5	2.5
E. coli	20.0	10.0	40.0	20.0	40.0

The same 3-keto-9a-azalide **45** was mentioned in a patent from Merck [63], in which the inventors described the synthesis of various 9-dihydro-9a-aza-homo-erythromycins and their 3-keto-derivatives as 3-decladinosyl-3-oxo-9a-aza 9a-N, 6-O-methylene-9a-homo-erythromycin-11,12-carbonate (**46**), and 3-decladino-syl-3-oxo-9a-aza -9a-homoerythromycin-11,12-carbonate-9a-N,6-O-carbamate (**47**). Also various 11,12-carbamates are mentioned, but without any antimicrobial data.

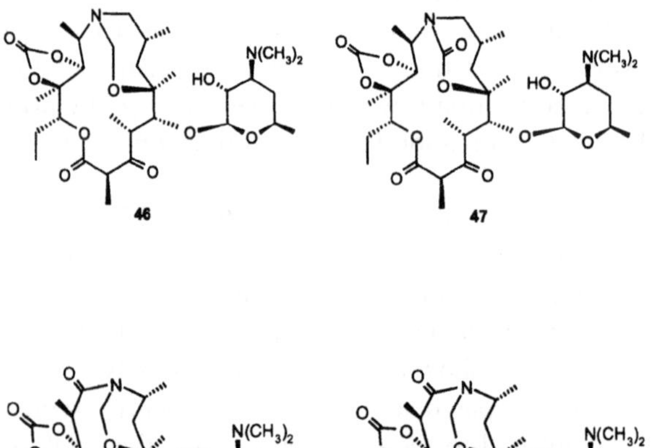

46 **47**

Figure 7. Structures of 3-oxo-9a-aza-9-dihydro-homoerythro-mycin-11,12-carbonate-6-O,9a-N-methylene or bridged carbo-nyl derivative.

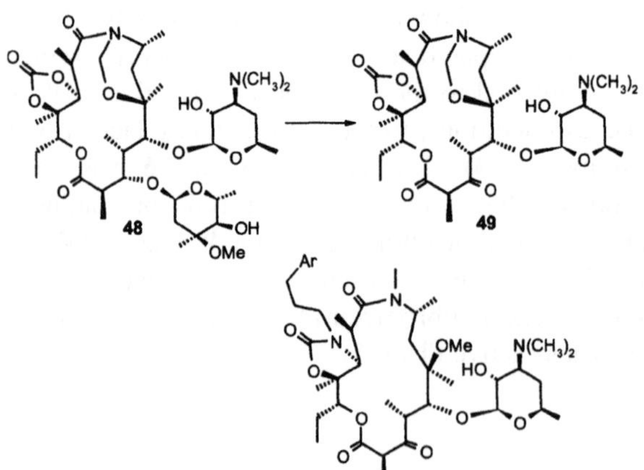

50

Scheme 12. Synthesis of 3-oxo-6,8a-methylene-8a-aza-homoerythromycin-11,12-car-bonate.

In another patent, Merck described broad derivatisation of 8a-lactam **11** [64]. They have prepared 8a-methyl or 8a-N,6-O-methylene-8a-aza-8a-homoerythromycin-11,12-carbonate (**48**), which was transformed in four steps to its 3-decladinosyl-3-keto derivative (**49**). Various combinations of 3-hydroxy substituted or 3-deoxy compounds have been prepared, but none of them showed antibacterial activity.

In the same patent application [64], various 3-oxo-arylalkyl-substituted 11,12-cyclic carbamates are claimed (**50**); aryl groups comprised phenyl-, naphthyl-, 4-quinolyl-, and pyridyl-imidazolyl groups. Starting from 6-O-methyl-erythromycin 9(E)- or (Z)- oxime, PLIVA researchers prepared 8a-lactam **51** and 9a-lactam **43** by Beckmann rearrangement, which were converted, *via* their 3-decladinosyl derivatives, to their corresponding 8a- and 9a-3-ketolactams **52** and **53** [65].

Antibacterial activity of 8a-lactam **51** was similar to azithromycin (**5**), while its 9a-isomer was less active. Ketolactam **52** was less active than **5** and more active than **53**, but it showed improved activity against inducible resistant *S.aureus*.

17-membered azalides

The 17-membered ring macrolides have been prepared from natural 16-membered macrolides, another large and important family of macrolide antibiotics. These are traditionally divided into sub-families based upon the substitution patterns of their aglycones [1]. The principal prototypes of this family can be represented by leucomycin, spiramycin, and tylosin. Tylosin is a representative of 16-membered macrolides, which possess a highly substituted aglycone with two double bonds (tylonolide) and a third saccharide substituent (β-D-mycinose) in addition to the disaccharide attached to the 5-hydroxyl group. Hydrolysis of mycarose from disaccharide yielded desmycarosyl-tylosin (desmycosin), which possesses the same antibacterial activity as tylosin.

The best known semi-synthetic derivative is tilmicosin, produced by reductive amination of the C-20-aldehyde group of desmycosin with 3,5-dimethylpiper-

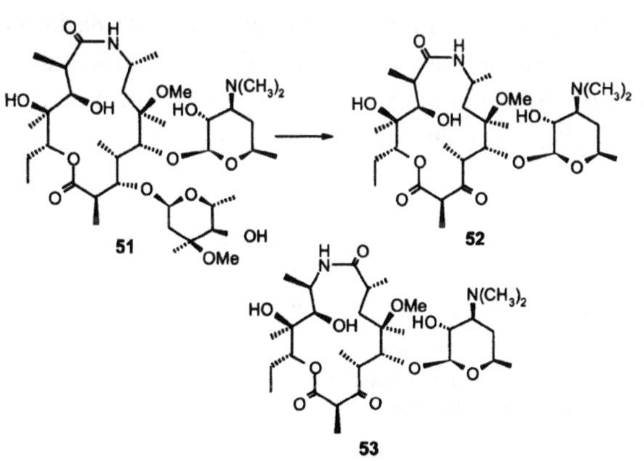

Scheme 13. Synthesis of 3-oxo-6(O)-methyl-8a-aza-8a-homoerythromycin (ketolactam).

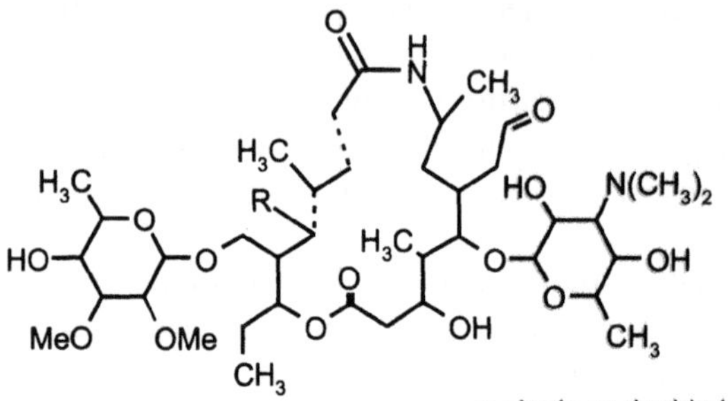

····· = single or double bond

54 R = H, OH

Figure 8. Structure of 8a-aza-homodesmycosins and its di- or tetrahydro derivatives.

idine, which is used in veterinary medicine [66]. The other possibilities in tylosin derivatisation were transformations of double bonds by catalytic reduction or epoxidation. Researchers at PLIVA have prepared many polyhydro derivatives of tylosin and desmycosin [67]; among them, 4'-deoxy-10,11,12,13-tetrahydro-desmycosin showed better activity than tylosin [68]. Oximes of tylosin and desmycosin and their polyhydro- derivatives have been prepared [69]. Most of the chemical transformations have been made on the desmycosin scaffold but have not achived significant improvement of biological activities.

Beckmann rearrangement of these compounds resulted in the corresponding 8a-aza-8a-homodesmycosins (**54**) with small amounts of 9a-aza isomers.

In an attempt to prepare 17-membered cyclic amines instead of lactams, 12,13-dihydro-13-hydroxy-desmycosin and 10,11,12,13-tetrahydro-13-hydroxy-desmycosin have been synthesised [70]. Beckmann rearrangement did not result in the desired imino-ethers, but 12,13-dihydro-13-hydroxy-8a-aza-8a-homodesmycosin, 10,11,12,13-tetrahydro-13-hydroxy-8a-aza-8a-homodesmycosin, and its 9a-aza-9a-homo regioisomers were formed [71].

Most 17-membered lactams showed very low antibacterial activity. In order to improve activity, a series of 20-deoxo-20-amino derivatives of 8a-aza-8a-homo-desmycosin (**55**) were prepared by reductive amination of the C-20 aldehyde.

Only a few newer compounds (**55a-e**) showed slight improvement in activity compared with other 20-deoxo-20-amino derivatives (Tab. 6).

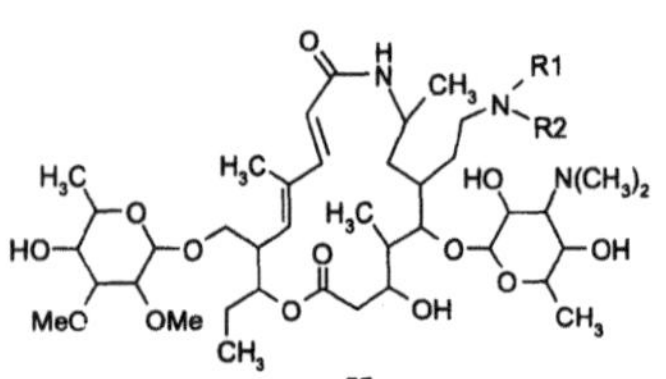

55

55a $R_1 = CH_3$, $R_2 = CH_2PH$

55b $R_1 = H$, $R_2 = (CH_2)_4PH$

55c $R_1 = H$, $R_2 =$ 3-chlorphenyl

55d $R_1 = H$, $R_2 =$ 3,5-dimethylpiperidin

55e $R_1 = CH_2Ph$, $R_2 = CH_2Ph$

Figure 9. Structure of 20-deoxo-20-amino-8a-aza-homo-desmycosins.

The activity of the 17-membered azalide 4'-demycarosyl-20-deoxo-20-(N,N-dibenzylamino)-8a-aza-8a-homotylosin (**55e**) was examined *in vitro* using five different human cell lines for their effects on proliferation [72]. At a concentration of 10^{-4} M, these azalides completely inhibited the growth of all cell lines examined and induced morphological changes such as cell shrinkage, condensation, and DNA fragmentation. This is observed typically in cells undergoing apoptosis.

Table 6. Antibacterial activity of some 20-amino derivatives of 17-membered azalides compared with desmycosin (MIC in µg/ml) [39]

Microorganism	**Compound**							
	Desmyc	**55a**	**55b**	**55c**	**55d**	**55e**	**56b**	**57b**
S. pneumoniae	0.5	128	32	8	32	32	64	64
S. aureus, Ery_S	1	32	32	4	64	2	8	8
S. aureus, Ery_{Rind}	1	ND	32	4	ND	4	8	ND
S. aureus, Ery_{Rcon}	128	128	128	128	128	128	128	128
S. faecalis	1	64	16	4	64	4	16	8
E. coli	128	128	128	128	128	128	128	128

In further synthetic work 3-oxo-derivatives (**56**) and 2,3-anhydro-derivatives (**57**) of 8a-aza-8a-homodesmycosin or its 20-dibenzylamino analogues have been prepared, but no improvement in antibacterial activity was demonstrated (Tab. 6).

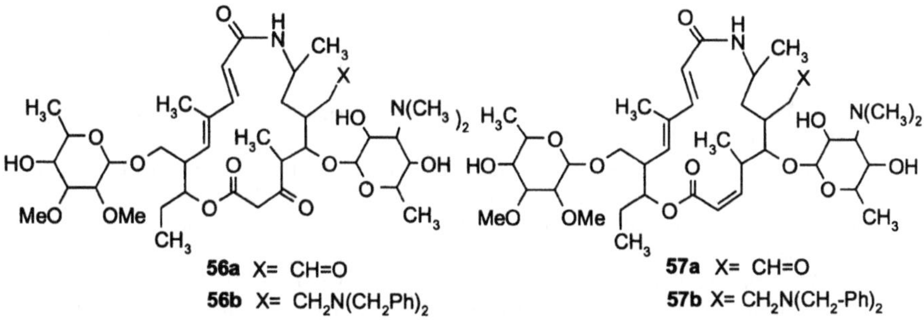

Figure 10. Structures of 3-oxo- and 2,3-anhydro- 20-dibenzylamino-8a-aza-homodemycosins.

Conclusion

Derivatisation of erythromycin by introduction of a nitrogen into the aglycone ring yields highly active antibacterial compounds with favourable pharmacokinetic, highly tolerable profile as exemplified by azithromycin. Ongoing derivatisation of various subclasses of azalides yielded active compounds; however, no clear rules for derivatisation so far could be established. Derivatisation lines successfully applied to erythromycin or other aglycones cannot easily be transferred to azalides, from a chemistry point of view as well as with regard to their antibacterial properties. Thus macrolide chemistry remains a difficult, resource-consuming task and requires a very specialised research team. However, the promising general biological features of this class and the tremendous opportunities for broad derivatisation offer a huge potential to identify novel antibiotics overcoming current resistance patterns.

References

1 a) Kirst HA (1990) Structural modification of macrolide antibiotics. *Recent progress in the chemical synthesis of antibiotics*. Springer-Verlag, Berlin-Heidelberg, 39–63
b) Kirst HA (1996) Expanding the role of macrolide compounds as therapeutic agents, Progress in medicinal chemistry, Harwood Academic Publisher, Amsterdam, 1: 1–47
c) Kirst HA (1998) Recent developments with macrolide antibiotics. *Exp Opin Ther Patents* 8: 111–120

2 a) Omura S (1984) Macrolide antibiotics. *Chemistry, biology and practice. Academic Press Inc.*, Orlando, FL
b) Neu HC, Young LS, Zinner SH, Acar JF (eds) (1995) *New macrolides, azalides and streptogramins in clinical practice*. Marcel Dekker, New York

3 Bryskier AJ, Agouridas C, Chantot J-F (1993) New insights into the structure-activity relationship of macrolides and azalides. In: AJ Bryskier, J-P Butzler, HC Neu, PM Tulkens; (eds): *Macrolides: Chemistry, pharmacology and clinical uses*. Arnette Blackwell, Paris, 3–30

4 Gasc JC, d'Ambrieres GS, Lutz A, Chantot JF (1991) New ether oxime of erythromycin A; a structure activity relationship study. *J Antibiotics* 44: 313–330

5 Counter FT, Ensminger PW, Preston DA, Wu C-YE, Greene JM, Felty-Duckworth AM, Paschal JW, Kirst HA (1991) Synthesis and antimicrobial evaluation of dirithromycin, a new macrolide antibiotic. *Antimicrob Agents Chemother* 35: 1116–1126

6 Watanabe Y, Morimoto S, Adachi T, Kashimura M, Asaka T (1993) Chemical modification of erythromycins IX. Selective methylation at the C-6 hydroxyl group of erythromycin A oxime derivatives and preparation of clarithromycin. *J Antibiot* 46: 647–660

7 Đokić S (1988) From erythromycin to azithromycin – From macrolides to azalides. *Saopćenja* 31: 3–39, Edition Pliva, Zagreb

8 Agouridas C, Denis A, Auger J-M, Beneddeti Y, Bonnefoy A, Bretin F, Chantot J-F, Dussarat A, Fromentin C, D'Ambriéres SG et al (1998) Synthesis and antibacterial activity of ketolides (6-O-methyl-3-oxoerythromycin derivatives): a new class of antibacterials highly potent against macrolide-resistant and -susceptible respiratory pathogens. *J Med Chem* 41: 4080

9 Ma Z, Clark RF, Wang S, Nilius AM, Flamm RK, Or Y (1999) Design, synthesis and characterization of ABT-773: A novel ketolide highly active against multidrug resistant pathogens. *39th ICAAC,* San Francisco, California, Abstr. F-2133
b) Or YS, Clark RF, Wang S, Chu DTW, Nilius AM, Flamm RK, Mitten M, Ewing P, Alder J, Ma Z (2000) Design, synthesis and antimicrobial activity of 6-O-substituted ketolides active against resistant respiratory tract pathogens. *J Med Chem* 43: 1045–1049

10 Đokić S, Tamburašev Z (1967) Erythromycin study: 9-amino-3-O-cladinosyl-6,11,12-trihydroxy-2,4,6,8,10,12-hexamethylpentadecane-13-olide. *Tetrahedron Lett* 17: 1645–1647

11 Tamburašev Z, Vazdar G, Đokić S (1967) Erythromycin series II: Acylation of erythromycin oxime and 9-amino-3-O-cladinosyl-5-O-desosaminyl-6,11,12-trihydroxy-2,4,6,8,10,12-hexamethylpentadecane-13-olide with ester chlorides of dicarboxylic acids. *Croat Chem Acta* 3: 273–276

12 Kobrehel G, Tamburašev Z, Đokić S (1977) Erythromycin series IV. Thin-layer of erythromycin, erythromycin oxime, erythromycylamine and their acyl derivatives. *J Chromatography* 133: 415–419

13 Kobrehel G, Đokić S (Pliva) (1981) Nouveaux derives de l'erythromycine A, procede pour leur preparation et leur utilisation comme substances antibacteriennes, Belg.P. 892 357, July 1, 1982, Prior.Yug. March 6,1981

14 Kobrehel G and Đokić S (Pliva) (1981) 11–Methyl-11-aza-4-O-cladinosyl-6-O-desosaminyl-15-ethyl-7,13,14-trihydroxy-3,5,7,9,12,14-hexamethyl-oxacyclopentadecane-2-one and derivatives thereof. USP 4 517 359, May 14, 1985, Prior.Yug March 6,1981

15 Kobrehel G, Radobolja G, Tamburašev Z and Đokić S (Pliva) (1982), 11-Aza-10-deoxo-10-dihydroerythromycin A and derivatives thereof as well a process for their preparation. USP 4 328 334

16 Đokić S, Kobrehel G, Lazarevski G, Lopotar N, Tamburašev Z, Kamenar B, Nagl A and Vicković I (1986), Erythromycin series. Part 11. Ring expansion of erythromycin A oxime by the Beckmann rearrangement. *J Chem Soc Perkin Trans I* 1881–1990

17 Đokić S, Kobrehel G, Lopotar N, Kamenar B, Nagl A, Mrvoš D (1988) Erythromycin series. Part 13. Synthesis and structure elucidation of 10-dihydro-10-deoxo-11-methyl-11-azaerythromycin A. *J Chem Research (S)* 1988: 152–153

18 Bright GM (Pfizer) (1984) Antibacterial N-methyl 11-aza-10-deoxo-10-dihydro-erythromycin A and pharmaceutically acceptable acid addition salts thereof, intermediates therefore, and processes for their preparation. USP 4 474 768, Oct. 2,1984, Prior. Nov. 15, 1982

19 Bright GM, Nagel AA, Bordner J, Desai KA, Dibrino JN, Nowakowska J, Vincent L, Watrous RM, Sciavolino FC, English AR et al (1988) Synthesis, *in vitro* and *in vivo* activity of novel 9-deoxo-9a-aza-9a-homoerythromycin A derivatives; a new class of macrolide antibiotics, the azalides. *J Antibiot* 41: 1029–1047

20 Allen DJM, Nepveux KM (Pfizer) (1989) Non-hygroscopic, azithromycin (9-deoxo-9a-aza-9a-methyl-9a-homoerythromycin) dihydrate and a process therefor. PCT US87 01612, Jan. 26, 1989, Prior. US July 9, 1987

21 Kamenar B, Nagl A, Mrvoš D (1987) Structural investigations of 11-methylaza-10-deoxo-10-dihydroerythromycin A (DCH_3). 10th Meeting of chemists of Croatia, Zagreb, Feb. 16–18, 1987, Abstr. No A-2, Abstr. book p. 29

22 Đokić S, Kobrehel G, Lazarevski G (1987) Erythromycin series XII. Antibacterial *in vitro* evaluation of 10-dihydro-10-deoxo-11-azaerythromycin A: synthesis and structure activity relationship of its acyl derivatives. *J Antibiot* 40: 1006–1015

23 Đokić S, Vajtner Z, Lopotar N, Mrvoš-Sermek D, Kamenar D, Nagl A (1995) Complexes of azithromycin with some divalent metal ions. *Croatica Chemica Acta* 68: 375–381

24 Retsema J, Girard A, Schelkly W, Manousos M, Anderson M, Bright G, Borovoy R, Brenan L, Mason R (1987) Spectrum and mode of action of azythromycin (CP-62,993), a new 15-membered-ring macrolide with improved potency against Gram-negative organisms. *Antimicrob Agent Chemother* 31: 1939–1947

25 Fiese EF, Steffen SH (1990) Comparism of the acid stability of azythromycin and erythromycin A. *J Antimicrob Chemother* 25: 39–47

26 Girard AE, Girard D, English AR, Gotz TD, Cimochowski CR, Faiella JA, Haskell SL, Retsema JA (1987) Pharmacokinetic and *in vivo* studies with azithromycin (CP-62,993), a new macrolide with an extended half life and excellent tissue distribution. *Antimicrob Agent Chemother* 31: 1948–1954

27 Foulds G, Shepard RM, Johnson RB (1990) The pharmacokinetics of azithromycin in human serum and tissues. *J Antimicrob Chemother* 25: 73–82

28 Schonwald S, Skerk V, Petricevic I, Car V, Majerus-Misic L, Gunjaca M (1991) Comparism of three-day and five-day courses of azithromycin in the treatment of atypical pneumonia. *Eur J Clin Microbiol Infect Dis* 10: 877–880

29 Drew R, Gallis H (1992) Azithromycin-spectrum of activity, pharmacokinetics and clinical applications. Pharmacotherapy 12: 161–173

30 Schentag J, Ballow C (1991) Tissue directed pharmacokinetics. Am J Med 91(suppl 3 A): 3–11

31 Lazarevski G, Vinković M, Kobrehel G, Đokić S, Metelko B and Vikić-Topić D (1993) Conformational analysis of azithromycin by nuclear magnetic resonance spectroscopy and molecular modelling. Tetrahedron 49: 721–730

32 Awann A, Brennan RJ, Regan AC, Barber J (1995) Conformational analysis of the erythromycin analogues azithromycin and clarithromycin in aqueous solution and bound to bacterial ribosomes. J Chem Soc, Chem Commun 1995: 1653–1654
33 Yang BV, Goldsmith M, Rizzi (1994) A novel product from Beckmann rearrangement of erythromycin A 9(E) oxime. Tetrahedron Lett 55: 3025–3028
34 Fattori R, Pelacini F, Romagnano S, Fronza G, Rallo R (1996) Unusual isoxaline formation by intramolecular cyclization of (9E)-erythromycin oxime. J Antibiot 49: 938–940
35 Wilkening RR, Ratcliffe RW, Doss GA, Mosley RT, Ball RG (1997) Novel transanular rearrangements of azalide iminoethers. Tetrahedron 53: 16923–16944.
36 Wilkening RR, Ratcliffe RW, Doss GA, Bartizal KF, Graham AC, Herbert CM (1993) The synthesis of novel- 8a-aza-8a-homoerythromycin derivatives via the Beckmann rearrangement of (9Z)-erythromycin A oxime. Bioorg Med Chem Lett 3: 1287–1292
b) Wilkening RR (Merck) (1993) 8a-Aza-8a-homoerythromycin lactams. USP 5,202,434, Apr. 13,1993, Prior. US Mar. 27, 1992.
37 Lazarevski G, Vinković M, Kobrehel G, Đokić S, Metelko B (1994) Conformational analysis of 9-deoxo-9a-aza-9a- and 9-deoxo-8a-aza-8a-homoerythromycin A 6,9-cyclic iminoethers. Tetrahedron 50: 12201–12210
38 Kamenar B, Mrvoš-Sermek D, Nagl A (1996) Crystal structure of 9-deoxo-9-dihydro-9a-(n-propyl)-9a-aza-9a-homo-erythronolide A, $C_{24}H_{47}NO_7$. *Zeitschrift für Kristallographie* 211: 415–417
39 Kujundžić N, Kobrehel G, Banić Z, Kelnerić Ž, Kojić-Prodić B (1995) Azalides: Synthesis and antibacterial activity of novel 9a-N-(N'-substituted carbamoyl and thiocarbamoyl) derivatives of 9-deoxo-9a-aza-9a-homoerythromycin A. Eur J Med Chem 30: 455–462
40 Sheldrick GM, Kojić-Prodić B, Banić Z, Kobrehel G, Kujundžić N (1995) Structure of 9-Deoxo-9a-N-(N'-(4'-pyridyl)-carbamoyl)-9a-Aza-9a-homoerythromycin A and conformational analysis of analogous 9a-aza 15-membered azalides in solid state. Acta Cryst B51: 358–366
41 Asaka TT, Misawa YT, Kashimura MT, Morimoto ST, Hatayama KT (Taisho) (1994) 5-O-Desosaminylerythronolide derivative. EP 0 619 320, 12 Oct. 1994, Prior. JP 27 Dec. 1991
42 Kobrehel G, Lazarevski G, Đokić S, Kolačni-Babić L, Kučišec-Tepeš N, Cvrlje M (1992) Synthesis and antibacterial activity of O-methylazithromycin derivatives. J Antibiot 45: 527–534
43 Waddell ST, Santorelli GM, Blizzard TA, Graham A, Occi J (1998) Synthesis and antibacterial activity of O-methyl derivatives of azalide antibiotics: I. 4", 11 and 12-O-Me derivatives via direct methylation. Bioorg Med Chem Lett 8: 549–554
44 Kamenar B, Košutić-Hulita N, Vicković I, Kobrehel G, Lazarevski G (1996) 11,12,4"-Tri-O-methylazythromycin monohydrate. Acta Cryst C52: 2566–2568
45 Waddell ST, Santorelli GM, Blizzard TA, Graham A and Occi J (1998) Synthesis and antibacterial activity of O-methyl derivatives of azalide antibiotics: II: 6-O-Me derivatives *via* clarithromycin. Bioorg Med Chem Lett 8: 1321–1326
46 Denis A, Agouridas C (1998) Synthesis of 6-O-methyl-azithromycin and its ketolide analogue via Beckmann rearrangement of 9(E)-6-O-methyl-erythromycin oxime. Bioorg Med Chem Lett 8: 2427–2432
47 Kobrehel G, Lazarevski G, Kelnerić Ž, Đokić S (1993) 9a, 11-Cyclic carbamates of 15-membered azalides. J Antibiot 46: 1239–1245
48 Wu YJ, Wons R, Durkin D, Goldsmith M, Su WG, Rainville J, Smyth K, Yang BV, Massa M, Kane J, et al (1998) Synthesis and in vitro activity of novel C-4 carbamates of 14- and 15-membered macrolides. 38th ICAAC, San Diego, California, Abstract F-123
49 Cheng H, Letavic MA, Ziegler CB, Dutra JK, Bertinato P, Bronk BS (Pfizer) (2000) C11 Carbamates of macrolide antibacterials. EP 0 984 019 A1, Mar. 8, 2000, Prior. US Aug. 19, 1988
50 Waddell ST, Blizard TA (1993) Chimeric azalides with simplified western portions. Tetrahedron Lett 34: 5385–5388
51 Waddell ST, Blizard TA (1992) Base catalysed ring opening reactions of erythromycin A. Tetrahedron Lett 33: 7827–7830
52 Waddell ST, Blizard TA (1993) Semisynthesis of linear fragments corresponding to the eastern portion of azalide antibiotics. Bioorg Med Chem Lett 3: 1757–1760

53 Lazarevski G, Kobrehel G, Naranđa A, Banić-Tomišić Z, Metelko B (1998) Acid catalised ring opening reactions of 6-deoxy-9-deoxo-9a-aza-9a-homoerythromycin 6,9-cyclic imino ether. J Antibiot 51(9): 893–896

54 Lazarevski G, Kobrehel G, Metelko B, Duddeck H (1996) Ring opening reactions of 6-deoxy-9-deoxo-9a-aza-9a-homoerythromycin 6,9-cyclic imino ether. J Antibiot 49(10): 1066–1069

55 Rafka RJ, Morton BJ , Ragan CB, Bertinato P, Dirlam JP, Blize AE, Ziegler CB (Pfizer) (2000) 13-Membered azalides and their use as antibiotic agents.PCT WO 00/31097, 2 June 2000, Prior. US 20 Nov. 1998.

56 Leclercq R, Courvalin P (1991) Bacterial resistance to macrolide, lincosamide and streptogramin antibiotics in bacteria. *Antimicrob Agents Chemother* 35: 1267–1272

57 Weisblum B (1995) Erythromycin resistance by ribosome modification. *Antimicrob Agents Chemother* 39: 577–585

58 Corbaz L, Ettlinger L, Gauman E, Keller W, Kradolfer F, Kyburz E, Neipp L, Prelog V, Reusser R, Zahner H (1955) Stoffwechselprodukte von Actinomyceten. Narbomycin. *Helv Chim Acta* 35: 935–942

59 Brockmann H, Henkel W (1951) Picromycin, ein bitter schmeckendes Antibioticum aus Actinomyceten. *Chem Ber* 84: 284–288

60 Allen N (1977) Macrolide resistance in *Staphylococcus aureus*: inducers of macrolide resistance. *Antimicrob Agents Chemother* 11: 669–674

61 Kobrehel G, Lazarevski G, Vinković M (Pliva) (1999) Novel 3,6-hemiketals from the class of 9a-azalides. Pat. WO-09920693, 29 Apr. 1999, Prior.HR 10 Sep. 1998

62 Denis A, Agouridas C, Auer J-M, Beneddeti Y, Bonnefoy A, Bretin F, Chantot J-F, Dussarat A, Fromentin C, D'Ambrieres SG et al (1999) Synthesis and antibacterial activity of HMR 3647, a new ketolide highly potent against erythromycin-resistant and susceptible pathogens. *Bioorg Med Chem Lett* 9: 3075–3080

63 Blizzard TA, Waddell ST, Santorelli GM (Merck) (1999) 9a-Aza-3-ketolides, compositions containing such compounds and methods of treatment. PCT 99/00125, 7 Jan. 1999, Prior US 27 June 1997

64 Blizzard TA, Santorelli GM (Merck) (1999) 8a-Azalides, compositions containing such compounds and methods of treatment. PCT 99/19331, 22 Apr. 1999, Prior US 16 Oct. 1997

65 Lazarevski G, Kobrehel G and Kelnerić Ž (Pliva) (1999) 15-Membered lactams ketolides with antibacterial activity. Patent WO-09951616, 14 Oct. 1999, Prior. HR 06 Apr. 1998

66 Debono M, Willard KE, Kirst HA, Wind JA, Crouse GO, Tao EV, Vicenzi JT, Counter FT, Ott JL, Ose EE, et al (1989) Synthesis and antimicrobial evaluation of 20-deoxo20-(3,5-dimethylpiperidin-1-yl)-desmycosin (tilmicosin, EL-870) and related cyclic amino derivatives. *J Antibiot* 42: 1253–1267

67 Naranda A, Šušković B, Kelnerić Ž and Đokić S (1994) Structure-activity relationship among polyhydro derivatives of tylosin. *J Antibiot* 47: 581–587

68 Naranda A, Kelnerić Ž, Kolačni-Babić L, Đokić S (1995) 10,11,12,13-Tetrahydro derivatives of tylosin. Synthesis, antibacterial activity and tissue distribution of 4'-deoxy-10,11,12,13-tetrahydrodesmycosin. *J Antibiot* 48: 284–253

69 Lopotar N, Đokić S (Pliva) (1990) Preparation and properties of some tylosine derivatives. EP 0410433B1, Prior. YU July 26, 1989

70 Naranda A, Lopotar N, Kelnerić Ž (1998) Synthesis of novel dihydro and tetrahydro desmycosin derivatives. *ICMASK 4, Fourth International Conference on the Macrolides, Azalides, Streptogramins and Ketolides,* Barcelona, Spain, Abstr. 1.29

71 Lopotar N, Naranđa A, Vela V, Đerek M, Maršić N (2000) Synthesis and microbiological activity of 17-membered azalides. *ICMAS-KO 5, Fifth International Conference on the Macrolides, Azalides, Streptogramins, Ketolides and Oxazolidinones*, Seville, Spain, Abstr. 1.01

72 Grdiša M, Lopotar N, Pavelić K (1998) Effect of a 17-member azalide on tumor cell growth. *Chemotherapy* 44: 331

Macrolide Antibiotics
ed. by W. Schönfeld and H. A. Kirst

Ketolides: novel antibacterial agents designed to overcome resistance to erythromycin A within gram-positive cocci

André Bryskier and Alexis Denis

Aventis Pharma Research Center, 102, route de Noisy, 93230 Romainville, France

Introduction

Erythromycin A [1] was discovered at a time when a new drug active against penicillinase-producing *Staphylococcus aureus* strains was needed. Penicillinase-producing resistant strains appeared in London hospitals very shortly after the early clinical use of penicillin G, and they soon spread worldwide [2]. Erythromycin use rapidly was limited by the development of other drugs active on penicillin G-resistant *S. aureus* isolates and by the fact that it shows only a bacteriostatic activity. In addition, erythromycin's pharmacokinetic behaviour is erratic, as the compound is unstable in acidic condition [3].

The outbreak of Legionnaire's disease at the end of the 1970s and the discovery of *Legionella pneumophila* [4] led to renewed interest in the macrolide class. In the meantime, microbiological research highlighted the crucial role of *Chlamydia trachomatis* in sexually transmitted diseases [5].

A second wave of erythromycin A derivatives, including roxithromycin [6], clarithromycin, [7] and azithromycin [8], was synthesized and designed to overcome instability in acidic environments, with the aim of obtaining compounds with good pharmacokinetic behaviour after oral administration.

The rapid spread of bacterial resistance within common pathogens involved in various infections has driven the synthesis of new antibacterial agents with new mechanism of action: ketolides, which were designed to overcome erythromycin A resistance within gram-positive cocci. [9]

Definition

Ketolides are defined by their chemical structure and their biological properties.

Ketolides are semisynthetic derivatives of erythromycin A, having a 3-keto function instead of an L-cladinose moiety. The name ketolide is derived from keto (3-keto group) and olide (lactone).

These compounds are unable to induce MLS_B resistance, and they are active against inducible *erm*-containing gram-positive cocci such as *S. aureus*, *Strepto-*

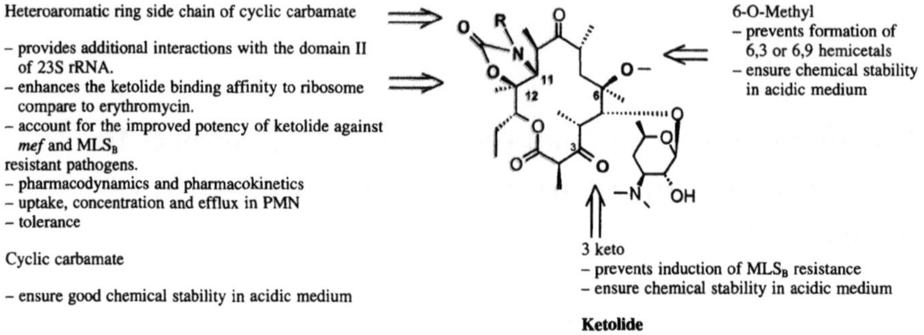

Figure 1.

coccus pneumoniae, and other streptococci. They display good antibacterial activity against gram-positive cocci harboring an efflux mechanism of resistance. They are stable in acidic conditions [10]. These properties result from the combination of three chemical features (Fig. 1).

Classification

Erythromycin A is a good substrate for chemical modifications. Addition of various substituents at C-6, C-9, C11–12, C-8, or the ring expansion of erythromycin derivatives yielded a group of compounds having an improved pharmacokinetic profile, a higher stability at acidic pH, or slightly better antibacterial activity in comparison with erythromycin A. These compounds are roxithromy-

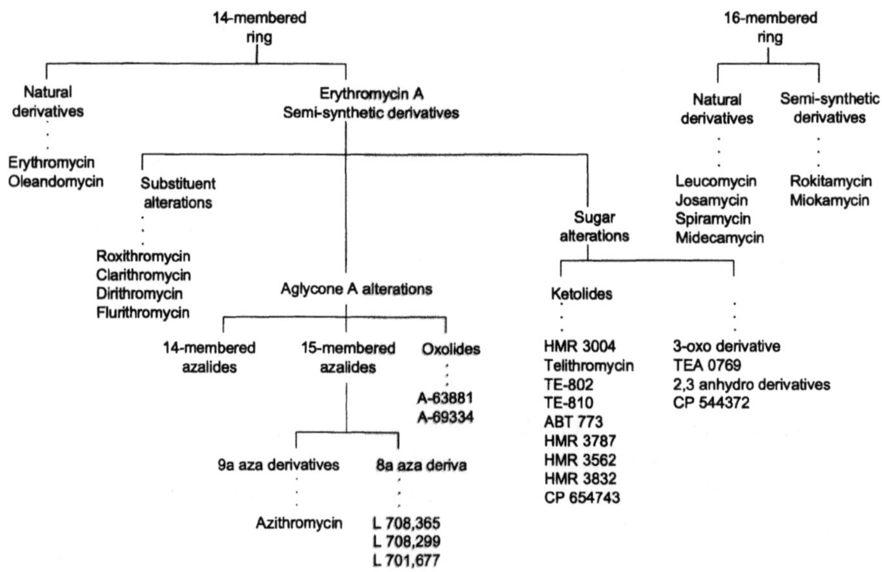

Figure 2.

cin, clarithromycin, azithromycin [8], flurithromycin, dirithromycin, and davercin.

All of these compounds exhibit an improved antibacterial activity against intracellular pathogens such as *Legionella pneumophila* and enhanced pharmacokinetic behaviour. However, all of them display cross-resistance with erythromycin A [10].

Recently, a new group of compounds including ketolides, have been obtained through L-cladinose removal. Two types of derivatives have been obtained: ketolides and a miscellaneous group of analogues [10] (Fig. 2).

Rationale for new macrolide derivatives

Despite recent significant advances in drug therapy and medical technology, pneumonia continues to present a challenge for physicians. The successful treatment of community-acquired pneumonia (CAP) relies on prompt antibacterial therapy, which leads to clinical improvement after 2 to 4 days. The aetiology of CAP is rarely defined at the time of presentation, and empirical therapy is the rule. An empirical therapy had been recommended by the American Thoracic Society and The Infectious Disease Society of America. Community-acquired pneumonia is the most serious of the respiratory infections requiring hospitalisation and carries a 5% to 15% mortality rate (featuring in the top 10 leaders of morbidity and mortality) [11].

In non-immunocompromised out-patients suffering from a lower or upper respiratory tract infection (RTI), the most common pathogens are *S. pneumoniae*, *Haemophilus influenzae*, and *Moraxella catarrhalis*. The role of atypical microorganisms like *Mycoplasma pneumoniae* or intracellular pathogens such as *Chlamydia pneumonial* or *L. pneumophila* as etiological pathogens in RTI is now well established. Other intracellular pathogens are responsible for CAP, such as *Chlamydia psittaci*, *Coxiella burnetii*, or more recently described parachlamydia. Other common pathogens are involved in this pathological process, either in specific frames, like whooping cough due to *Bordetella pertussis*, *B. parapertussis*, or *Bordetella holmesii*, or non specific with *Pasteurella* spp, *Neisseria meningitidis*, and some anaerobic gram-negative rods (*Prevotella* spp, *Porphyromonas* spp).

Antibacterial resistance among respiratory tract pathogens has become an increasing worldwide problem during the last 15 years.

Until the 1970s, *S. pneumoniae* infections were successfully treated with β-lactams. Since then, however, increasing resistance to penicillin G and erythromycin A has been reported on a worldwide scale.

North American survey has found that 11.1% of the *S. pneumoniae* isolates have a decreased susceptibility to amoxicillin and a decreased suseptibility of 8.3% to cefotaxime-ceftriaxone. Co-trimoxazole resistance is seen alongside penicillin G resistance (27.8%), as well as tetracycline (20.4%) and chloramphenicol (11%) resistance. Today resistance to fluoroquinolones remains low, i.e., less than 1% of the clinical isolates. The production of β-lactamase in *H. influenzae* is a widespread problem, with an incidence rate of 10% to 40% of β-lactamase producing strains. The average incidence of β-lactamase producing *H. influenzae* was 33.5% in the USA in 1997. Today, for *M. catarrhalis* almost 95% of the clinical isolates are resistant to ampicillin by producing TEM-1 or BRO-1, BRO-2 or BRO-3 enzymes.

The need to combat resistance, particularly to provide activity against penicillin G and/or erythromycin A-resistant *S. pneumoniae* clinical isolates has driven the development of new compounds designed to overcome multi-drug-resistant *S. pneumoniae*. Among those new compounds resulting from intensive research for novel antibacterials is the ketolide class of antibacterial agents. [9]

History of a discovery

In our effort to overcome erythromycin A-resistance and to develop a new macrolide derivative without MLS_B inductibility potential, we have rediscovered two natural 14-membered-ring, 3-keto macrolides: narbomycin [12] and pikromycin [13]. Actually, these compounds are natural ketolides.

It was known since 1974 that narbomycin and pikromycin as well as their 3-keto and 3-hydroxy erythromycin A oxime analogues (compounds **1** and **2**) were both inactive but unable to induce MLS_B resistance within macrolides [14–18]. Furthermore, it was also demonstrated that chemical modifications and removal or replacement of this sugar in position 3 produced 14-membered ring macrolides able to increase or suppress the MLS_B resistance within the macrolide class [19–21]. It was long thought from all these studies that the L-cladinose sugar was crucial for the antibacterial activity and resistance-inducibility properties of erythromycin A. Although the 3-keto macrolide narbomycin was also considered

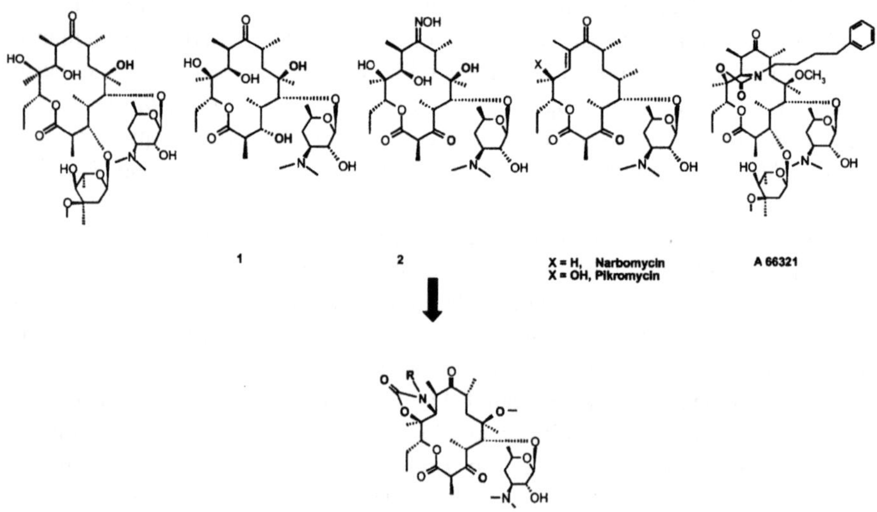

Figure 3.

Table 1. *In vitro* evaluation of narbomycin

	MIC μg/ml				
compd	*S. aureus* 011UC4	*S. aureus* EryRi 011GO25i	*S. aureus* EryRc 011CB20	*S. pneumoniae* EryRc 030SJ1	*S. pneumoniae* EryRi 030SJ5i
Narbomycin	1.25	2.5	> 40.0	10.0	20.0
ERY	0.3	> 40.0	> 40.0	> 40.0	> 40.0

EryS= erythromycin A susceptible, EryRc= constitutively erythromycin A resistant, EryRi= inducibly erythromycin A resistant

inactive, we concluded that the activity of 3-keto macrolides should be re-examinated carefully (Fig. 3). Thus, narbomycin was tested against some erythromycin A-resistant, gram-positive cocci and shown to display a weak but significant *in vitro* antibacterial activity (Tab. 1).

When considering these results, we concluded that the synthesis of 3-keto macrolides could be an innovative starting point for the synthesis of new agents addressing the problem of erythromycin A resistance (Fig. 3). Starting from the 3-keto-6-O-methyl erythromycin A, numerous compounds were synthesized, giving rise to a new class of semi-synthetic erythromycin A derivatives named "ketolides" for 3-keto-erythromycin A.

This series has culminated with the introduction of a C11–12 carbamate side chain, leading to the discovery of the innovative carbamate ketolide telithromycin, which is currently under clinical introduction worldwide. [22, 23]

Synthesis of ketolides

The first targeted molecule was the previously described [15] 3-keto-6-hydroxy-9-oxime derivative of erythromycin A **2**. However, following the published experimental protocols , it was found that structure **2** was incorrect and was actually the hemiacetal **3** (Fig. 4). Therefore, the 6-OH function was protected by using 6-O-methyl analogue of erythromycin A as a starting material to avoid the 6–3 cyclization. The cladinose was removed in acidic medium to give the corresponding 3-hydroxy intermediate, which was efficiently converted into the corresponding ketone by using

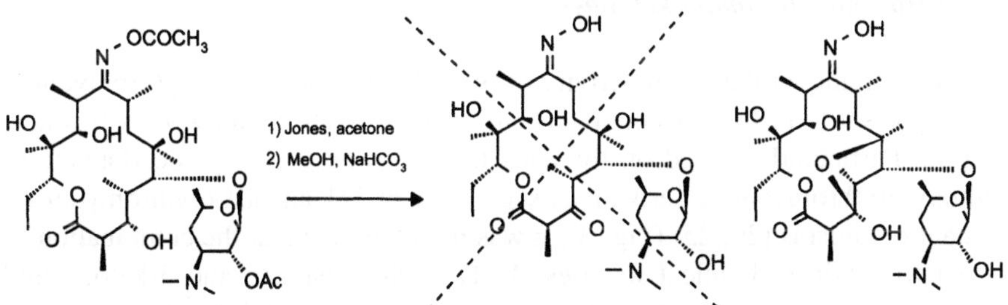

2 3

Figure 4. Attempted synthesis of 9-oxime-3-keto-erythromycin.

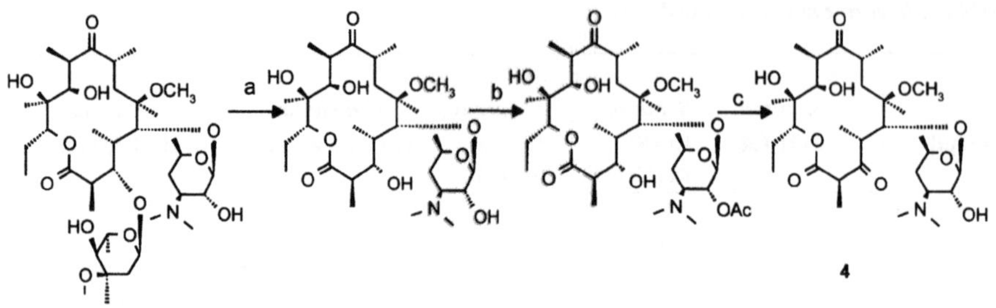

a) HCl/H_2O (76%), b) Ac_2O/K_2CO_3, acetone (82%), c) EDC,HCl, DMSO, Pyridinium trifluoroacetate, CH_2Cl_2, then MeOH (70%)

Figure 5. Synthesis of the first ketolide, 6-O-methyl-3-keto-erythromycin.

the modified Pfitzner-Moffat procedure (1-(3-dimethylaminopropyl)-3-ethylcarbodiimide hydrochloride (EDC,HCl) – DM SO, pyridinium trifluoroacetate) to give the first ketolide ever synthesized **4** [24] (Fig. 5).

Whereas the 6,3 hemiacetal compound **3** was completely inactive, the 3-keto-O-methyl-erythromycin A **4** was as active as erythromycin A against sensitive strains but in contrast exhibited a moderate activity (MICs ranging from 1.2 to 20 mg/l) against erythromycin A-resistant (MLS_B inducible) strains of *S. aureus*, *Staphylococcus epidermidis*, and *S. pneumoniae* (Tab. 2)

Table 2. *In vitro* evaluation of the first ketolide

	MIC mg/l							
	S. aureus	***S. aureus***	***S. epidermidis***	***S. aureus***	***S. pneumoniae***	***S. pneumoniae***	***S. pneumoniae***	***E. coli***
compd	**011UC4**	**EryRi 011GO25i**	**EryRi 012GO11i**	**EryRc 011CB20**	**EryRc 030SJ1**	**EryRi 030SJ5i**	**032UC1**	**250UC5**
4	0.3	**10.0**	**5.0**	> 40.0	> 40.0	**20.0**	0.15	> 40.0
3	> 40.0	> 40.0	> 40.0	> 40.0	> 40.0	> 40.0	> 40.0	> 40.0
ERY	0.3	> 40.0	> 40.0	> 40.0	> 40.0	> 40.0	0.08.0	> 40.0

EryS= erythromycin A susceptible, EryRc= constitutively erythromycin A resistant, EryRi= inducibly erythromycin A resistant

Discovery of telithromycin and HMR 3004. Synthesis of 11, 12 carbamate and hydrazono-carbamate ketolides

The encouraging antibacterial activity of the 3-keto-6-O-methyl-erythromycin A **4**, prompted us to further explore the chemical modifications allowed by this new scaffold. Particularly, based on the activities of some 11,12-cyclocarbamate-6-methoxy-erythromycin A derivatives such as A-66321 against erythromycin A-resistant organisms [20, 25] (Fig. 3), it was hypothesised that the combination of these two original chemical features, 11,12-cyclocarbamate and 3-keto, could generate new 11,12-carbamate and hydrazono-carbamate ketolides with improved antibacterial activities against erythromycin A-resistant, gram-positive cocci strains [23, 24].

Synthesis of 11,12-carbamate ketolides

The synthesis of the 12-acyl-imidazolyl ketolide **5** was carried out in three steps from 6-O-methyl-erythromycin A (Fig. 6). The 11-hydroxy group was first removed by treatment with $(MeSO_2)_2O$ and with DBU in acetone. The remaining 12-hydroxy group was acylated by treatment with NaH in DMF at –10°C followed by addition of 3 equivalents of carbonyldiimidazole. Stirring **5** in CH_3CN/H_2O with various amines at 60°C yielded the desired 11,12-cyclocarbamate ketolides **6–18** in a 24% to 64% yield (Figs. 6, 8; Table 3) [23, 24]. The reaction with ammonia gave a 2/1 mixture of 10-methyl epimers yield, whereas introduction of bulky amino groups yielded the single natural 10 (R) isomer (Fig. 7).

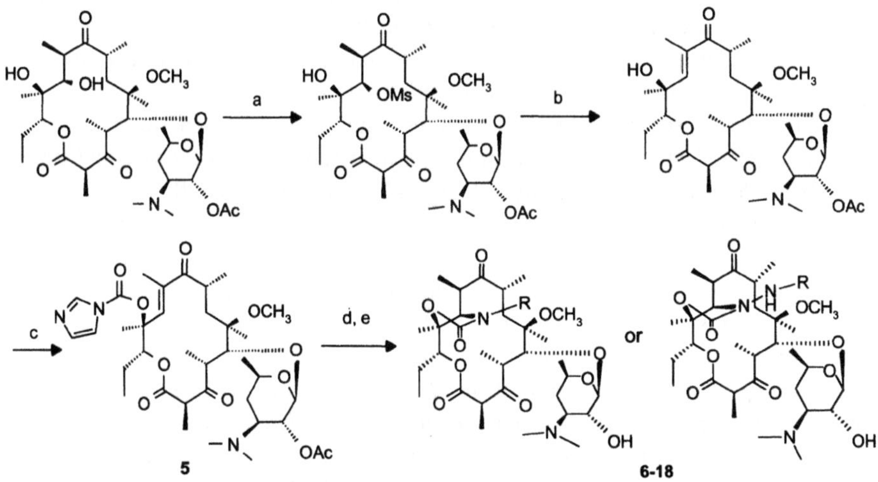

a) $(MeSO_2)_2O$, pyridine; b) DBU, acetone,rt; c) NaH/DMF or DBU/THF, carbonyldiimidazol; d) RNH_2 or e) NH_2NH_2, RCHO, $NaBH_3CN$, CH_3CO_2H, MeOH

Figure 6. General synthesis of carbamate and hydrazono-carbamate ketolides.

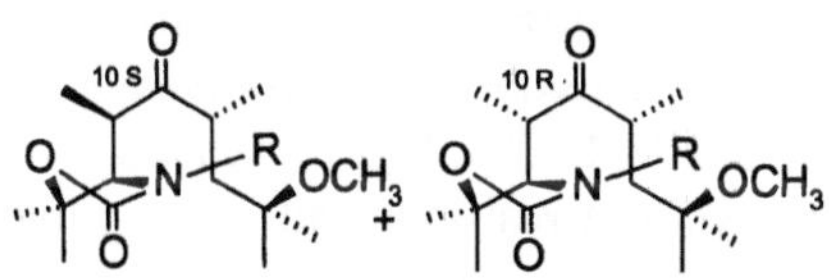

	10(R)/10(S) > 95/5
R= H	2/1
R= NH2	1/1
R= alkyl	100/0

Figure 7. Stereochemistry of 11,12 cyclocarbamatation.

Synthesis of 11,12-hydrazono-carbamate ketolides

By comparison with the reactivity of ammonia, it was expected that hydrazine would react identically with the acyl-imidazole intermediate to generate an 11,12-hydrazono-carbamate.

When **5** was heated at 60°C in CH_3CN with 4 equivalents of $NH_2NH_2.H_2O$, the two epimeric hydrazono-ketolides were obtained in a 1:1 ratio (Fig. 7) [23, 26]. The 10(R)-hydrazono-ketolide **7** was selected as starting material to introduce aryl-alkyl side chains similar to those of some of the carbamates. This was carried out by reductive alkylation of the hydazono function by $NaBH_3CN$/AcOH in MeOH with the corresponding aldehydes (Figs. 6, 8) [24].

Structure-activity relationship (Tab. 3)

All the compounds obtained were inactive against *E. coli* and the erythromycin A-resistant *S. aureus* 011CB20 (MLS_B constitutive type) strains (MIC > 40 mg/l). The non-substituted ketolides **6** and **7** were weakly active against erythromycin A-resistant strains, their 10-epimeric counterparts (Fig. 7) being inactive. The introduction of an aryl-alkyl side chain resulted in a dramatic increase of antibacterial activity against erythromycin A-resistant, gram-positive cocci strains and *H. influenzae* as shown by **10** and **11** compared with **8**. In contrast to clarithromycin and azithromycin that were inactive (MICs > 40 mg/l) against erythromycin A-resistant strains whatever the phenotype, all the MICs of **10** and **11** against erythromycin A-resistant strains ranged from 0.04 to 5 mg/l to 1.2 to 2.5 mg/l against *H. influenzae*. The hydrazono-carbamate **11** was slightly less active than its carbamate counterpart against the MLS_B constitutively resistant *S. pneumoniae* 030SJ1. The length of the chain was also critical, as exemplified by phenylbutyl derivative **10** (4 atoms between the carbamate and the aryl group), which clearly exhibited higher *in vitro* activity than its propyl counterpart **9**. Introduction of heteroatoms in the side chains resulted in a loss of activity against MLS_B constitutively resistant *S. pneumoniae* (MICs 5 to 40 mg/l for **12**). A second improvement was achieved with the introduction of heteroatoms in the aryl moiety of both series.

In the carbamate series, the antibacterial activity of the quinoline compound **15** was within the range of the phenyl compound **10** against gram-positive organisms. However, it showed comparable *in vitro* activity to azithromycin against *H. influenzae*. The hydrazono-carbamate **16** (HMR 3004, Fig. 8) was now even more potent against gram-positive, erythromycin A-resistant and -susceptible cocci (MICs 0.02 to 0.15 mg/l) and more active than azithromycin against *H. influenzae*.

According to these results, we hypothesised that introduction of an additional heterocyclic nitrogen would be beneficial for enhancing the antibacterial activity. The phenylimidazole compounds **13** and **14** were shown to be less active than the quinoline compounds against the MLS_B constitutively resistant *S. pneumoniae* 030SJ1 (MIC ~2.5 to 5 mg/l). Finally, the introduction of an imidazolo-pyridyl

Table 3. *In vitro* evaluation of 11,12-carbama and carbaza ketolides

		MIC mg/l								
N°	R=	*S. a.* 011UC4	*S. a.* EryRi 011GO25i	*S. e.* EryRi 012GO11i	*S. a.* EryRc 011CB20	*S. p* EryRc 030SJ1	*S. p.* EryRi 030SJ5i	*S. p.* 032UC1	*S. pyo.* 02A1UC1	*H. i.* 351HT3
6	**H**	0.6	0.6	10	40	5	2.5	0.02	0.04	5
7	**NH_2**	1.2	1.2	1.2	40	40	40	0.08	0.15	10
8	**$(CH_2)CH_3$**	1.2	5	40	40	40	40	0.04	0.15	40
9	**$(CH_2)_3C_6H_5$**	1.2	2.5	1.2	40	40	20	0.3	0.15	40
10	**$(CH_2)_4C_6H_5$**	0.08	0.15	0.04	40	0.15	0.3	0.02	0.02	1.2
11	**$NH(CH_2)_3C_6H_5$**	0.08	0.15	0.15	40	5	0.15	0.02	0.02	1.2
12	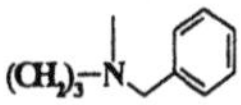	0.15	0.6	0.15	40	10	0.3	0.02	0.04	5
13	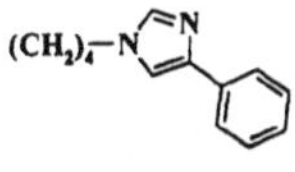	0.04	0.15	0.6	40	5	0.04	0.02	0.02	1.2
14	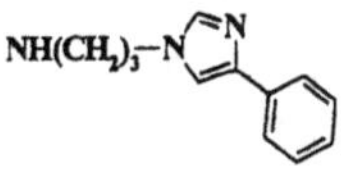	0.08	0.3	0.6	40	2.5	0.15	0.02	0.04	1.2
15	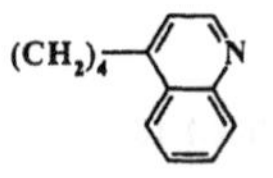	0.04	0.08	0.15	40	1.2	0.02	0.02	0.02	1.2
16 (HMR 3004)	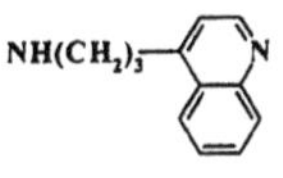	0.02	0.08	0.04	40	0.15	0.02	0.02	0.02	0.6
17	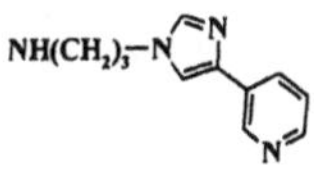	0.08	0.08	0.08	40	0.6	0.04	0.02	0.04	2.5
18 (telithromycin)	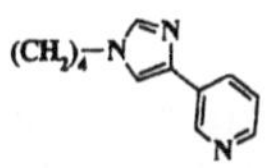	0.04	0.08	0.04	40	0.08	0.02	0.02	0.02	1.2
A 66321		0.3	20	40	20	10	1.2	0.02	0.04	2.5
CLA		0.3	40	40	40	40	40	0.04	0.08	5
AZI		0.3	40	40	40	40	40	0.15	0.6	1.2

S. a.: *Staphylococcus aureus; S.e.*: *Staphylococcus epidermidis; S. p.*: *Streptococcus pneumoniae; S. pyo.*: *Streptococcus pyogenes; H. i.*: *Haemophilus influenza; E. c.*: *Escherichia.coli.* EryS= erythromycin susceptible, EryRc= constitutively erythromycin resistant, EryRi= inducibly erythromycin resistant; CLA: clarithromycin; AZI: azithromycin.

group in the side chain of the carbamate resulted in a dramatic increase of activity against the MLS_B constitutively resistant *S. pneumoniae* 030SJ1 (MIC = 0.08 mg/l). The improvement of activity culminated with **18** (telithromycin, Fig. 8), which was the most active compound synthesized in the series; **18** was very potent against both erythromycin A-resistant and -susceptible gram-positive cocci (MICs between 0.02 and 0.08 mg/l) and was comparable to azithromycin against *H. influenzae*.

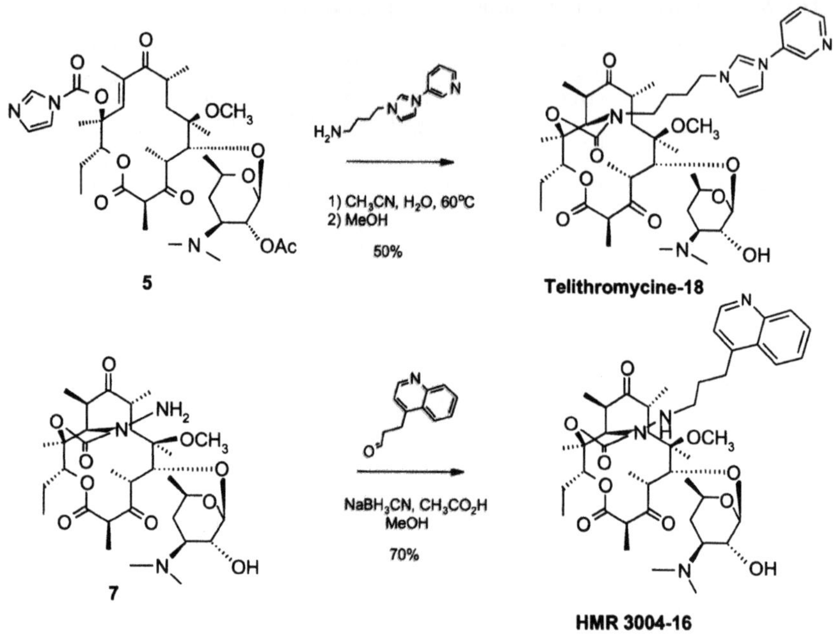

Figure 8. Synthesis of telithromycin and HMR 3004.

Structure-activity relationship within the 11,12-carbamate ketolide series

Chemical modifications in positions 2, 3, and 6

Using telithromycin as a template, several chemical modifications were made to investigate the relative importance of positions 2, 3, and 6 for the overall antibacterial activity of ketolides and particularly the role of the 3-keto function relative to its cladinosyl or 3-hydroxy counterparts. The chemical reactivity of the β keto-ester function of ketolides also was exploited to introduce in position 2 different electrophiles such as halogen atoms or a methyl group. The 3-cladinosyl **21**, 6-deoxy **19**, and 2,3 anhydro **23** analogues of telithromycin were synthesized by reacting their corresponding acyl-imidazole intermediate [25, 27–31] with (4-(3-pyridyl)-1H-imidazo)-1-butyl amine. The 3-OH analogue was obtained from **20** by hydrolysis of the cladinose [30] (Fig. 9).

Fluorination at C-2 was achieved [31] by reacting the 2'-protected silylated telithromycin with tBuOK and N-fluorosulfonimide (NSFI) to give stereospecifically the desired 2(S)-fluoro ketolide (Fig. 10). The chlorine atom was introduced by radical chlorination using N-chlorosuccinimide with AIBN (Fig. 10) [31]. Methylation at C-2 was carried out by phase-transfer catalysis alkylation of telithromycin with methyl iodide (Fig. 10). In addition, the enolate intermediate also may be converted into stable 2, 3 enol-ether derivatives by O-alkylation with a known chloromethylether (Fig. 10) [31].

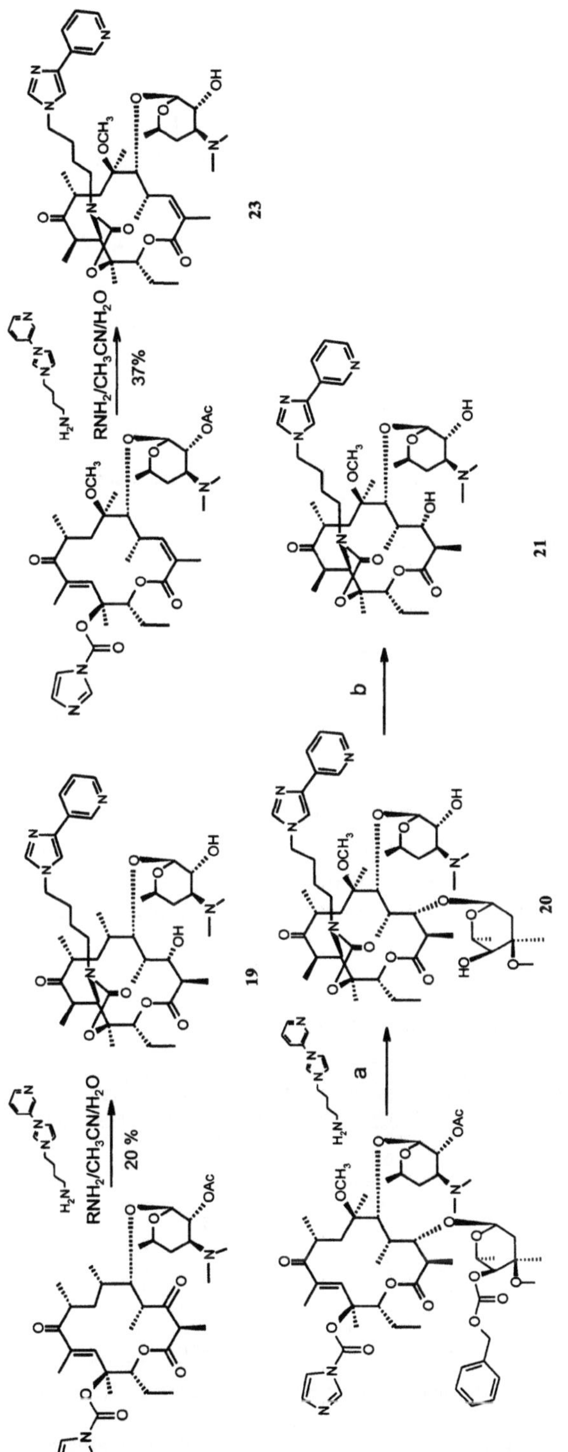

a) RNH$_2$/CH$_3$CN/H$_2$O then H$_2$/Pd/C/MeOH, 20%; b) HCl, EtOH, 53%

Figure 9. Synthesis of 6-deoxy, 2,3 anhydro, 3-cladinosyl and 3-hydroxy analogues of telithromycin.

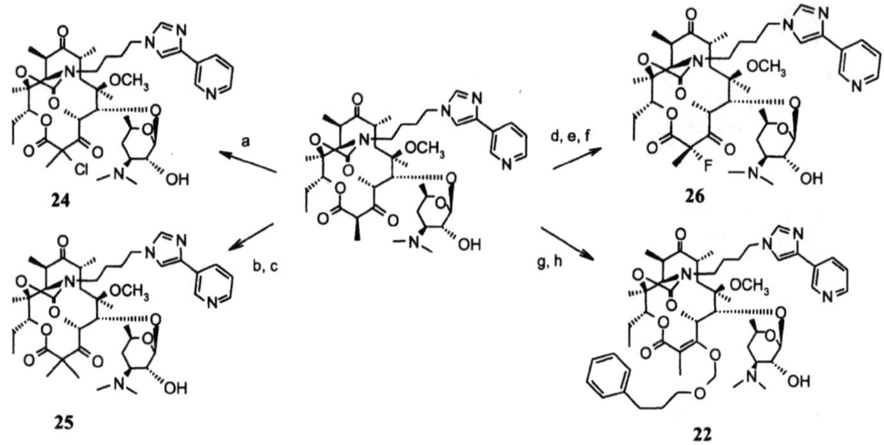

a) N-chlorosuccinimide/AIBN/CCl_4/40°C, b) MeI/NaOH/ $Bu_4N^+HSO_4^-$/CH_2Cl_2, c) MeOH, d) $(TMS)_2NH$/imidazole/THF, e) tBuOK/NSFI/THF/-10°C, f) $N^+Bu_4F^-$/THF, g) NaH/DMF/ /$C_6H_5(CH_2)_3OCH_2Cl$, f) MeOH

Figure 10. Synthesis of 2 and 2–3 substituted ketolides.

In vitro *and* in vivo *antibacterial activities (Tab. 4)*

The cladinosyl counterpart of telithromycin **20** (RU 69874) was less active against erythromycin A-resistant strains with a complete loss of activity against the inducibly resistant *S. aureus* (MIC > 40 mg/l), whereas the 3-hydroxy analogue **21**, which was generally less active (factor 4–6) against erythromycin A-susceptible strains and inactive against MLS_B constitutively resistant strains, was weakly active against the erythromycin A-resistant (inducible MLS_B) strains (MIC = 5 mg/l). These observations were in agreement with the involvement of

Table 4. *In vitro* activity of 2, 3 and 6 modified ketolides MIC (mg/l)

	S. a. EryS 011UC4	*S. a.* EryRi 011GO25i	*S. a.* EryRc 011CB20	*S. pyo.* EryS 02A1UC1	*S. p.* EryS 032UC1	*S. p.* EryRc 030PW23c	*S. p.* EryRc 030SJ1	*S. p.* EryRi 030SJ5i	*H. i.* 351HT3 (β lactamase +)
19	5.0	> 20.0	> 40.0	0.15	0.3	20.0	20.0	5.0	> 20.0
20	0.15	> 40.0	> 40.0	0.08	0.02	0.3	0.6	0.3	2.5
21	2.5	5.0	> 40.0	0.15	0.02	> 40.0	> 40.0	5.0	10.0
22	5.0	> 40.0	> 40.0	0.15	0.8	20.0	20.0	20.0	> 40.0
23	0.08	0.3	> 40.0	0.02	0.02	0.3	10.0	2.5	2.5
24	0.6	> 40.0	> 40.0	0.04	0.04	1.2	5.0	0.6	2.5
25	0.6	1.2	> 40.0	0.02	0.02	2.5	2.5	0.6	2.5
26	0.02	0.08	> 40.0	≤ 0.02	≤ 0.02	≤ 0.02	≤ 0.02	≤ 0.02	1.2
TEL	0.04	0.08	> 40.0	≤ 0.02	≤ 0.02	0.04	≤ 0.02	≤ 0.02	1.2
AZI	0.3	> 40.0	> 40.0	0.6	0.15	> 40.0	> 40.0	> 40.0	1.2
CLA	0.3	> 40.0	> 40.0	0.08	0.04	> 40.0	> 40.0	> 40.0	5.0

AZI= azithromycin; CLA: clarithromycin; TEL: telithromycin; EryS = susceptible; EryRc = constitutive MLS resistance;
EryRi = inducible MLS resistance. *S. a. = Staphylococcus aureus; S. pyo. = Streptococcus pyogenes; S. p. = Streptococcus pneumoniae; H. i. = Haemophilus influenzae.*

Table 5. *In vivo* efficacy of 2-fluoro ketolide I

	ED_{50} (mg/kg)*				
	S. a.	*S. p.*	*S. p.*	*S. p.*	*H. i.*
	EryS	**EryS**	**EryRc**	**EryRi**	**AmpR**
	011HT17	**032UC1**	**030MV2**	**030SJ5i**	**351RD7**
					(β lactamase +)
CLA	12	2	> 50	> 50	> 150
AZI	72	4.5	> 50	> 50	94
26	9	1.5	2	4.3	56

*Effective dosage that protect 50% of mice from lethal infection after oral administration; AmpR = ampicillin resistant.

the cladinose moiety in the induction of MLS_B resistance and were later confirmed by induction experiments.

Surprisingly, removal of the 6-OCH_3 group has a dramatic impact on the antibacterial activity, the 6-deoxy analogue of telithromycin **19** being almost inactive against most of the strains tested.

The planar derivative **22** was generally poorly active against most of the strains tested with a complete loss of activity against gram-positive organisms resistant to erythromycin A (MICs > 2.5 to 40 mg/l). In contrast, the anhydrolide **23** retained activity against erythromycin A-susceptible and MLS_B-inducible, erythromycin A-resistant *S. aureus* strains. However, it was poorly active against erythromycin A-resistant *S. pneumoniae*. The 2-chloro **24** and 2-methyl analogues **25** were both less active than the parent compound; particularly, they were almost ineffective against MLS_B-inducible erythromycin A-resistant *S. aureus* and less active against erythromycin A-resistant *S. pneumoniae*.

The replacement of a C2-hydrogen atom for a fluorine gave a C-2 fluoro analogue of telithromycin (HMR 3562) that demonstrated good antibacterial activities against gram-positive cocci isolates susceptible to erythromycin A and against MLS_B inducibly resistant *S. aureus* and *S. pneumoniae*, as well as against MLS_B constitutively resistant *S. pneumoniae*. Furthermore this 2-fluoro-ketolide **26** exhibited comparable *in vitro* activity to azithromycin and telithromycin against *H. influenzae* (Tab. 4). *In vivo*, **26** showed an excellent anti-pneumococcal efficacy in infections induced by erythromycin A-resistant *S. pneumoniae* and also was shown to exhibit a two-fold improvement in efficacy over azithromycin against *H. influenzae* (Tab. 5).

From these observations it can be concluded that within the ketolide class

- position 2 needs to remain tetrahedral, and tolerates only very small substituents such as fluorine (F > Cl > > Me),
- the 3-keto analogues are more active than the 3-hydroxy or the 3-L-cladinosyl analogues (C=O> OH> Cladinose) against erythromycin A-resistant gram-positive cocci, and
- position 6 needs at least an alkoxy substituent.

Telithromycin, a novel ketolide

Telithromycin is C11–12 carbamate ketolide that is characterised by the butyl imidazolyl pyridyl side chain substituting the carbamate residue (Fig. 11).

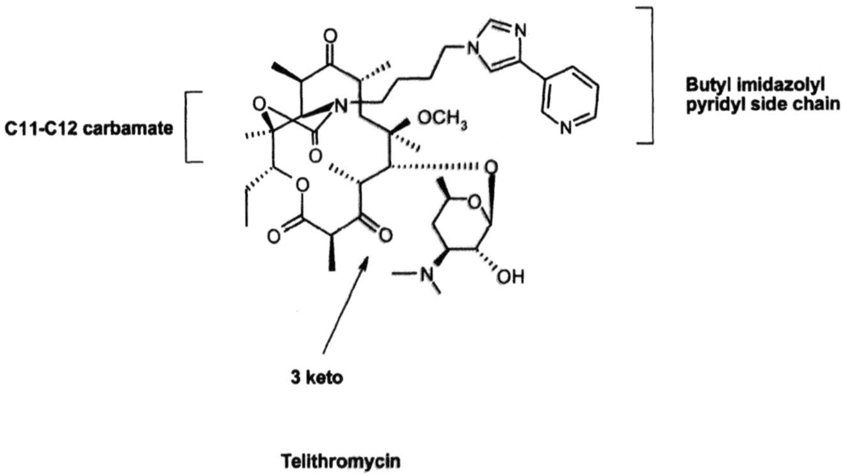

Figure 11. Telithromycin structure.

Physico-chemical properties

The physico-chemical properties of telithromycin are listed in Table 6.

Table 6. Physicochemical properties of ketolide

	Empirical formula	Molecule weight (Daltons)	pK	Log P	Melting point (°C)
Telithromycin	$C_{43} H_{64} N_5 O_{10}$	812.0	5.1; 3.0; 8.7	3.1	177

Acid stability

Ketolides are more stable in acidic conditions than clarithromycin, roxithromycin, and azithromycin. It was shown that the latter compounds were degraded in acidic conditions by transformation into a descladinosyl derivative, with 3-OH group on the lactone ring [32–34].

The ketolides, which are 3-keto derivatives, are highly acid stable. They retain *in vitro* activity at very low pH (pH 1.2) for more than 6 h. In contrast, at pH 1.2, clarithromycin and azithromycin are devoid of any *in vitro* activity after 1 h of contact (Fig. 12). This stability results from a combination of 6-O-methyl and

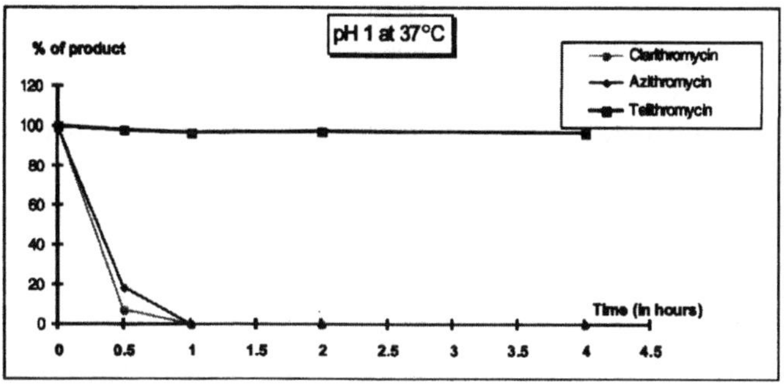

Figure 12. Acid stability of telithromycin
a:% of remaining product after stirring the tittle compounds at pH=1 (0.2 M KCl/0.2M HCl) at 37°C for 4 h. Based upon HPLC titration with a Purecil C_{18} column-5μ; elution: MeOH/Na_2HPO_4 0.02M 75/25; detection UV 220 nm.

11,12 carbamate, or hydrazono-carbamate, which both suppress the formation of the classical 6,9 ketal or 12, 9, 6 spiroketal [32] and the 3-keto which replaces the instable cladinose.

Antibacterial activity

Telithromycin is two to four times more active than clarithromycin against gram-positive cocci susceptible to erythromycin A and retains activity against gram-positive cocci isolates having an underlying mechanism of resistance to erythromycin A [22].

Streptococcus pneumoniae [35–41]

Telithromycin is one of the most active antibacterial agents against *S. pneumoniae*, irrespective of susceptibility or resistance to other antibacterial agents.

Telithromycin was tested against more than 5000 *S. pneumoniae* isolates collected worldwide, using clarithromycin as the comparator. Against fully susceptible *S. pneumoniae* isolates, MIC_{50} values for telithromycin ranged from 0.004 to 0.06 mg/l and MIC_{90} values were 0.004 to 0.125 mg/l.

Against isolates showing intermediate susceptibility to penicillin G (MIC 0.12 to 1.0 mg/l), telithromycin MIC_{50} values were 0.015 to 0.03 mg/l, and MIC_{90} values were 0.03 to 0.25 mg/l. Telithromycin was up to 10 times more active than clarithromycin.

Telithromycin MIC_{50} values for *S. pneumoniae* isolates resistant to penicillin G (MIC > 1 mg/l) were 0.015 to 0.125 mg/l, and MIC_{90}values were 0.015 to 2.0 mg/l. In contrast, clarithromycin and azithromycin activities delineate two populations of *S. pneumoniae* isolates, one population remaining sensitive and the second being totally resistant. This finding is mainly attributable to a combination of penicillin G- and erythromycin-A resistance.

Telithromycin was also active (MIC_{50} 0.015 to 0.06 mg/l, MIC_{90} 0.015 to 2 mg/l) against erythromycin A-resistant strains harboring an MLS_B mechanism of resistance (*erm B*). Against isolates resistant to erythromycin A, clarithromycin and azithromycin are inactive whether the mechanism of resistance is MLS_B, efflux, or a mutation in ribosomal proteins L4 or L22.

Telithromycin antibacterial activity was investigated against 114 *S. pneumoniae* isolates of M-phenotype (erythromycin-A-resistant and clindamycin susceptible). MIC_{50} values for telithromycin ranged from 0.015 to 0.25 mg/l, and MIC_{90} values from 0.12 to 0.5 mg/l. Clarithromycin exhibited lower *in vitro* activity than telithromycin, with MIC_{50} values ranging from 0.5 to 8.0 mg/l and MIC_{90} values from 4.0 to 16 mg/l.

It was demonstrated that telithromycin is more active against *S. pneumoniae* isolates (including resistant strains) than 14-, 15-, and 16-membered ring macrolides, fluoroquinolones, and other antibacterial agents tested.

In a comparative study, 400 *S. pneumoniae* isolates were tested for their susceptibility to 15 antibacterial agents, including telithromycin. Results for selected agents are summarized in Table 7.

Telithromycin was more active than the fluoroquinolones tested, 16 times more active than quinupristin/dalfopristin, and 60 times more active than linezolid.

Telithromycin was active against ofloxacin-resistant *S. pneumoniae* ($MIC_{50/90}$ 0.03 mg/l) and other fluoroquinolones. All the strains tested were susceptible to telithromycin, irrespective of the underlying mechanism of resistance to fluoroquinolone. This included multiple drug-resistant strains and strains containing *par C* and *par E* mutations in topoisomerase IV.

A total of 39 isolates of *S. pneumoniae* harboring different genes conferring erythromycin-A resistance and 20 erythromycin A-susceptible isolates were tested for their susceptibility to telithromycin and 6 comparative compounds. Telithromycin was 4 times more active than clarithromycin against erythromycin A-susceptible *S. pneumoniae* isolates and 16 times more active than clarithromycin against *S. pneumoniae* isolates harboring the *mef E*$^+$ gene (efflux). Telithromycin remained active against isolates harboring an *erm B*$^+$ gene, whereas clarithromycin was inactive. Telithromycin was 4 times more active than clarithromycin or ampicillin and 30 times more active than cefdinir against erythromycin-A-susceptible strains. These results are summarized in Table 8.

Table 7. *In vitro* activity of antibacterial agents against *S. pneumoniae* isolates

Antibacterial agent	MIC (mg/l)	
	MIC_{50}	MIC_{90}
Telithromycin	0.015	0.12
Levofloxacin	1.0	1.0
Trovafloxacin	0.06	0.12
Sparfloxacin	0.12	0.25
Quinupristin/dalfopristin	0.25	0.5
Linezolid	1.0	1.0

Table 8. *In vitro* activity of antibacterial agents against *S. pneumoniae* Ery-S and Ery-R (*mef E*+ and *erm B*+)

Antibacterial agent	MIC (mg/l)					
	Ery-S (N = 20)		**Ery-R** *mef E*+ (N = 21)		**Ery-R** *erm B*+ (N = 18)	
	MIC_{50}	**MIC_{90}**	**MIC_{50}**	**MIC_{90}**	**MIC_{50}**	**MIC_{90}**
Telithromycin	0.008	0.008	0.06	0.12	0.03	0.125
Erythromycin A	0.03	0.06	2.0	2.0	32.0	> 128.0
Clarithromycin	0.016	0.03	1.0	2.0	16.0	> 128.0
Azithromycin	0.12	0.125	2.0	4.0	64.0	> 128.0
Ampicillin	0.03	0.25	1.0	2.0	0.03	2.0
Cefdinir	0.125	4.0	4.0	8.0	0.25	16.0
Levofloxacin	1.0	2.0	1.0	1.0	1.0	2.0

Note: N = number of isolates. Ery-R = erythromycin A-resistant, Ery-S = erythromycin A-susceptible.

Against 15 tetracycline-resistant *S. pneumoniae* strains, the $MIC_{50/90}$ value for telithromycin was 0.015 mg/l. In this same study, the MIC_{50} was 0.003 mg/l, and the MIC_{90} was 0.007 mg/l against 20 cotrimoxazole-resistant strains.

Telithromycin is bactericidal against *S. pneumoniae* (including strains resistant to penicillin G, erythromycin A, and cefotaxime) (Fig. 13).

In disseminated murine infections, telithromycin displayed oral *in vivo* activity against pneumococcal infections due to erythromycin A-resistant isolates. In contrast, clarithromycin and azithromycin were inactive (Protective Dose 50 [PD_{50}] > 50 mg/kg). Telithromycin was also more active than clarithromycin against *S. pneumoniae* strains susceptible to erythromycin A.

Telithromycin exhibits a good efficacy in murine models of pneumococcal pneumonia. Efficacy remained in murine pneumonia induced with *S. pneumoniae* strains resistant to erythromycin A and/or penicillin G. In these models, the *in vivo* efficacy of telithromycin was greater than that of clarithromycin, azithromycin, or cefdinir.

The intracellular anti-pneumococcal activity of telithromycin was evaluated after polymorphonuclear neutrophil (PMN) phagocytosis of *S. pneumoniae*. Telithromycin was very active intracellularly against *S. pneumoniae*, irrespective of susceptibility to penicillin G or erythromycin A. Telithromycin at four times MIC reduced intracellular growth by 1.8 to 3.0 $\log_{10}$ cfu at 24 hours, irrespective of the strain.

It has been shown that *S. pneumoniae* can enter and survive within human lung alveolar carcinoma cells (Type 2 pneumocytes, A I49 cells). *S. pneumoniae* isolates may persist in tissue, despite exposure to adequate antibacterial concentrations [42]. Telithromycin killing activity was compared with that of azithromycin and three fluoroquinolones in human lung alveolar carcinoma cells against *S. pneumoniae* 14.8 and *S. pneumoniae* ATCC 49619 (MIC 0.002 mg/l). It was found that moxifloxacin, trovafloxacin, and telithromycin were most active, but only telithromycin killed all

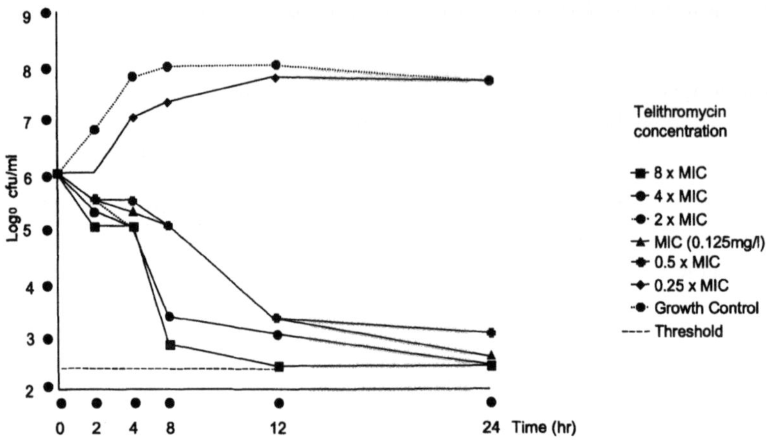

Figure 13. Telithromycin: Bactericidal activity against *S. pneumoniae* resistant to erythromycin A (*erm* B).

intracellular pneumococci. This finding appears to be related, at least in part, to a high intracellular concentration of telithromycin in addition to its potent bactericidal activity against *S. pneumoniae* [43].

Haemophilus influenzae [35, 37, 38, 44, 45]

H. influenzae is involved in respiratory tract infections such as community-acquired pneumonia, acute bacterial exacerbations of chronic bronchitis, and acute bacterial maxillary sinusitis. In recent years, there has been an increase in the incidence of ampicillin-resistant *H. influenzae* isolates due to beta-lactamase production. Non-enzymatic resistance to beta-lactams is a second mechanism of resistance, with a lower incidence than beta-lactamase production.

MIC values against *H. influenzae* are strongly influenced by the experimental medium. NCCLS for antibacterial susceptibility testing recommends use of the microbroth dilution technique in the Haemophilus Test Medium (HTM). The HTM tends to give higher MIC values than those obtained in other parts of the world with other methods. MIC values also can vary with incubation atmosphere, with higher MIC values occurring in 6% CO_2.

The *in vitro* activity of telithromycin was tested against approximately 2300 isolates collected worldwide, irrespective of the resistance profile to ampicillin. MIC_{50} values for telithromycin ranged from 0.25 to 2.0 mg/l and MIC_{90} values from 0.5 to 4.0 mg/l. Telithromycin was shown to be slowly bactericidal against *H. influenzae*.

Studies in mouse models of experimental murine pneumonia due to *H. influenzae* showed that telithromycin 50 mg/kg had a faster onset of activity against *H. influenzae* than azithromycin 100 mg/kg. Lung bacterial clearance was comparable for the two compounds at 24 h.

Moraxella catarrhalis [44]

More than 90% of *M. catarrhalis* clinical isolates produce beta-lactamases.

Telithromycin was tested against approximately 1100 isolates of *M. catarrhalis*, against which it displayed *in vitro* activity comparable with clarithromycin. The MIC_{50} values for telithromycin ranged from 0.02 to 0.25 mg/l, and MIC_{90} values from 0.03 to 0.5 mg/l. The MIC_{50} values for clarithromycin ranged from 0.03 to 0.25 mg/l, and MIC_{90} values from 0.06 to 0.25 mg/l. Telithromycin, like 14- and 15-membered ring macrolides, is slowly bactericidal against *M. catarrhalis*.

Bordetella *species*

Bordetella pertussis and *B. parapertussis* are the etiologic agents of whooping cough, and 14- and 15-membered ring macrolides are reference antibacterial agents for this infection. The *in vitro* activity of telithromycin was investigated against 133 isolates of *B. pertussis*. Results showed that MIC_{50} values for telithromycin were 0.01 to 0.03 mg/l, and MIC_{90} values were 0.01 to 0.06 mg/l. The MIC_{50} values for clarithromycin were 0.01 to 0.06 mg/l, and MIC_{90} values were 0.03 to 0.06 mg/l.

The MIC_{50} and MIC_{90} values for telithromycin against 31 *B. parapertussis* isolates were 0.12 mg/l, and 0.25 mg/l respectively [46].

Streptococcus pyogenes *and other streptococci [35, 38, 47]*

S. pyogenes (Lancefield Group A streptococci) and Lancefield Group C and G streptococci are responsible for tonsillitis.

Telithromycin displayed good *in vitro* activity against β-hemolytic Lancefield Group A, B, C, G, and F streptococci isolates. For telithromycin, MIC_{50} values were $\leq$ 0.008 to 0.03 mg/l and MIC_{90} values were 0.015 to 0.06 mg/l against erythromycin A-susceptible strains. Telithromycin showed comparable *in vitro* activity to clarithromycin.

When an efflux mechanism of resistance to erythromycin A was involved, $MIC_{50/90}$ values for telithromycin could rise to 2.0 mg/l. Against isolates in which an *erm B* gene was the underlying mechanism of resistance to erythromycin A, MIC values for telithromycin could reach > 16 mg/l. For *erm TR*-containing *S.pyogenes*, MIC values ranged from 0.03 to 0.25 mg/l.

Telithromycin showed bactericidal activity at four times MIC and at 6 h against *S.pyogenes* erythromycin A-susceptible isolates and against erythromycin A-resistant (M-phenotype) isolates. Telithromycin was highly active against other β-hemolytic streptococci (Group C, G, and F) ($MIC_{50/90} \leq$ 0.015 to 0.06 mg/l). For Lancefield Group B streptococci, MIC_{50} values for telithromycin were 0.008 to 0.06 mg/l and the MIC_{90} values were 0.015 to 0.12 mg/l.

Intracellular concentration of telithromycin in polymorphonuclear neutrophils (PMN) (Fig. 14)

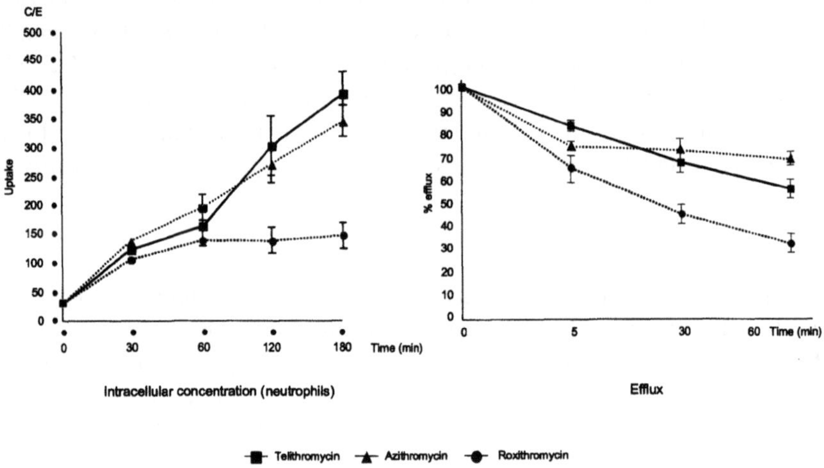

Figure 14. Intracellular accumulation in neutrophils of telithromycin.

Telithromycin, like macrolides, fluoroquinolones, tetracycline, and clindamycin, concentrates in various types of cells.

The *in vitro* uptake of [^{3}H]-telithromycin was investigated using a velocity gradient centrifugation technique. Telithromycin (extracellular concentration of 2.5 mg/l) was gradually concentrated by PMN with an intracellular/extracellular concentration ratio reaching 27.0 ± 8.1 at 5 min and 348 ± 27.1 at 180 min.

Telithromycin was located mainly in the granule fraction of PMN (56 ± 10.9%). Telithromycin was gradually released from drug-loaded PMN placed in a drug-free medium. In the first 5 min, approximately 20% of telithromycin was effluxed from the cell; after 5 min, the efflux slope was slower, with approximately 60% telithromycin remaining in the cell at 1 h. The uptake of telithromycin was temperature dependent [48, 49].

Activity against atypical or intracellular pathogens involved in lower respiratory tract infections

Three intracellular or atypical pathogens commonly are associated with infections known as atypical parenchymal lower respiratory tract infections: *Chlamydia (Chlamydophila) pneumoniae*, *Legionella pneumophila*, and *Mycoplasma pneumoniae*. *Chlamydia psittaci* and *Coxiella burnetii* are also responsible for lung parenchymal infections, but to a lower extent.

Chlamydia pneumoniae [50, 51]

C. pneumoniae is an obligate intracellular pathogen.

Telithromycin exhibits good *in vitro* and bactericidal activity against *C. pneumoniae*, with MIC range from 0.01 to 0.25 mg/l and MCC (minimum Chlamycidal concentration) from 0.03 to 2.0 mg/l).

Legionella pneumophila [52]

- Telithromycin was tested against approximately 140 strains of *L. pneumophila*. The resulting $MIC_{50/90}$values were 0.03 to 0.12 mg/l in buffered yeast extract agar (BYE). However, in buffered charcoal yeast extract (BCYE α), $MIC_{50/90}$ values increased to 2 mg/l. The presence of charcoal in BCYE α is known to impair the *in vitro* activity of several antibacterial agents.
- The post-antibiotic effect (PAE) of telithromycin on *L. pneumophila* was 4.6 h, recorded at two times MIC, compared with a PAE of 1.0 h with erythromycin A.
- Using broth-dilution techniques, bactericidal synergy of telithromycin was shown in combination with rifampin.
- Telithromycin was active against intracellular *L. pneumophila* F2111 and F889 (guinea pig alveolar macrophages).
- The bactericidal activity of telithromycin was assessed against *L. pneumophila* serogroup 1 (strain CB 81–13) within monocyte-derived macrophages.

For a low extracellular concentration (0.05 mg/l) of telithromycin, an inhibition of intracellular multiplication of *L. pneumophila* has been demonstrated.

Telithromycin *in vivo* was more effective than erythromycin A against *L. pneumophila* investigated in Dunkin-Hartley strain male guinea pig models of infections, being able to sterilize the infected guinea pig lungs.

Mycoplasma pneumoniae [53]

Telithromycin was very active against *M. pneumoniae*. Against 90 isolates, $MIC_{50/90}$ values ranged from 0.001 to 0.005 mg/l.

Other intracellular organisms

Telithromycin displays *in vitro* activity against *Chlamydia psittaci* 4521UC1 strain (MIC and MCC values: 0.006 mg/l) and against *C. psittaci* 1058 strain (MIC 0.25 mg/l and MCC 0.5 mg/l).

The bacteriostatic activity of telithromycin was determined against three strains of *C. burnetii:* the Nine Mile strain (reference strain in acute infections), the Q-212 strain, and the Priscilla strain (reference strains in chronic infections). Assays were conducted using human fibroblasts (HEL) [54].

Telithromycin exhibited *in vitro* activity against *C. burnetii* (MIC of 1.0 mg/l), while erythromycin A was inactive (MIC > 8 mg/l).

Telithromycin exhibits a good antibacterial activity against *Rickettsia* spp [54], *Franciscella tularensis*, [55] *Bartonella* spp [54], *Borrelia* spp, and *Leptospira* spp.

Staphylococcus *spp [35, 37, 56]*

Telithromycin demonstrated activity against more than 2000 *S. aureus* isolates with different patterns of resistance to methicillin and erythromycin A. The MIC_{50} values ranged from 0.06 to 0.12 mg/l, and MIC_{90} values ranged from 0.12 to 0.25 mg/l, irrespective of susceptibility to oxacillin (methicillin). For an *S. aureus* isolate harboring an inducible MLS_B mechanism of resistance, MIC_{50} and MIC_{90} values remained in the range 0.06 to 0.25 mg/l. However, when an isolate of *S. aureus* harbored a constitutive MLS_B mechanism of resistance, MIC_{50} values were above 16 mg/l.

Irrespective of the species of coagulase-negative staphylococci, telithromycin $MIC_{50/90}$ values were 0.03 to 0.25 mg/l with isolates susceptible to erythromycin A. When a constitutive MLS_B mechanism of resistance was present, the telithromycin $MIC_{50/90}$ value was above 16 mg/l. In contrast, when an inducible MLS_B mechanism of resistance was present, $MIC_{50/90}$ values were of the same magnitude as those observed for erythromycin A-susceptible strains.

Enterococcus *species [35]*

Telithromycin exhibits *in vitro* activity against enterococci in the absence of underlying mechanisms of resistance (vancomycin, gentamicin, ampicillin). Telithromycin was active against *E. faecalis* (MIC_{50} 0.12 to 1.0 mg/l and MIC_{90} 2.0 to 8.0 mg/l) and *Enterococcus* species ($MIC_{50/90} \leq 0.03$ to 0.06/0.06 to 8.0 mg/l), with a bimodal population distribution. Telithromycin also exhibited bimodal *in vitro* activity against *E. faecium* ($MIC_{50/90} \leq 0.03/4.0$ mg/l).

Anaerobes [57–60]

Telithromycin has been tested against numerous genera and species of anaerobic bacteria.

Telithromycin was active against the following gram-positive cocci and bacilli: *Propionibacterium* (MIC_{50} was 0.015 mg/l), *Peptostreptococcus* spp (MIC_{50} was 0.004 to 0.12 mg/l), and *Clostridium difficile* (MIC_{50} was 0.06 to 1.0 mg/l).

The activity of telithromycin against gram-negative anaerobes was shown to be more species-dependent than against gram-positive species. Telithromycin was active against *Prevotella* spp ($MIC_{50} < 0.008$ to 0.25 mg/l) and *Porphyromonas* spp (MIC_{50} 0.008 to 0.06 mg/l). Telithromycin MIC_{50}s were 4.0 and 1.0 to > 32 mg/l for *B. fragilis* and *Fusobacterium* spp, respectively.

Other bacterial species

Telithromycin exhibits good *in vitro* activity against other gram-positive bacilli and gram-negative cocci (Tab. 9).

Telithromycin is very active against gram-positive bacteria and gram-negative cocci. Additionally, against *Mycoplasma hominis*, MIC_{50} values for telithromycin

Table 9. Summary of telithromycin *in vitro* activity against various other pathogens

Species/group studied			MIC (mg/l)	
	N	**Range**	**MIC_{50} range**	**MIC_{90} range**
Viridans group streptococci	1141	–	≤ 0.003–0.25	≤ 0.003–0.5
Corynebacterium diphtheriae	442	–	0.004	0.008
Listeria spp.	181	–	0.03–0.12	0.03–0.25
Lactobacillus spp.	124	–	0.007–0.03	0.03–0.12
Pediococcus spp.	40	–	0.007–0.03	≤ 0.03
Leuconostoc spp.	91	–	≤ 0.03	≤ 0.03–0.25
Erysipelothrix rhusopathiae	10	≤ 0.015–0.03	–	–
Micrococcus spp.	191	–	≤ 0.03	≤ 0.03
Stomatococcus spp.	63	–	≤ 0.03	≤ 0.03
Rhodococcus equi	31	≤ 0.015–0.25	–	–
Coryneforms	162	-	≤ 0.01–0.25	≤ 0.01 – > 128
Bacillus spp	14	0.03–0.06	-	-
Neisseria meningitidis	448	–	0.015–0.12	0.03–0.25
Saprophytic *Neisseria* spp.	50	–	0.06–0.12	0.25–4.0

were 2 to 32 mg/l, and MIC_{90} values were 4 to 32 mg/l. The corresponding MIC_{50} and MIC_{90} values for clarithromycin were > 32 to > 64 mg/l. Telithromycin exhibited bimodal activity against *Corynebacterium jeikeium* and *C. urealyticum* and good activity against other coryneforms [61, 62]. Telithromycin exhibited good antibacterial activity against *Neisseria* spp [62] and against *Bacillus anthracis* (MIC_{50}: 0.25 mg/l).

Telithromycin is inactive against *Enterobacteriaceae* and non-fermentative gram-negative bacilli (e. g., *Pseudomonas aeruginosa* [MIC range 32 to > 128 mg/l], *Acinetobacter baumannii* [MIC range 2 to > 128 mg/l]). Telithromycin exhibits moderate *in vitro* activity against *V. cholerae*.

Telithromycin exhibited good *in vitro* activity against *Helicobacter pylori* [63].

Postantibiotic effect (PAE) of telithromycin [64]

A PAE is the suppression of bacterial growth that persists after short exposure to an antibacterial agent.

Several laboratories have investigated the PAE of telithromycin. Although methodology varied between laboratories, all studies clearly demonstrated a PAE for telithromycin. Telithromycin exhibited a PAE against *S. pneumoniae* of 1.5 to 3.8 h a PAE of 0.3 to 2.4 h against *S. aureus*, and a PAE of 0.4 to 2.7 h against *S.pyogenes*.

Mode of action [65–69]

Erythromycin A, clarithromycin, and azithromycin prevent bacterial protein synthesis by binding to specific sites in the bacterial ribosome and interfering with the elongation of nascent polypeptide chains. In addition, these compounds interfere with a second cellular process, the formation of the 50S ribosomal subunit.

Ribosomes are the functional units of translation. Bacterial ribosomes consist of ribonucleoprotein particles having a sediment coefficient of 70 S. The 70 S ribosome is composed of two subunits: 30 S and 50 S particles. The 30 S subunit is made up of 16S ribosomal ribonucleic acid (rRNA) and 21 different proteins. The 50 S subunit consists of 2 rRNA molecules, 23S rRNA and 5S rRNA, and 33 proteins. The main function of the 50 S ribosomal subunit is to promote peptide-bond formation. Six distinct structural domains have been found in the 23S rRNA, and 5S rRNA forms a structural link between domain II and domain V. Further, 5S rRNA may help in the proper juxtaposition of domain II and V in the ribosomal tertiary structure.

Telithromycin binds approximately 6- to 10-fold more tightly than erythromycin A or clarithromycin to wild type *E. coli* ribosome [65, 66]. However, while the presence of an A-2058 G mutation in the 23S rRNA (domain V) reduces binding of erythromycin A and clarithromycin to bacterial ribosomes by over 10,000 fold, the binding of telithromycin is also lowered by this mutation, but to a smaller extent, and remains more than 20-fold higher than erythromycin A [66] (Fig. 15).

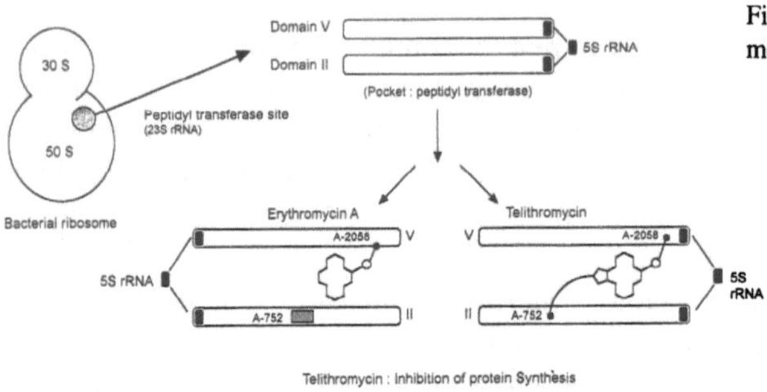

Figure 15a. Telithromycin mode of action.

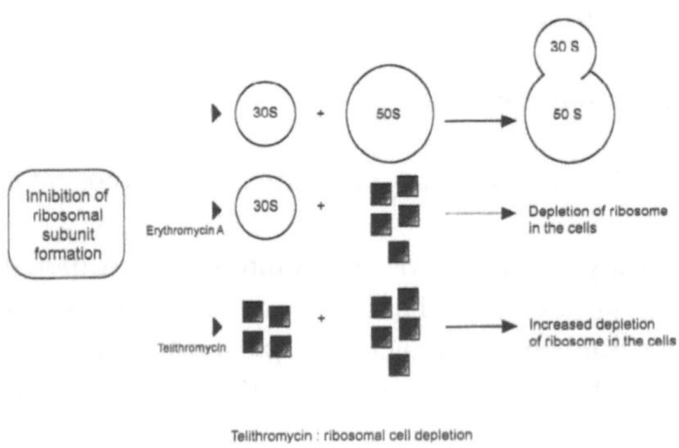

Figure 15b.

The higher affinity of telithromycin for the ribosome depends on the C11–C12 side chain. In contrast to erythromycin A, telithromycin interacts with an additional binding site located near the A752 residue in hairpin 35 of domain II of the ribosomal RNA.

The interaction with domain II may explain telithromycin's enhanced antibacterial activity reflected in lower MIC values and superior activity against bacteria harboring an MLS_B mechanism of resistance.

Telithromycin versus resistance to erythromycin A [70–73]

All 14- and 15-membered ring macrolides derived from erythromycin A share the same mechanism of resistance. The mechanisms of resistance to erythromycin A are complex and can be divided into three main patterns:

- housekeeping,
- defensive, and
- preventive.

"Housekeeping"

Efflux mechanism of resistance
In gram-positive cocci, efflux pumps for erythromycin A have been described for *S. aureus* (*msr A*), coagulase-negative staphylococci (*msr A, msr B*), *S pyogenes* (*mef A*), *S. pneumoniae* (*mef E*), *S. agalactiae* (*mef A* and *E*, *mre A*), and viridans group streptococci (*mef E* and *mef A*). These pump proteins bind to erythromycin A and pump molecules out of the bacterial cells, resulting in reduced intracellular concentrations of erythromycin A.

The mef mechanism of efflux: The *mef* gene has been found in various gram-positive bacteria including, *Streptococcus* spp, *Micrococcus* spp, *Corynebacterium* spp, and *Enterococcus* spp. Strains harboring a *mef* mechanism of resistance are also known as M-phenotype.

In streptococci, two genes encode for efflux pump proteins: *mef* for all streptococci and *mre* A for *S. agalactiae*. The most important *mef* gene with respect to *S. pneumoniae*, and therefore telithromycin, is *mef E*. Telithromycin MIC_{50} values may increase more against *S. pneumoniae* isolates carrying a *mef* E gene than others, but they remain within the likely therapeutic range. Against *S. mitis*/*S. oralis* isolates harboring a *mef* E^+ gene, telithromycin MICs were 0.06 to 1.0 mg/l, and against 18 isolates of *S. agalactiae* with the M-phenotype (*mef* A^+ or *mef* E^+), telithromycin MICs ranged from 0.1 to 0.2 mg/l, in comparison with an MIC of 0.02 mg/l for erythromycin A-susceptible isolates.

The *mef A* gene has been described in a variety of bacterial species, including *S.pyogenes; S. agalactiae*; viridans group streptococci (*S. mitis*, *S. milleri*); Lancefield group C, F, and G streptococci; *Micrococcus* spp; *Listeria* spp;

Corynebacterium jeikeium; and *Enterococcus faecium*. The *mef A* gene appears to be inducible by 14- and 15-membered ring macrolides but not by 16-membered ring macrolides. Further, 16-membered ring macrolides are not good substrates for Mef A protein.

For telithromycin, an analogous effect to the pneumococcal MefE pump was shown for *mef A* in *S.pyogenes*. Strains expressing this gene could exhibit higher telithromycin MICs compared with wild strains; however, the MICs remained within the therapeutic range.

The mre A mechanism of efflux: A putative efflux pump Mre A from a *Streptococcus agalactiae* strain conferred resistance to 14-, 15-, and 16-membered ring macrolides. Telithromycin retained good activity against *S. agalactiae* harboring the *mre A* gene. $MIC_{50/90}$ values for telithromycin were ≤ 0.015 mg/l in comparison with clarithromycin, for which MIC values ranged from 0.5 to 4.0 mg/l.

The msr A mechanism of efflux: Msr A protein is a member of the ABC superfamily of efflux pumps and is specific to 14- and 15-membered ring macrolides and streptogramin B. The gene *msr A* has been sequenced from *S. epidermidis* and *S. aureus*. The 14- and 15-membered ring macrolides and telithromycin (but not 16-membered ring macrolides) act as inducers of *msr* genes. However, the ketolides are poor substrates for Msr pumps.

Bottle brush

Erythromycin A resistance can be conferred by short pentapeptides with specific amino acid sequences. The synthesis of pentapeptides is due to translation of mini-gene sequences within 23S rRNA. This mechanism of resistance is also known as "bottle brush".

In bottle brush resistance, the newly synthesized pentapeptide actively displaces the macrolides or ketolides from the ribosome. After the compound is removed, the ribosome either can initiate synthesis of new polypeptides or can bind another molecule of macrolide or ketolide.

Defensive mechanism of resistance

The second mechanism of resistance for bacterial cells to xenobiotics is to render the ribosomal targets (the peptidyl transferase site) inaccessible. Two main mechanisms have been described: 1) blockade of the binding site of erythromycin A by mono- or dimethylation (*erm* gene system) or 2) transformation of the binding site by *in situ* mutation or indirectly by mutation on certain ribosomal proteins that modify the peptidyltransferase site.

Mono- or dimethylated ribosome: the erm *gene system*

MLS_B resistance is the consequence of induction of the synthesis of 23S rRNA methylase activity. This adds one or two methyl groups to a single adenine residue

(A-2058) on the N^6 amino group of adenine, or to one of the adjacent residues A-2057 or A-2059 in the peptidyltransferase loop of domain V of the 23S rRNA. This prevents access of erythromycin A to its binding site on ribosome.

MLS_B resistance may be constitutively expressed or induced by sub-inhibitory MIC concentrations of 14- and 15-membered ring macrolides. MLS_B resistance is due to *erm* (**e**rythromycin **r**esistance **m**ethylase) genes.

A total of 20 different *erm* genes have been described. *S. pneumoniae* isolates resistant to erythromycin A by an MLS_B mechanism of resistance harbor the *erm B* gene. *S.pyogenes* isolates resistant to erythromycin A harbor *erm B* or *erm TR* genes. The *erm A* and *erm C* genes are found in *S. aureus* and coagulase-negative staphylococci. The *erm C* gene is found mainly in animal staphylococci. Many *erm* genes are often associated with other antibiotic resistant genes, especially tetracycline-resistant genes. The *erm F* gene is often linked with the *tet Q* gene.

Telithromycin retains activity against *S. aureus* resistant isolates when an inducible mechanism of resistance is involved ($MIC_{50/90}$ 0.12 and 0.25 mg/l), but not when MLS_B resistance is constitutively expressed (MIC > 128 mg/l).

Against *S. pneumoniae*, telithromycin retains good *in vitro* and *in vivo* activity, as demonstrated in animal models (lung infections) and clinical trials. There is no correlation between MIC values for telithromycin (from 0.002 to 1.0 mg/l) and the expression of the *erm* gene in bacterial cells. Epidemiological surveys, showed that *S. pneumoniae* isolates for which telithromycin exhibited MIC > 2 mg/l are rare, with an incidence of approximately 0.001%.

For *S.pyogenes*, two *erm* genes are involved: *erm B* and *erm TR*. The *in vitro* activity of telithromycin differs according to the genes that are expressed. For *erm TR*-containing *S.pyogenes*, MIC values for telithromycin ranged from 0.03 to 0.25 mg/l, and for *erm* B-containing strains, MIC values for telithromycin ranged from 0.5 to 64 mg/l.

Mutations

Resistance to erythromycin A can be achieved by mutation affecting 23S rRNA sequences or the amino acid sequences of at least two ribosomal proteins, L4 and L22.

Mutations on 23S rRNA: A-2058→G mutation on 23S rRNA has been described in some bacterial species, rendering them resistant to erythromycin A and its derivatives. These mutations have been described in *Helicobacter pylori*, *Mycoplasma pneumoniae*, *Treponema pallidum*, *Propionibacterium acnes*, and *Mycobacterium avium* complex.

The ribosomal affinity of both erythromycin A and clarithromycin are lowered 10^4-fold by A-2058→G mutation. The binding affinity of telithromycin also is lowered by the A-2058→G mutation, but to a lesser extent. Telithromycin activity remains at least 20- to 60-fold greater than that of erythromycin A and clarithromycin.

Mutations on protein ribosomal L4 and L22: Clinical isolates of *S. pneumoniae* and *S. pyogenes* isolates containing ribosomal mutations in proteins have been reported in Bulgaria, Slovakia, Croatia and Poland. Against 19 *S. pneumoniae* isolates resistant to erythromycin A (MIC > 64 mg/l) but susceptible to clindamycin and streptogramin B, a mutation on protein L4 at $_{69}$GTG $_{71}$→$_{69}$ TPS$_{71}$ was reported. Footprinting experiments in ribosome from the *E. coli* L4 mutants revealed that the conformation of 23S rRNA in domain II (A-789, G-799, and U-1255) and domain V (A-2572) is altered relative to wild-type strain. Telithromycin retained activity against these isolates.

Preventive mechanism of resistance

The degradative enzymes produced by micro-organisms that are known to inactivate macrolide antibiotics are the glycosylases and phosphorylases. However, this mechanism is limited to bacterial species such as *Nocardia* spp. These enzymes fix a glucose moiety or a phosphate on the 2'OH substituent of the D-desosamine moiety, an amino sugar at position 5 of the erythronolide A ring. By this mechanism, erythromycin A, its derivatives, and telithromycin are inactivated to various degrees. The same enzymes also render *Nocardia* spp resistant to telithromycin. Although of interest scientifically, these are of little relevance to the potential clinical use of telithromycin.

The erythronolide A ring may be hydrolyzed by esterases I or II from *E. coli*, but this enzymatic activity is not known for telithromycin.

Mechanism of resistance to telithromycin

Telithromycin is inactive against *S. aureus* isolates harboring an *erm* gene of constitutive type. MIC values for telithromycin are above 32 mg/l. Within *S.pyogenes* isolates resistant to erythromycin A and harboring an *erm B* gene, telithromycin MIC values for some isolates are > 16 mg/l.

Other potential mechanisms of resistance have been reported from mutants obtained in the laboratory: L4 protein and L22 ribosomal mutants, 23S rRNA mutants, and K-peptide.

Two types of L4 mutations have been observed. For a mutation at $_{69}$GTG$_{71}$ leading to $_{69}$TPS$_{71}$, increases in telithromycin MIC values of 8-fold have been recorded in *S. pneumoniae* (MIC 0.03 to 0.1 mg/l *versus* MIC 0.006 mg/l for wild type). In type II mutants ($_{63}$KPW RQK GTG *REK GTC* RAR$_{74}$), increases in telithromycin MIC values up to 500-fold have been recorded (MIC 1.56 to 3.13 mg/l *versus* MIC 0.006 mg/l for the wild type).

A mutation in ribosomal protein L22 produces an increase in telithromycin MIC values of about 10-fold. However, the activity of telithromycin remains within the therapeutic range.

Mutations of the 23S rRNA, which may increase MICs for telithromycin, have been artificially created by mutation selection in the laboratory. Summarized below are the mutations characterized to date. At this time, these remain laboratory curiosities and their likelihood of arising in the clinic is not known.

- A novel mutation at U 2609→C has been described, which confers resistance to telithromycin but increases bacterial cell susceptibility to erythromycin A. This mutation appears to be located within the compound binding site and may directly affect interaction of the telithromycin molecule with the ribosome.
- One mutant selected by clarithromycin, resistant to 14- and 15-membered ring macrolides (MIC > 32 mg/l), and with decreased susceptibility to telithromycin (MIC 4 mg/l) had a single base deletion (A-752) in domain II.
- The C-2611→U mutation confers mild macrolide-ketolide resistance that does not extend to other members of the MLS group. This has been characterized in laboratory studies.
- In laboratory studies, mutations at A-2058/2059 of domain V of 23S rRNA yielded three different mutations: A-2058→T, A-2059→G, and A-2058→G. Telithromycin *in vitro* activity decreased in comparison with wild type.
- Mutation in the hairpin 35 at U 754→A renders bacterial cells resistant to low concentrations of erythromycin A and telithromycin.
- K-peptide, a specific pentapeptide acting as a bottle brush, which cleans the ribosome from the bound antibiotic, confers resistance to the ketolides.

Selection of mutants [74]

The ability of sequential subcultures in subinhibitory concentrations of telithromycin, azithromycin, roxithromycin, clindamycin, and pristinamycin to select for resistance was investigated. The study was performed in five erythromycin A-susceptible and six erythromycin A-resistant *S. pneumoniae*, the latter group including three examples of each containing *mefE* or *ermB* genes.

Overall, 54 mutants were derived with increased MICs to at least one of the antibiotics. Of these only three exhibited telithromycin MICs of > 1 mg/l. This compared to 34 mutants and 28 exhibiting MICs of > 1 mg/l to azithromycin and clarithromycin, respectively.

While exposure to telithromycin did select for pneumococcal mutants with increased MICs, the MICs nevertheless remained within the proposed susceptibility range, and, furthermore, telithromycin selected mutations in the least number of strains, compared with the other MLS agents.

In summary, telithromycin was shown to have good *in vitro* activity against strains containing *mefE* and *ermB* genes and against *in vitro*-selected mutants resistant to 14- and 15-membered ring macrolides, clindamycin, and pristinamycin.

Non-induction of MLS_B resistance [75]

It has been shown that ketolides, which lack L-cladinose at position 3 of the erythronolide A ring, are unable to induce MLS_B resistance. The ability to induce MLS_B resistance was investigated for telithromycin and its L-cladinose counterpart (**20**-RU 69874), and 14- and 15-membered ring macrolides with and without

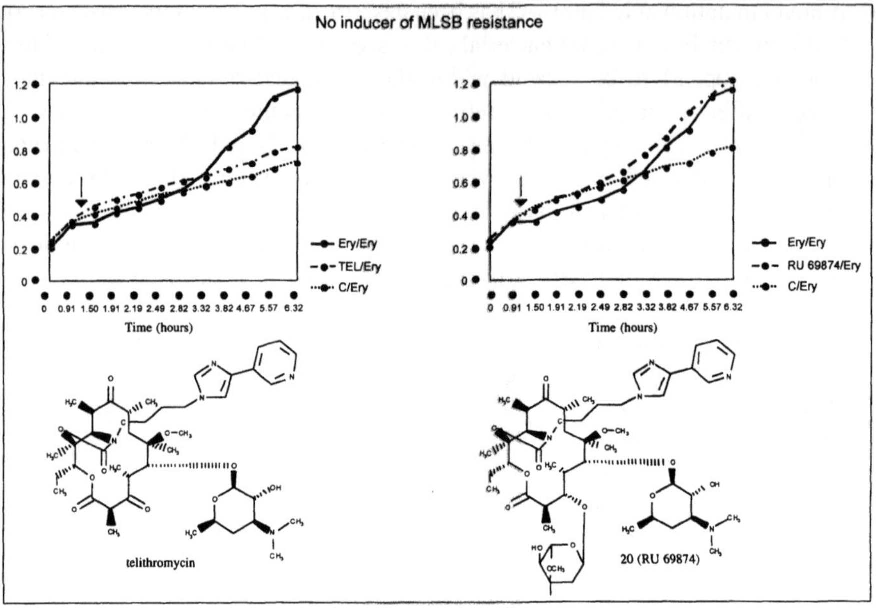

Figure 16. Non-inducing properties of ketolides.

L-cladinose. Erythromycin A, azithromycin, clarithromycin, and RU 69874 (all bearing a 3–α-L-cladinose moiety) were strong inducers of MLS_B resistance in erythromycin A-inducible resistance strains. In contrast, telithromycin (with no L-cladinose moiety) was unable to induce resistance to erythromycin A. The presence of a keto function instead of a sugar in position 3 clearly suppresses the possibility to induce an MLS_B resistance and can account for the antibacterial activity of this new class against the activity against the inducibly erythromycin A-resistant pathogens. (Fig. 16)

Pharmacodynamics

Effect on normal microflora

The effect of telithromycin on oral and faecal flora were investigated in healthy volunteers after 800 mg once a day for 10 days.

The mean peak concentration of telithromycin was 3.05 mg/l and 514 mg/kg in saliva and faeces, respectively.

Telithromycin is responsible for a selective reduction in oral (saliva) and faecal microflora (mainly *E. coli* and *E. faecium*). None of the volunteers was carrying *Clostridium difficile* [76].

Animal model

Using the mouse thigh model in neutropenic and non-neutropenic mice challenged with *S. pneumoniae* and *S. aureus* with different pattern of resistance to erythromycin A and/or penicillin G, it was demonstrated that telithromycin efficacy is concentration-dependent and allowed a once-daily regimen [77].

Pharmacokinetics [22, 78]

In open single or multiple dose studies, telithromycin was given orally to 12 healthy volunteers at the dose of 800 mg once-daily. Telithromycin was assayed in plasma by using a validated HPLC method with detection by fluorimetry. Limit of quantification was 0.005 mg/l in plasma and 0.5 mg/l in urine.

The results are summarised in Table 10.

Table 10. Pharmacokinetics of telithromycin after single and multiple oral dose of 800 mg

	Day 1	Day 11
	(n*=18)	(n*=18)
Cmax (mg/l)	1.90 ± 0.8	2.27 ± 0.71
Tmax (h)	1.0 (1–2)	2.0 (0.5–3.0)
$C_{24\,h}$ (mg/l)	0.029 ± 0.013	0.07 ± 0.05
$AUC_{0-24\,h}$ (mg.h/l)	8 ± 2.6	12.5 ± 5.4
T½ γ (h)	7.16 ± 1.3	12.5 ± 5.4
Urinary elimination% (0–72 h)	12.66 ± 4.2	17.7 ± 4.7
Cl_{REN} (l/h)	12.32 ± 2.1	12.5 ± 4.3

*n: number of volunteers

Following multiple administration of 800 mg once a day, steady state was reached after two days of dosing. The overall accumulation ratio after multiple dosing is about 1.42.

The rate and extent of absorption of telithromycin is unaffected by food intake.

In vitro binding to human serum albumin is 45% to 49% at concentrations up to 2.44 mg/l. The percentage binding to α_1-acid glycoprotein is about 30% for a concentration of 0.07 mg/l. The total percentage binding to plasma protein is about 70% at concentration up to 1.02 mg/l.

The absolute bioavailability after 800 mg telithromycin was 57%.

Telithromycin distribution in lung tissue has been assessed after a single oral dose of 800 mg of telithromycin. Results are summarised in Table 11.

In elderly volunteers after single or repeated oral doses of 800 mg telithromycin once a day, the accumulation ratio is about 1.17 in: comparison with 1.45 in young volunteers. Steady-state was reached after two days of dosing. At steady-state

Table 11. Lung distribution of telithromycin

Time of sampling	N	Plasma (mg/l)	Bronchial Mucosa (mg/kg)	ELF* (mg/l)	Alveolar macrophages (mg/l)
1–3	5	1.07	0.68	5.4	65.0
6–8	6	0.61	2.2	4.2	100.0
24	6	0.07	3.5	1.17	41.0
48	6	LOQ	LOQ	0.30	2.15

Cmax and AUC were two times higher in elderly subjects. Renal clearance decreased with age. However, it was recommended not to change the daily dose and the rhythm of administration of telithromycin in elderly patients. (Tab. 12).

Twelve patients with hepatic impairment with a Child Pugh score ≥ 6 and ≤ 13 (A, B, and C) were enrolled in a pharmacokinetics study in comparison with 20 healthy volunteers. After a single oral dose of 800 mg telithromycin, the pharmacokinetic behaviour of telithromycin was moderately altered in patients with impaired liver function (Tab. 13). The decrease of telithromycin metabolic clearance is partially compensated by a 50% increase in renal clearance.

Table 12. Telithromycin pharmacokinetics in elderly subjects

	Elderly		Young	
	Day 1	Day 10	Day 1	Day 10
Cmax (mg/l)	3.0	3.6	1.99	1.84
Tmax (h)	0.5	0.75	1.0	2.0
$C_{24\,h}$ (mg/l)	0.057	0.142	0.025	0.046
$AUC_{0-24\,h}$ (mg·h/l)	11.56	17.2	7.25	8.49
$t_{1/2}$ (h)	11.46	14.23	10.64	13.4
Urinary elimination% (0–72 h)	10.9	18	12.0	14.5
Cl_{REN} (l/h)	7.35	7.83	13.07	12.98

Telithromycin pharmacokinetics was investigated after a single oral dose of 800 mg telithromycin in 40 patients with varying degrees of renal impairment (Tab. 14). Peak plasma concentrations and AUC increased by 1.4- to 1.5-fold respectively in renal impaired patients in comparison with healthy volunteers. The apparent elimination half-life increased slightly in renal impaired patients in comparison with healthy volunteers.

Telithromycin metabolism is mediated by CYP3A4 and CYP2D6. Four metabolites have been described. Three of them retained antibacterial activity, and one is considered inactive.

Table 13. Telithromycin pharmacokinetics in hepatic impaired patients

	Hepatic impaired patients	**Healthy volunteers**
N	12	20
Cmax (mg/l)	1.99	2.32
Tmax (h)	0.75	1.0
$C_{24\,h}$ (mg/l)	0.087	0.039
$AUC_{0-\infty\,(mg\cdot h/l)}$	11.1	10.1
Urinary elimination% (0–72 h)	22.4	13.1
Cl_{REN} (l/h)	17.3	10.78

Table 14. Telithromycin pharmacokinetics in renal impaired patients after a single oral dose of 800 mg

	Creatinine clearance (ml/min)			
	> 80	80–41	40–11	≤ 10
N	10	10	10	10
Cmax (mg/l)	2.25	3.0	3.25	2.13
Tmax (h)	1.15	1.30	1.10	1.35
$C_{24\,h}$ (mg/l)	0.029	0.055	0.066	0.05
$AUC_{0-\infty\,(mg\cdot h/l)}$	10.09	14.31	16.0	10.79
t½ β (h)	10.66	11.41	12.58	14.64
Cl_{REN} (l/h)	9.34	5.71	2.63	0.36*
Urinary elimination%	10.96	9.57	5.51	0.46*

N: number of patients * 2 patients

Clinical efficacy [79]

Four different clinical studies have been conducted to assess the clinical efficacy and safety of telithromycin at the oral doses of 800 mg once a day.

In all studies performed, the clinical cure rate is above 87%. A good efficacy of telithromycin was recorded in pneumococcal bacteriemic patients, irrespective of the susceptibility of *S. pneumoniae* to penicillin G and erythromycin A.

HMR 3004 [9, 36, 64, 80]

HMR 3004 is a ketolide derivative that bears a cyclic hydrazano carbamate at the C11–12 positions of the erythronolide A ring on which a quinoline moiety is linked by a propyl side chain (Fig. 17).

HMR 3004 was more active than clarithromycin against erythromycin A-susceptible isolates (MIC_{50}: 0.01 mg/l) and retained activity against inducible (MLS_B) resistant *S. aureus* (MIC_{50}: 0.04 mg/l), but it is inactive against constitutively MLS_B erythromycin A-resistant strains. Against enterococci, HMR 3004 is highly active irrespective to their susceptibility to vancomycin (MIC_{50}: 0.01 to 0.06 mg/l). HMR 3004 exhibited good activity against β-haemolytic streptococci, including *S. pyogenes* (MIC_{50}: 0.06 mg/l) isolates resistant to erythromycin A.

HMR 3004 also shows high activity against the viridans group of streptococci (MIC_{50} ~ 0.001 mg/l). Against *Streptococcus pneumoniae* isolates susceptible (MIC_{50}: 0.016 mg/l) or resistant to erythromycin A (MIC_{50}: 0.06 mg/l), HMR 3004 displays good activity. It exerts strong and identical *in vitro* activity against S. *pneumoniae* isolates susceptible or intermediately susceptible to penicillin G (MIC_{50}: 0.016 mg/l), but slightly lower activity has been noted against penicillin G-resistant strains (MIC_{50}: 0.06 mg/l); clarithromycin can be considered inactive (MIC_{50}: 2 mg/l) [12, 13]. The available macrolides are poorly active or inactive against anaerobes as a whole [14]. Compared to metronidazole, HMR 3004 shows enhanced activity against *Bacteroides fragilis* (MIC_{50} ~ 0.5 mg/l). It is four times more active than metronidazole against *B. thetaiotamicron* (MIC_{50}: 0.15 mg/l). It is respectively two and eight times more active than clarithromycin and azithromycin against *Fusobacteria* spp. (MIC_{50}: 0.06 mg/l).

HMR 3004 is highly active against *Clostridium spp.* and *Peptostreptococcus* spp. It is more active than clarithromycin against *H. influenzae* (MIC_{50} ~ 1 mg/l) and shows activity identical to that of Clarithromycin against *Moraxella catarrhalis* (MIC_{50}: 0.12 mg/l). Unusual among the macrolides is the strong activity against *Neisseria meningitidis* (MIC_{50}: 0.007 mg/l). Preliminary results show that HMR 3004 is effective against *Chlamydia* spp and *Legionella* spp. One interesting characteristic is the good *in vitro* activity of HMR 3004 against *Mycoplasma hominis* (MIC ~ 0.2 mg/l) and *M. fermentans* (MIC: 0.2 mg/l), which are usually resistant to 14-membered-ring macrolides. It is effective against *M. pneumoniae* (MIC: 0.01 mg/l) and respectively 5 × and 100 × more active against *Ureaplasma urealyticum,* whatever the resistance to tetracycline (MIC: 0.01 mg/l).

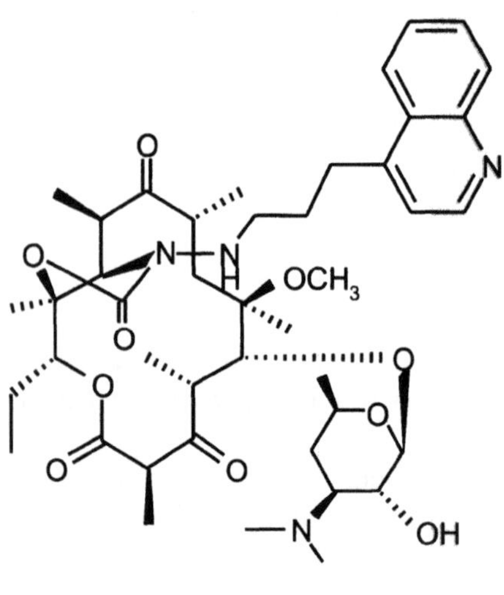

Figure 17. HMR 3004 structure.

The *in vivo* antibacterial activity of HMR 3004 was explored comparatively to that of erythromycin, clarithromycin, azithromycin, and pristinamycin. In murine septicemia due to erythromycin-susceptible *S. aureus*, HMR 3004 shows comparable activity to clarithromycin ($PD_{50:}$ 20 mg/kg – MIC value 0.01 mg/l), but it shows good *in vivo* activity against erythromycin-resistant *S. aureus* by an inducible mechanism (PD_{50}: 13 mg/kg), whereas clarithromycin was totally inactive (PD_{50} < 100 mg/kg). It is also more active (PD_{50}: 17 mg/kg) than clarithromycin (PD_{50}: 30 mg/kg) against *S. aureus* resistant to erythromycin by an inducible mechanism and oxacillin.

Against *S. pneumoniae*, whatever the susceptibility of the isolate to erythromycin, HMR 3004 shows good activity. PD_{50}s range between 15.8 mg/kg (erythromycin-susceptible strain) and 42 mg/kg (erythromycin-resistant, isolate-constitutive mechanism). Against erythromycin-resistant isolates, whatever the mechanism of resistance, other tested macrolides were inactive (PD_{50} < 50 mg/kg). HMR 3004 displays good *in vivo* activity against *S. pyogenes* (PD_{50}: 16 mg/kg) and *S. agalactiae* (PD_{50}: 36 mg/kg). It is more active than pristinamycin against enterococci, with PD_{50} between 11 mg/kg *(E. faecium* erythromycin-R and Van-R) and 22 mg/kg *(E. faecium* erythromycin-R).

In experimental murine septicemia induced by *H. influenzae,* HMR 3004 shows an *in vivo* activity close to that of azithromycin. PD_{50}s ranged between 142 mg/kg (ampicillin-S) and 410 mg/kg (ampicillin-R, β-lactamase neg).

Experimental pneumonia was induced in Swiss mice by intratracheal inoculation of virulent *S. pneumoniae* isolates that were either susceptible to erythromycin A *(S. pneumoniae* 4241) or constitutively erythromycin-resistant (*S. pneumoniae* 6254). The drug administration started at 6 h and 18 h after challenge. Two regimens have been given intraperitoneally: 50 and 100 mg/kg. MIC values for HMR 3004 were 0.01 and 0.5 mg/l for erythromycin A-susceptible and erythromycin-resistant isolates, respectively. When administered every 6 h or 24 h, survival rates were 92% and 54%, respectively. Comparatively, there was no survival with erythromycin. C5 + BV6 mice were intratracheally infected with *H. influenzae* type b (10^8 CFU). Bacterial lung clearance was assayed after a single oral dose of 100 mg/kg of HMR 3004 or 50 mg/kg of azithromycin, administered 16 h after challenge. Both compounds exhibit identical activities with a -2.5 log CFU reduction in burden compared to control. Initial clearance (at 6 h) was more efficient with HMR 3004 than with azithromycin [24].

HMR 3004 is highly accumulated in polymorphonuclear neutrophils, with a ratio of extracellular/intracellular above 400. HMR 3004 uptake occurred rapidly, and in approximately 5 minutes, intracellular concentration reaches a plateau. HMR 3004 is different from telithromycin and similar to that of HMR 3562 and HMR 3787, which rapidly concentrate but to a lower level than HMR 3004 (Fig. 18) [80, 81].

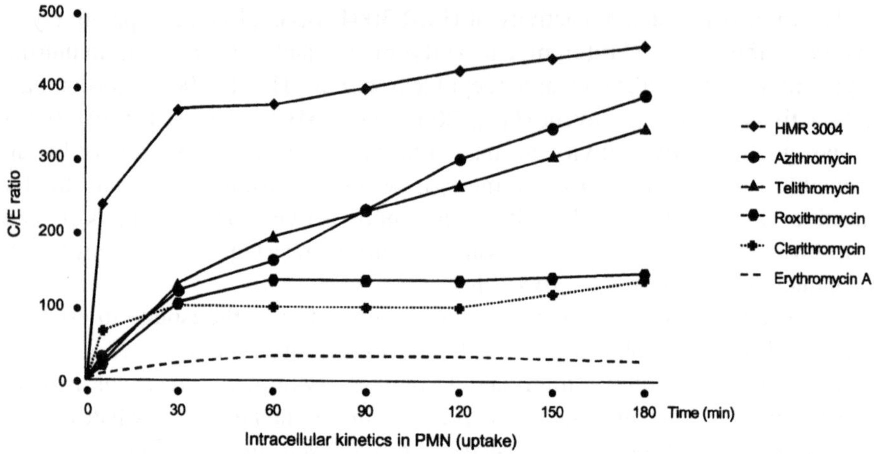

Figure 18. Intracellular kinetics in PMN (uptake) of HMR 3004.

HMR 3832 [82] (Fig. 19)

HMR 3832 is a C11–C12 carbamate that differs from telithromycin by having an amino phenyl moiety instead of a pyridinyl moiety on the C11–C12 side chain.

In vitro activity of HMR 3832 was investigated. HMR 3832 exhibited comparable activity to clarithromycin against erythromycin A-susceptible, gram-positive cocci but retained activity against gram-positive cocci isolates harboring a mechanism of resistance to erythromycin A. HMR 3832 exhibited better *in vitro* activity than clarithromycin against *H. influenzae* ($MIC_{50/90:}$ 2.0 and 4.0 mg/l), but MIC values increased two times when incubated in 5% to 6% CO_2. Against *Moraxella catarrhalis* and *Bordetella pertussis*, MIC_{90} values were 0.12 mg/l for both species. Against *H. pylori* MIC_{90} values were 0.25 and 0.03 mg/l for

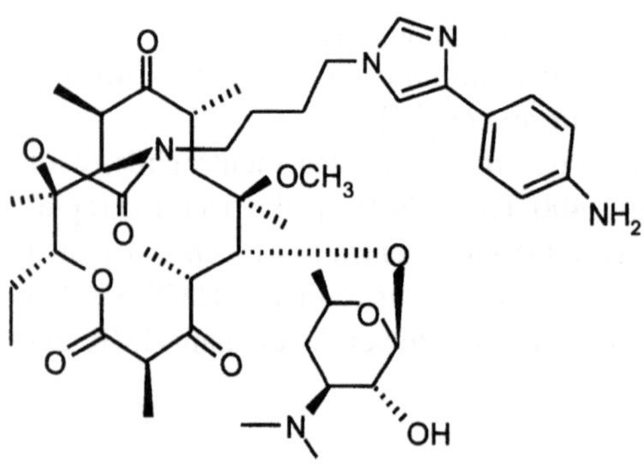

HMR 3832

Figure 19. HMR 3832 structure.

HMR 3832 and clarithromycin, respectively. HMR 3832 was inactive against *Mycobacterium tuberculosis* (MIC > 64 mg/l). Against *Clostridium difficile*, *Peptostreptococcus*, *Clostridium perfringens*, *B. fragilis*, *Porphyromonas* spp, *Prevotella* spp, and *Fusobacterium* spp, MIC_{50} values were 0.06, 0.03, 0.12, 8, 1.0, 0.06 and 1.0 mg/l respectively.

For gram-positive bacteria, HMR 3832 *in vitro* activity in comparison to that of clarithromycin is summarized in Table 15.

Table 15. *In vitro* activity of HMR 3832 against gram-positive bacteria [81]

		MIC (mg/l)			
	N	HMR3832		Clarithromycin	
S. aureus ery-S	22	0.12	0.12	0.12	0.12
Coagulase negative staphylococci	22	0.12	0.12	0.12	0.12
S. pyogenes	23	0.03	1.0	0.01	8.0
S. agalactiae	23	0.03	0.03	0.01	0.03
Lancefield group C and G streptococci	44	0.03	0.03	0.03	0.03
Viridans Streptococci	35	0.06	0.25	1.0	> 64.0
S. pneumoniae	21	0.03	0.06	0.01	0.01
S. pneumoniae ery-R	20	0.06	0.25	> 64	> 64.0
E. faecalis	21	0.06	0.06	0.25	0.25
C. diphtheriae	20	0.008	0.01	0.004	0.004
L. monocytogenes	26	0.06	0.06	0.12	0.12

HMR 3562 and HMR 3787 [31, 83–88]

Both HMR 3562 and HMR 3787 are 2-fluoro ketolides. They differ by the side chain substituting the C11–C12 carbamate residue.

HMR 3562 is the 2-fluoro counterpart of telithromycin, and HMR 3787 has bicyclic moiety (imidazolo pyridyl) links to the C11–12 carbamate residue through a butyl side chain.

HMR 3562 and HMR 3787 are strongly concentrated by human polymorphonuclear neutrophils with a C/E ratio greater than 100 within the first 5 minutes, HMR 3562 being greater concentrated than HMR 3787. Both are located in the granule compartment of PMN, and they are moderately released from loaded PMN (Fig. 20).

HMR 3787

HMR 3787 (Fig. 21) exhibits comparable activity to telithromycin against *S. pneumoniae* isolates susceptible to erythromycin A, with $MIC_{50/90}$ values of 0.008 and 0.015 mg/l, respectively. HMR 3787 also retains activity against *S. pneumo-*

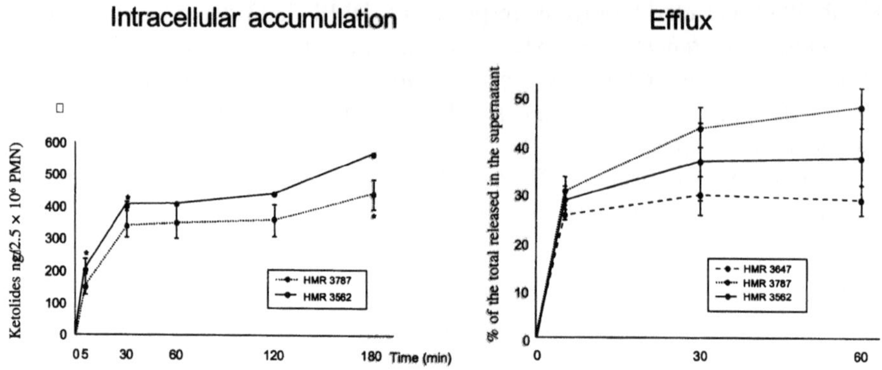

Figure 20. Intracellular concentration and efflux of HMR 3787 and HMR 3562.

niae isolates harbouring an underlying mechanism of resistance to erythromycin A, i.e., MLS_B (*erm* B), efflux (*mef* E), or ribosomal protein mutation (L4 and L22).

After 6 and 12 hours of contact, irrespective of the mechanism of resistance to erythromycin A, HMR 3787 exhibits a bactericidal activity with a reduction above 3 $\log_{10}$ cfu/ml at low concentration (MIC or two times MIC).

HMR 3787 is highly active against *S. pyogenes* susceptible to erythromycin A (MIC mode: 0.015 mg/l). Against *S. pyogenes* harbouring *erm* TR or *mef* A genes as a mechanism of resistance to erythromycin A, HMR 3787 is two times more active than telithromycin. Against *erm* B, only isolates for which erythromycin A exhibits an MIC > 64 mg/l were chosen to investigate the potential of HMR 3787 against these strains. Half of the isolates range in the intermediate zone of susceptibility for HMR 3787 if considering the resistant break-point for telithromycin (MIC > 2 mg/l). HMR 3787 $MIC_{50/90}$ values are 2.0/2.0 mg/l against *H. influenzae*.

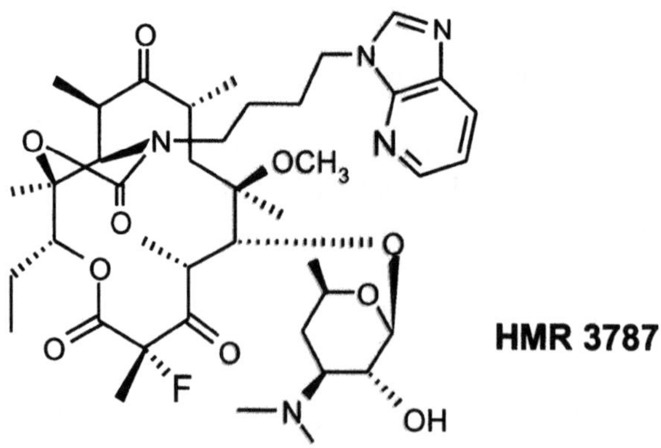

Figure 21. HMR 3787 structure.

HMR 3787 exhibits activity comparable to telithromycin against *S. aureus* susceptible to erythromycin A, or slightly higher (MIC_{50}: 0.06 mg/l versus 0.12 mg/l for telithromycin), which is a reflection of the data obtained in exploring the mechanism of action [89].

HMR 3787 seems to be the most active ketolide against *C. pneumoniae* and *L. pneumophila*, with an MIC value range of 0.06 to 0.12 mg/l and 0.004 to 0.004 mg/l respectively. This excellent activity is correlated with intracellular concentration of HMR 3787.

HMR 3787 is extremely active against *Mycoplasma pneumoniae*, with $MIC_{50/90}$ values of 0.0005 to 0.0005 mg/l.

In conclusion: HMR 3787 exhibits good *in vitro* activity against all the pathogens involved in respiratory tract infections, comparable to or higher than that of telithromycin, especially against *S. pyogenes*.

HMR 3562

HMR 3562 (Fig. 22) exhibited comparable activity to HMR 3787 against *S. aureus* strains susceptible to erythromycin A ($MIC_{50/90}$: 0.06 / 0.06 mg/l). Against erythromycin A-resistant isolates, like HMR 3787 and telithromycin, the anti-staphylococcal activity is delineated in MLS_B inducible and MLS_B constitutive strains, being active only against inducible MLS_B strains.

HMR 3562 retained good anti-pneumococcal activity against erythromycin A-resistant isolates ($MIC_{50/90}$: 0.03/0.06 mg/l) and against all streptococci. HMR 3562 also exhibited good activity against gram-positive bacilli. It is a bactericidal compound against *S. pneumoniae* (Fig. 23).

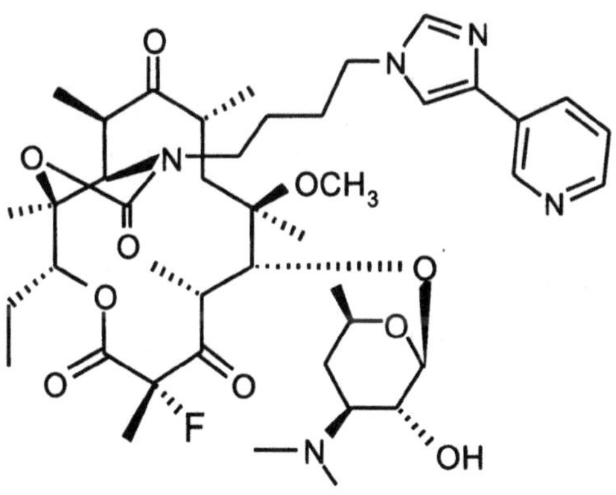

HMR 3562

Figure 22. HMR 3562 structure.

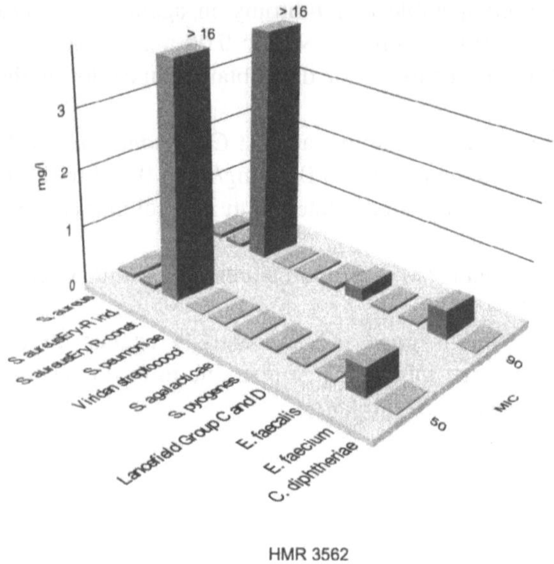

	MIC(mg/l)	
	50	90
S. aureus	0.06	0.06
*S. aureus*Ery-R ind.	0.06	0.06
*S. aureus*Ery R-const.	> 16	> 16
S. peumoniae	0.015	0.015
S. agalacticae	0.03	0.03
Viridan streptococci	0.03	0.06
S. pyogenes	0.03	0.25
Lancefield Group C and D	0.03	0.03
E. faecalis	0.03	0.03
E. faecium	0.50	0.50
C. diphtheriae	0.002	0.008

Figure 23. *In vitro* activity of HMR3562.

References

1 McGuire JM, Bunch PL, Anderson RC et al (1982) Ilotycin, a new antibiotic *Antibiot Chemother* 2: 281–282

2 Bryskier A, Labro MT (1994) Macrolides: nouvelles perspectives thérapeutiques *La Presse Med.* 23: 1762–1766

3 Bryskier A, Agouridas C, Chantot JF (1993) Acid stability of new macrolides *J Chemother 5 (Suppl 1)*: 158–159

4 Blackmon J, Hicklin MD, Chandler JF (1978) Legionnaires' disease: pathological and historical aspect of a new disease *Arch Pathol Lab Med* 102: 337–343

5 Kirst HA, Sides GD (1989) New directions for macrolide antibiotics *Antimicrob Agents Chemother* 33: 1419–1422

6 Chantot JF, Bryskier A, Gasc JC (1986) Antibacterial activity of roxithromycin, a laboratory evaluation *J Antibiot* 39: 660–668

7 Morimoto S., Takahashi Y, Watanabe Y, Omara S (1984) Chemical modification of erythromycin. Synthesis and antibacterial activity of 6-O-methyl erythromycin A. *J Antibiot* 37: 187–189

8 Bryskier A, Agouridas C (1993) Azalides: a new medicinal chemical family *Curr Opin Invest Drugs* 2: 687–694

9 Bryskier A, Agouridas C, Chantot JF (1997) Ketolides: new semi-synthetic 14-membered ring macrolides In: SH Zinner, LS Young, JF Acar, HC Neu (eds): *Expanding indications for the new macrolides, azalides and streptogramins.* Marcel Dekker, New York, 39–50

10 Bryskier A, Agouridas C, Chantot JF (2000) Ketolides: novel antibacterial agents designed to overcome erythromycin A resistance In: SH Zinner, LS Young, JF Acar, C Ortiz-Neu (eds): *New consideration for macrolides, azalides, streptogramins and ketolides*. Marcel-Dekker, New-York, 79–102

11 Bryskier A (1999) Respiratory fluoroquinolones myth or reality *Curr Opin Anti-infect Invest Drugs* 1: 413–427

12 Corbaz L, Ettlinger L, Gäumann E, Keller W, Kradolfer F, Kyburz E, Neipp L, Prelog V, Reusser R, Zähner H (1955) Stoffwechselprodukte von Actinomyceten. Narbomycin. *Helv Chimi Acta* 35: 935–942

13 Brockmann H, Henkel W (1951)Pikromycin ein bitter schmeckendes Antibioticum aus Actinomyceten. *Chem. Ber. 84:* 284–288

14 Allen N (1978) Macrolide resistance in *Staphylococcus aureus*: inducers of macrolide resistance. *Antimicrob. Agents Chemother.* 11: 669–674.

15 LeMahieu R, Carson M, Kierstead RW, Fern LM, Grunberg DE (1974) Glycoside cleavage reactions on erythromycin A. Preparation of erythronolide A. *J Med Chem* 17*:* 953–956

16 Pestka S, Lemahieu RA (1974) Effect of erythromycin analogues on binding of [^{14}C]erythromycin to *Escherichia coli* ribosomes. *Antimicrob Agents Chemother* 6: 479–488

17 Pestka S, Lemahieu RA, Miller P (1974) Correlation of effect of Erythromycin analogues on intact bacteria and on [^{14}C]erythromycin binding to *Escherichia coli* ribosomes. *Antimicrob Agents Chemother* 6: 489–491.

18 Pestka S, LeMahieu R (1974) Inhibition of [^{14}C]chloramphenicol binding to *Escherichia coli.* ribosomes by erythromycin derivatives. *Antimicrob Agents Chemother* 6: 39–45.

19 Pestka S, Vince R, LeMahieu R, Weiss F, Fern L, Unowsky J (1976) Induction of erythromycin resistance in *Staphylococcus aureus* by erythromycin derivatives. *Antimicrob Agents Chemother* 9*:* 128–130

20 Fernandes PB, Baker WR, Freiberg LA, Hardy DJ, McDonald EJ (1989) New macrolides active against *streptococcus pyogenes* with inducible or constitutive type of macrolide-lincosamide-streptogramin B resistance. *Antimicrob Agents Chemother* 33: 78–81

21 Morimoto S, Misawa Y, Kondoh H, Watanabe Y, Omura S (1990) Synthesis and antibacterial activity of 4"-O-methyl derivatives of erythromycin A 11,12-cyclic carbonate. *J Antibiotics* 43: 566–569

22 Bryskier A (2000) Telithromycin, an example of a new class of antibacterial agent *Clin Microbial Infect* 6: 661–669

23 Denis A, Agouridas C, Auger JM, Benedetti Y, Bonnefoy A, Bretin F, Chantot JF, Dussarat A, Fromentin C, Gouin et al (1999) Synthesis and antibacterial activity of HMR 3647- a new ketolide highly potent against erythromycin-resistant and susceptible pathogens. *Bioorg Med Chem Lett* 3075–3080

24 Agouridas C, Denis A, Auger JM, Benedetti Y, Bonnefoy A, Bretin F, Chantot JF, Dussarat A, Fromentin C, Gouin D'Ambrières S et al (1998) Synthesis and antibacterial activity of ketolides (6-O-methyl-3-oxo-erythromycin derivatives). A new class of antibacterials highly potent against macrolide-resistant and susceptible respiratory pathogens. *J Med Chem* 41: 4080–4100

25 Baker WR, Clark JD, Stephens RL, Kim KH (1988) Modifications of macrolide antibiotics. Synthesis of 11-deoxy-11-(carboxyamino)-6-O-methylerythromycin A 11,12-(cyclic esters) via intramolecular Michael reaction of O-carbamates with an α, β-unsaturated ketone. *J Org Chem* 53*:* 2340–2345

26 Griesgraber G, Or YS, Chu DTW, Nilius AM, Johnson PM, Flamm RK, Henry RF, Plattner JJ (1996) 3-keto-11,12-carbazate derivatives of 6-O-methylerythromycin A synthesis and *in vitro* activity. *J Antibiotics* 49: 465–477

27 Agouridas C, Chantot JF (1996) New erythromycin derivatives. EP Patent 7160093 A1

28 Denis A, Auger JM (2000) Preparation of 6-deoxy-erythromycins as antibiotics. WO Patent 0005239 A1

29 Elliott R L, Pireh D, Griesgraber G, Nilius AM, Ewing PJ, Ha Bui M, Raney PM, Flamm RK, Kim K, Henry RF, Chu DTW, Plattner JJ, Sun Or Y (1998) *J Med Chem* 41: 1651–1659

30 Agouridas C, Chantot JF (1997) New erythromycin derivatives. WO Patent 9731929 A1

31 Denis A, Bretin F, Fromentin C, Bonnet A, Piltan G, Agouridas C, Bonnefoy A (2000) β-Keto-ester chemistry and ketolides. Synthesis and antibacterial activity of 2-halogeno, 2-methyl and 2,3 enol-ether ketolides. *Bioorg Med Chem Lett* 2019–2022

32 Kurath P, Jones PH, Egan RS, Perun TJ (1971) Acid degradation of erythromycin A and erythromycin B. *Experentia* 27*:* 362

33 Fiese EP, Steffen SH (1990) Comparison of the acid stability of azithromycin and eythromycin A. *J Antimicrob Chemother* 25 (suppl A): 39–47

34 Puri SK, Lassman HB (1987) Roxithromycin: pharmacokinetic review of a *macrolide J Antimicrob Chemother* 20 (suppl B): 89–100

35 Schülin T, Wennersten EB, Moellering RC Jr, Eliopoulos GM (1998) *In vitro* activity of the new ketolide antibiotic HMR 3647 against gram-positive bacteria. *J Antimicrob Chemother* 42: 297–301
36 Reinert RR, Bryskier A, Lütticken R (1998) *In vitro* activities of the new ketolides antibiotics HMR 3004 and HMR 3647 against *Streptococcus pneumoniae* in Germany. *Antimicrob Agent Chemother* 42: 1509–1511
37 Boswell FI, Andrews JM, Ashby JP, Fogarty NP, Brenwald NP, Wise R (1998) The *in vitro* activity of HMR 3647, a new ketolide antimicrobial agent *J Antimicrob Chemother* 42: 703–709
38 Barry AL, Fuchs PC, Brown SD (1998) *In vitro* activities of the ketolide HMR 3647 against recent gram-positive clinical isolate and *Haemophilus influenzae Antimicrob Agent Chemother* 42: 2138–2140
39 Pankuch GA, Visalli HA, Jacobs HP, Appelbaum PC (1998) Susceptibilities of penicillin and erythromycin-susceptible and -resistant pneumococci to HMR 3647 (RU 66 647), a new ketolide compared with susceptibilities to 17 other agents. *Antimicrob Agent Chemother* 42: 462–650
40 Okamoto H, Miyazaki S, Tateda K, Ishii Y, Yamaguchi K (2000) Comparative *in vitro* activity of telithromycin (HMR 3647), three macrolides, amoxicillin, cefdinir and levofloxacin against gram-positive clinical isolates in Japan. *J Antimicrob Chemother* 46: 797–802
41 Inoue M, Sato Y, Kuga A, Okamoto R (1998) The novel ketolide HMR 3647 shows high activity against gram-positive cocci. *38th Interscience Conference on Antimicrobial Agents and Chemotherapy*, Abstract E-138
42 Talbot UM, Paton AN, Paton JC (1996) Uptake of *Streptococcus pneumoniae* by respiratory epithelial cells. *Infect Imm* 64: 3772–3777
43 Mandell GL, Coleman EJ (2000) Activities of antimicrobial agents against intracellular pneumococci. *Antimicrob Agent Chemother* 44: 2561–2563
44 Pankuch GA, Hoellman DB, Lin F, Bajaksouzian S, Jacobs MR, Appelbaum PC (1998) Activity of HMR 3647 compared to those of five agents against *Haemophilus influenzae* and *Moraxella catarrhalis* by MIC determination and time kill. *Antimicrob Agent Chemother* 43: 3032–3034
45 Piper KE, Rouse MS, Steckelberg TM, Wilson WA, Patel R (1999) Ketolide treatment of *Haemophilus influenzae* experimental pneumonia. *Antimicrob Agents Chemother* 43: 708–710
46 Hoppe JF, Bryskier A (1998) *In vitro* susceptibilities of *Bordetella pertussis* and *Bordetella parapertussis* to ketolides (HMR 3004 and HMR 3647), four macrolides (azithromycin, clarithromycin, erythromycin A, and roxithromycin), and two ansamycins (rifampicin and rifapentine). *Antimicrob Agent Chemother* 42: 965–966
47 Bemer-Melchior P, Juvin ME, Tassin S, Bryskier A, Schito GC, Drugeon H (2000) *In vitro* activity of the new ketolide telithromycin compared with those of macrolides against *Streptococcus pyogenes*: influence of resistance mechanism and methodological factors. *Antimicrob Agent Chemother* 44: 2999–3002
48 Vazifeh D, Bryskier A, Labro MT (2000) Effect of pro-inflammatory cytokines on the interplay between roxithromycin, HMR 3647, HMR 3004 and human polymorphonuclear neutrophils. *Antimicrob Agent Chemother* 44: 511–521
49 Vazifeh D, Preira A, Bryskier A, Labro MT (1998) Interactions between HMR 3647, a new ketolide, and human polymorphonuclear neutrophils. *Antimicrob Agents Chemother* 42: 1944–1951
50 Roblin PM, Hammerschlag MR (1998) *In vitro* activity of a new ketolide antibiotic, telithromycin against *Chlamydia pneumoniae. Antimicrob Agent Chemother* 42: 1515–1516
51 Gustafsson I, Hjelm E, Cars O (2000) *In vitro* pharmacodynamics of the new ketolides HMR 3004 and HMR 3647 (telithromycin) against. *Chlamydia pneumoniae. Antimicrob Agent Chemother* 44: 1846–1849
52 Edelstein PM, Edelstein MA (1999) *In vitro* activity of the ketolide HMR 3647 (RU66 647) for *Legionella* spp. Its pharmacokinetics in guinea pigs and use of the drug to treat guinea pigs with *Legionella pneumophila. Antimicrob Agent Chemother* 43: 90–95
53 Bébéar CM, Renaudin H, Bryskier A, Bébéar C (2000) Comparative activities of telithromycin (HMR 3647), levofloxacin, and other antimicrobial agents against human mycoplasmas. *Antimicrob Agent Chemother* 44: 1980–1982
54 Rolain JM, Maurin M, Bryskier A, Raoult D (2000) *In vitro* activities of telithromycin (HMR 3647) against *Rickettsia rickettsii, Rickettsia conerii, Rickettsia africae*, Rickettsia *typhi, Rick-*

ettsia prouvazekii, Coxiella burnetii, Bartonela henselae, Bartonella quintona, Bartonella bacilliformis, Ehrhichia chaffeensis. Antimicrob Agent Chemother 44: 1391–1393

55 Maurin M, Mersali NF, Raoult D (2000) Bactericidal activities of antibiotics against intracellular *Franciscella tularensis. Antimicrob Agent Chemother* 44: 3428–3431

56 Hamilton-Miller J, Shah S. (1998) Comparative *in vitro* activity of ketolide HMR 3647 and four macrolides against gram-positive cocci of known erythromycin susceptibility isolates. *J Antimicrob Chemother* 41: 649–653

57 Bryskier A (2001) Anti anaerobic activity of antibacterial agents. *Exp Opin Invest Drugs* 10: 239–267

58 Edlund C, Sillerstrom E, Wahland E, Nord CE (1998) *In vitro* activity of HMR 3647 against anaerobic bacteria. *J Chemother* 10: 280–284

59 Goldstein EJC, Citron DM , Merriam CV, Warren Y, Tyrrell K (1999) Activities of telithromycin (HMR 3647, RU 66 647) compared to those of erythromycin, azithromycin, clarithromycin, roxithromycin, and other antimicrobial agents against unusual anaerobes. *Antimicrob Agent Chemother* 43: 2801–2805

60 Dekerman G, Schaumann R, Pless B, Claros MC, Rodloff AC (2000) *In vitro* activity of telithromycin (HMR 3647) and seven other antimicrobial agents against anaerobic bacteria. *J Antimicrob Chemother* 46: 115–119

61 Zarazaga M, Saenz T, Portillo A, Tenerio C, Ruiz-Larrea F, Del Campo R, Baquero F, Torres C (1999) *In vitro* activities of ketolide HMR 3647, macrolides and other antibiotics against *Lactobacillus, Leuconostoc*, and *Pediacoccus* isolates. *Antimicrob Agents Chemother* 43: 3039–3041

62 Saez-Nieto JA, Vazquez JA (1999) *In vitro* activity of ketolides HMR 3647, and HMR 3004 against *Neisseria* spp and *Moraxella catarrhalis. Antimicrob Agent Chemother* 49: 983–984

63 Engstrand GL, Cars O (2001) *In vitro* pharmacodynamic studies of activities of ketolides HMR 3647 (telithromycin) and HMR 3004 against extracellular or intracellular *Helicobacter pylori. Antimicrob Agents Chemother* 45: 353–355

64 Munckhof WJ, Borlace G, Turnidge JD (2000) Post antibiotic suppression of growth erythromycin A-susceptible and -resistant gram-positive bacteria by the ketolides telithromycin (HMR 3647) and HMR 3004. *Antimicrob Agent Chemother* 44: 1749–1753

65 Hansen LH, Mauvais P, Douthwaite S (1999) The macrolide-ketolide antibiotic binding site is formed by structures in domain II and V of 23S ribosomal RNA. *Mol Microbio* 31: 623–631

66 Douthwaite S, Hansen LH, Mauvais P (2000) Macrolide-ketolide inhibition of MLS-resistant ribosomes is improved by alternative drug interaction with domain II of 23S rRNA. *Mol Microbiol* 36: 183–193

67 Champney JW, Tober CL (1998) Inhibition of translation and 50S ribosomal subunit formation in *Staphylococcus aureus* cells by 11 different ketolides antibiotics. *Current Microbiol* 37: 418–425

68 Khaitovich P, Mankin AS (1999) Effects of antibiotics on large ribosomal subunit apparently reveals possible function of 5S rRNA. *J Mol Biol* 291: 1025–1038

69 Xiong L, Shah S, Mauvais P, Mankin AS (1999) Ketolide resistance mutation in domain II of 23S rRNA reveals proximity of hair pie 35 of the peptidyl transferase centre. *Mol Microbio* 31: 633–639

70 Arpin C, Daube N, Tessier F, Quentin C (1999) Incidence of *mef* A and *mef* E genes in viridans group streptococci. *Antimicrob Agent Chemother* 43: 2335–2336

71 Arpin C, Canron MH, Maugein J, Quentin C (1999) Incidence of *mef* A and *mef* E genes in *Streptococcus agalactiae. Antimicrob Agent Chemother* 43: 944–946

72 Weisblum B (1998) Macrolide resistance. *Drug Res Update* 1: 29–41

73 Tait-Kamradt A, Davies T, Cronan M, Jacobs MR, Appelbaum PC, Sutcliffe J (2000) Mutations in 23S rRNA and ribosomal protein L4 account for resistance in pneumococci strains selected *in vitro* by macrolide passage. *Antimicrob Agent Chemother* 44: 2118–2225

74 Davies TA, Dewasse BE, Jacobs MR, Appelbaum PC (2000) *In vitro* development of resistance to telithromycin, four macrolides, clindamycin, and pristinamycin in *Streptococcus pneumoniae. Antimicrob Agent Chemother* 44: 414–417

75 Bonnefoy A, Girard AM, Agouridas C, Chantot JF (1998) Ketolides lack inducibility properties of MLS_B resistance phenotype. *J Antimicrob Chemother* 40: 85–90

76 Edlund C, Alván G, Barkholt L, Vacheron F, Nord CE (2000) Pharmacokinetics and comparative effects of telithromycin (HMR 3647) and clarithromycin on the oropharyngeal and intestinal microflora. *J Antimicrob Chemother* 46: 741–749
77 Vesga O, Bonnat C, Craig WA (1998) *In vivo* pharmacodynamic activity of HMR 3647 a new ketolide In program and abstract of the 38th Intersci. Conf Antimicrob. Agent Chemother. – Toronto – American Soc. Microbiol. Washington DC – F255: 189
78 Namour F, Wessels DH, Pascual MH, Reynolds D, Sultan E, Lenfant B (2001) Pharmacokinetics of the new ketolide telithromycin (HMR 3647) administered in ascending single and multiple doses. *Antimicrob Agent Chemother* 45: 170–175
79 Carbon C (2000) Telithromycin, a once-a-day ketolide in the treatment of community-acquired pneumonia. *Presse Med* 29: 2042–2043
80 Vazifeh D, Abdelghaffar H, Labro MT (1997) Cellular accumulation of the new ketolide RU 64004 by human neutrophils: comparison with that of azithromycin and roxithromycin. *Antimicrob Agents Chemother* 41: 2099–2107
81 Labro MT, Vazifeh D, Bryskier A (2000) Uptake of two new fluoroketolides, HMR3562 and HMR3787 by human neutrophils (PMN) *in vitro* compared with telithromycin (HMR3647) Abstracts of the 40th Interscience Conference on Antimicrobial Agents and Chemotherapy, Toronto, American Society for Microbiology – Washington DC, 1819: 214
82 Felmingham D, Robbins MJ, Mathias IL, Dencer C, Salman H, Ridgway GL, Bryskier A (2000) *In vitro* activity of the ketolide, HMR3832, against clinical bacterial isolates Abstracts of the 40th Interscience Conference on Antimicrobial Agents and Chemotherapy, Toronto, American Society for Microbiology – Washington DC, 2172: 183
83 Bonnefoy A, Denis A, Bretin F, Fromentin C, Agouridas C (1999) *In vivo* antibacterial activity of two ketolides HMR 3562 and HMR 3787 highly active against respiratory pathogens. Abstracts of the 39th Interscience Conference on Antimicrobial Agents and Chemotherapy, San Francisco, American Society for Microbiology – Washington DC, 2156: 351
84 Levasseur P, Vallee E, Bonnefoy A, Garry L, Agouridas C, Bryskier A, Carbon C (1999) Activity of ketolides HMR 3562 and HMR 3787 against erythromycin-sensitive (Ery-S) and -resistant (Ery-Rc) pneumococci in murine pneumonia models Abstracts of the 39th Interscience Conference on Antimicrobial Agents and Chemotherapy, San Francisco, American Society for Microbiology – Washington DC, 2158: 352
85 Drugeon H, Bryskier A, Bemer-Melchior P, Juvin ME (2000) New fluoreketolides-HMR3562 and HMR3787 bactericidal activity against *Streptococcus pneumoniae* Abstracts of the 40th Interscience Conference on Antimicrobial Agents and Chemotherapy, Toronto, American Society for Microbiology – Washington DC, 1818: 213
86 Champney WS, Tober CL (2000) Structure-activity relationship for six ketolide antibiotics Abstracts of the 40th Interscience Conference on Antimicrobial Agents and Chemotherapy, Toronto, American Society for Microbiology – Washington DC, 1820: 214
87 Bryskier A (1999) Novelties in the field of antibacterials. *Clin Infect Dis* 29: 632–658
88 Felmingham D, Robbins MJ, Mathias I, Bryskier A (1999) *In vitro* activity of two ketolides, HMR 3562 and HMR 3787, against clinical bacterial isolates. Abstracts of the 39th Interscience Conference on Antimicrobial Agents and Chemotherapy, San Francisco, American Society for Microbiology – Washington DC , 2154: 351
89 Champney SW, Tober CL (2001) Structure-activity relationships for six ketolide antibiotics. *Curr Microbiol* 42: 203–210

Macrolide Antibiotics
ed. by W. Schönfeld and H. A. Kirst

Novel macrolide derivatives active against resistant pathogens

Ly T. Phan[1] and Zhenkun Ma[2]

[1]*Enanta Pharmaceuticals, Inc., 500 Arsenal Street, Watertown, MA 02472, USA*
[2]*Abbott Laboratories, 200 Abbott Park Road, Abbott Park, IL 60064–3537, USA*

Introduction

Macrolide antibiotics are widely prescribed for the treatment of upper and lower respiratory tract infections. Erythromycin is the first member of this class and has been in clinical used for over four decades. To overcome some of the drawbacks of erythromycin, including acid instability [1], gastro intestinal (GI) irritation [2], and poor pharmacokinetic properties, second-generation macrolides such as clarithromycin [3] and azithromycin [4] were developed. Clarithromycin addresses the acid instability by methylating the 6-hydroxyl group and thus preventing the 6,9-ketal formation, while azithromycin addresses the problem by transforming the 9-ketone into a ring-expanded analog *via* Beckman rearrangement of the corresponding 9-oxime. Other drugs such as roxithromycin [5] and dirithromycin [6] solve the acid instability by converting the 9-keto group of erythromycin into 9-oxime and 9-amino derivatives respectively.

Over the past decade, the increasing emergence of antibiotic-resistant bacteria has resulted in a need to discover new agents [7]. In the mid-1980s, a series of erythromycin 11,12-carbamate derivatives (**4**) was introduced by Baker et al. [8] that exhibited modest activity against MLS_B resistance. Compared with the corresponding carbonate [9], the cyclic carbamate provided better stability and potential for derivatization. Recently, Roussel-Uclaf researchers have demonstrated that the cladinose moiety was not essential for biological activity when replaced by a 3-keto group [10]. This new class of macrolides, known as ketolides

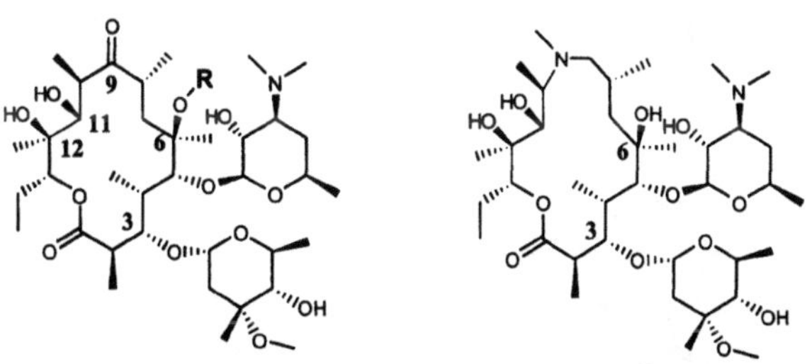

1 Erythromycin (R = H)
2 Clarithromycin (R = Me)

3 Azithromycin

Figure 1.

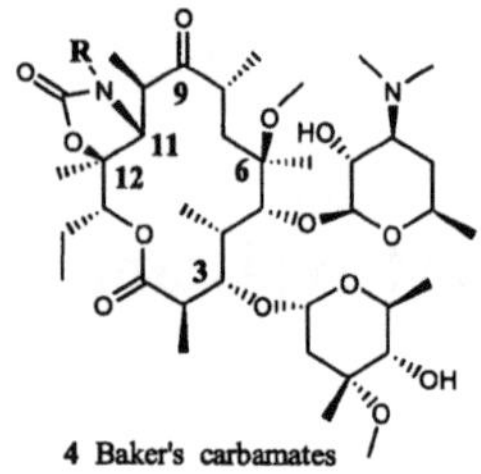

4 Baker's carbamates

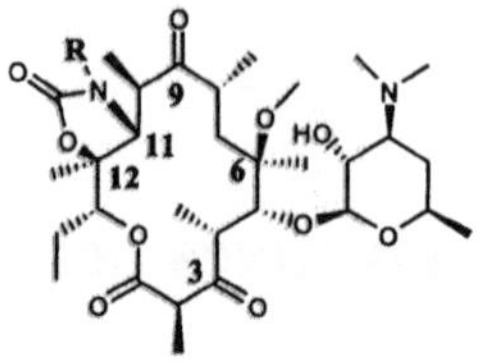

5 Ketolides

Figure 2.

(5), has shown improved activity against MLS_B-resistant bacteria. This review will summarize the research efforts at Abbott since 1995 aimed at developing a next generation of macrolide antibacterial agents to overcome the increasing antibiotic resistance [11].

3-deoxy derivatives of clarithromycin

3-deoxy analogs of clarithromycin (**7**) were prepared by a tributyltin hydride radical reduction of a 3-O-xanthyl intermediate of **6** [12]. Various 9-oxime, 11,12-carbonate, 11,12-carbamate, and tricyclic 3-deoxy (**9**) derivatives have been prepared from **7**. The phenyl butyl carbamate derivative (**8**) was the best compound in this series. Compound **8** was slightly less active than erythromycin against erythromycin-susceptible bacteria but was more potent against inducible and efflux-resistant strains. It was interesting to note that 3-hydroxy clarithromycin analog (**6**) was inactive, while 3-deoxy clarithromycin (**7**) displayed modest activity but was less active than erythromycin. A direct comparison of 3-deoxy compounds with the corresponding ketolides (**5**) indicated that the 3-keto group is essential for the potent antibacterial activity.

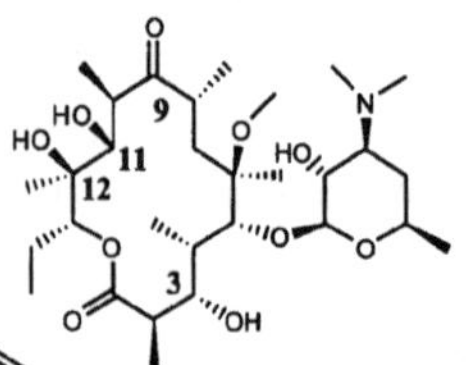

6

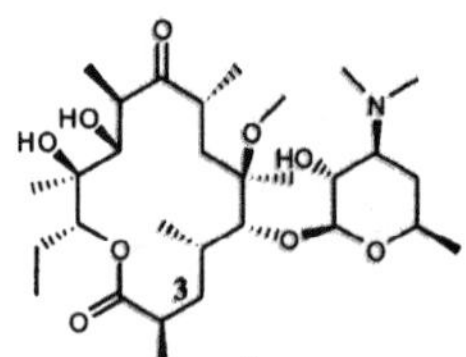

7

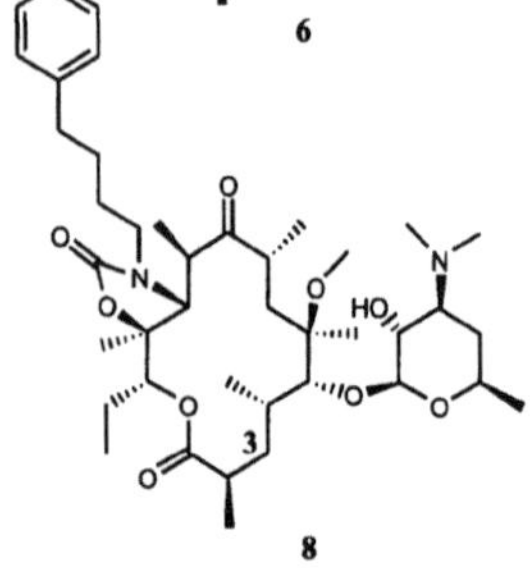

8

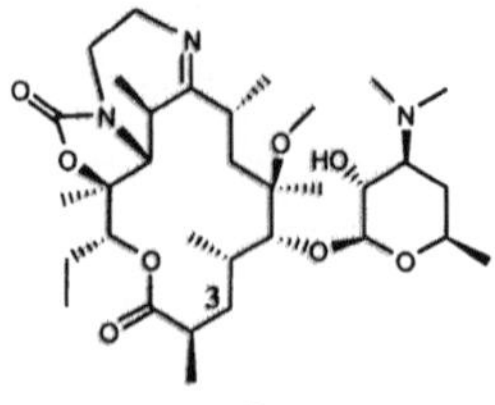

9

Figure 3.

2,3-anhydrolides

A series of 2,3-dehydrated derivatives, known as anhydrolides [13, 14], was prepared in an effort to maintain an sp^2 center at C-3 analogous to the ketolides.

Both 11,12-carbamate [13] and 11,12-carbazate [14] anhydrolides exhibited improved activity relative to erythromycin and similar activities to the corresponding ketolides against both susceptible and resistant bacteria. In general,

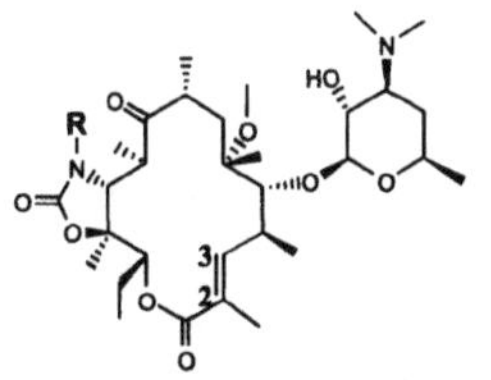

10a R = 4-bromophenyl$(CH_2)_2$-
10b R = 2-napthyl-O-$(CH_2)_3$-

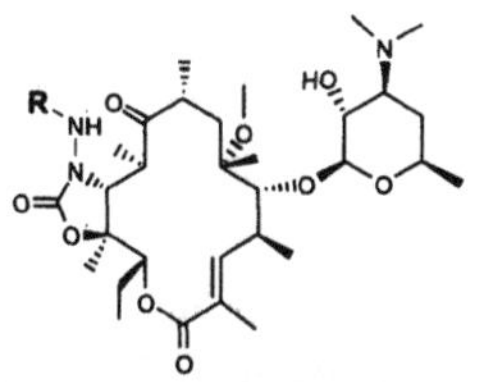

11a R = 4-quinolyl-$(CH_2)_3$-
11b R = 4-aminophenylCH=CHCH$_2$-

Figure 4.

carbamate analogs (**10a-b**) were more active against MLS$_B$-resistant streptococci (MICs 3.1 to 16 μg/ml) than the carbazate analogs (**11a-b**, MICs > 100 μg/ml). However, the carbazate analogs possessed better activity against *H. influenzae* (MICs 2 μg/ml) as compared with the carbamates (MICs 16 to 64 μg/ml) and erythromycin (MIC 4 μg/ml). In mouse protection tests, the carbamate analogs showed poor to moderate *in vivo* efficacy, while carbazate **11b** provided efficacy, comparable to clarithromycin. Corresponding C-10 epimers of the carbamate and carbazate anhydrolides also were tested and were found to be inactive [15].

Two classes of tricyclic anhydrolides also were investigated with the intent of imposing additional conformational constraint on the 14-membered macrolide ring. Both 5- and 7-membered ring systems linked between C-9 and C-11 were prepared. The 5-membered pyrazoline analog (**12a**) and pyrazolidine derivatives

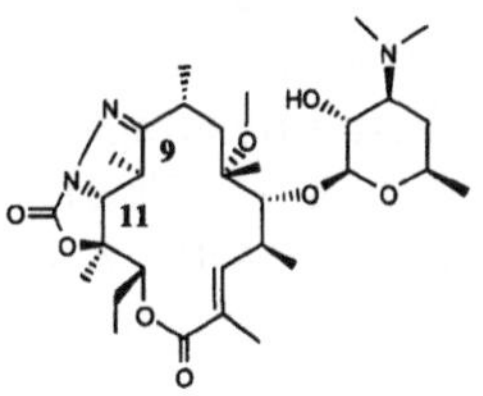

12a

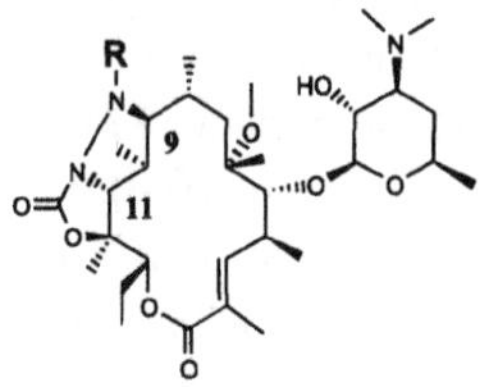

12b

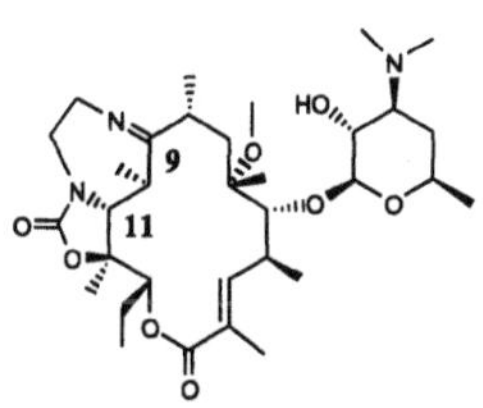

13a

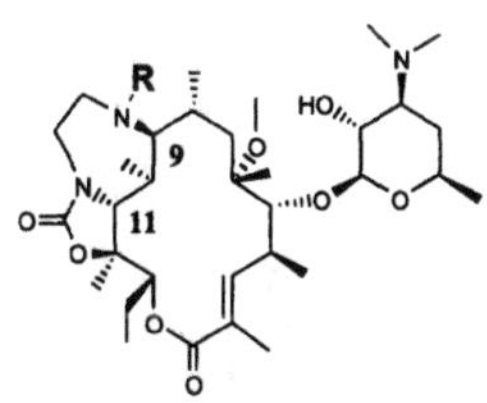

13b

Figure 5.

(**12b**) were not active. Although the 7-membered ring analog (**13a**) was slightly less potent than erythromycin against erythromycin-susceptible bacteria (MIC 0.78 *versus* 0.2 μg/ml), it was 4- to 16-fold more potent against the inducible and efflux-resistant strains. Furthermore, compound **13a** exhibited four-fold reduced activity against *H. influenzae* as compared with erythromycin and lacked *in vivo* efficacy in the mouse protection test. In general, the 9-amino derivatives (**13b**) displayed weaker activity relative to **13a**.

Tricyclic ketolides

TE-802 (**14**) [16], a tricylic ketolide developed by Taisho, has been shown to possess good *in vitro* and *in vivo* activity. Compared to clarithromycin, TE-802 showed two to three-fold improvements in *in vivo* efficacies against *S. aureus* and *S. pneumoniae* in the mouse protection test. The lack of activity against MLS_B-resistant bacteria and weak activity against *H. influenzae* were the major drawbacks associated with TE-802. Based on earlier macrolide SAR information, the presence of an aromatic group on the macrolide was important for activity against MLS_B-resistant bacteria. The aromatic moiety was thought to provide additional binding affinity of the macrolide for methylated ribosome. Therefore, aromatic substitutents were introduced to the diazapene ring of TE-802 at position C-16 or C-17 or both (**15**) in search for enhanced activity against MLS_B-resistant bacteria.

In general, aryl substituted TE-802 derivatives exhibited improved activity relative to TE-802 [17]. Both the regio- and stereochemistry of the aromatic substituent affected the activity. Aryl alkyl substitution at position C-16 gave better activity, particularly against *H. influenzae* (**16–17**, MICs 2 μg/ml), whereas substitution at position C-17 (**18a-c**) resulted in reduced activity (MICs 32 μg/ml). Conversely, substitution at position C-17 (**18a-c**) provided two to three-fold improvements in *in vivo* efficacy as compared with clarithromycin and exhibited similar efficacy relative to TE-802. Compounds **16–17** with substitutions at C-16 gave poor *in vivo* efficacy relative to clarithromycin. Various functional groups in the C-16 linker such as ether, amino, ester, thio, carbamate, amide, and urea were well tolerated. The ether (**16b**) and ester (**17**) provided the best activity against MLS_B-resistant streptococci (MICs 4 to 16 μg/ml) and *H. influenzae* (MICs 2 μg/ml). Disubstituted analog **19a** was less active against *H. influenzae* (MICs 8 μg/ml) but showed enhanced activity against MLS_B constitutively resistant *S. aureus*

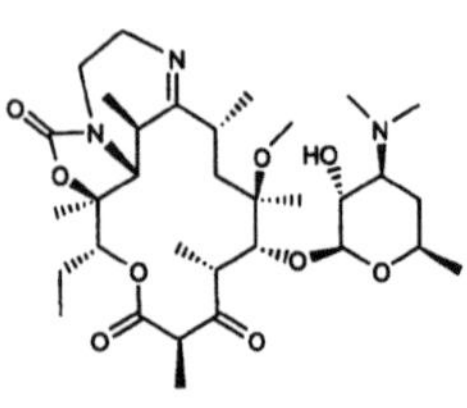

14 TE-802

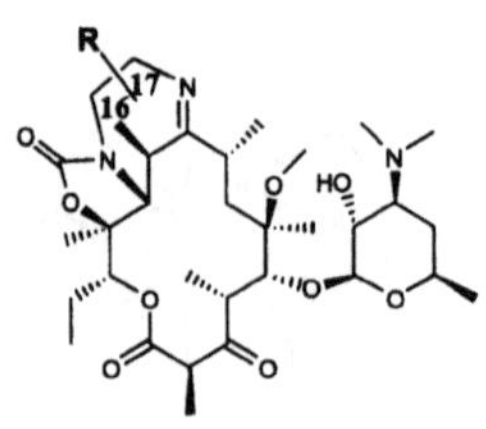

15

Figure 6.

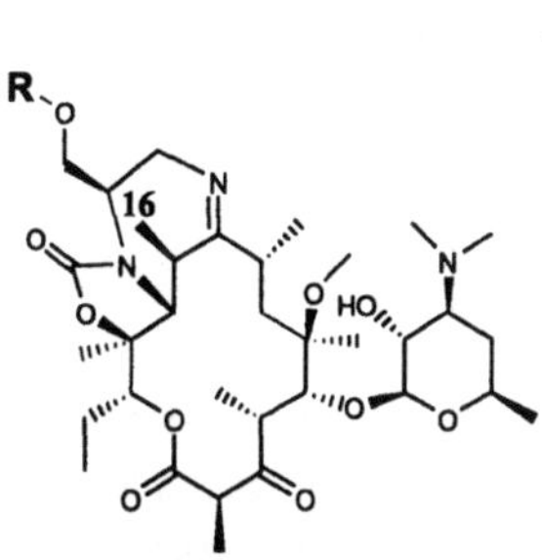

16a R = benzyl
16b R= (4-quinolyl)CH2-
17 R= (4-quinolyl)C(O)-

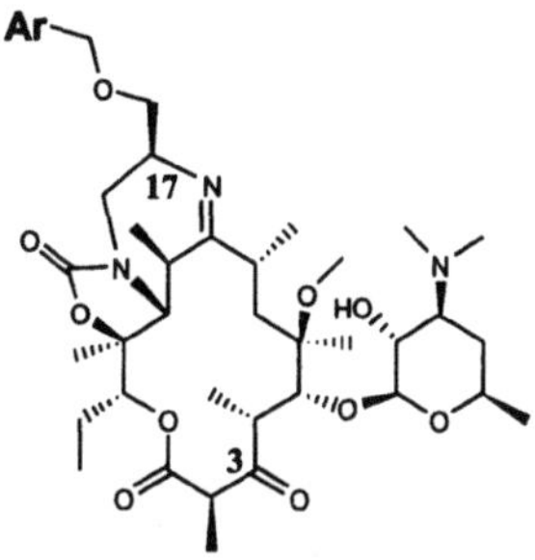

18a Ar = phenyl
18b Ar = 4-pyridyl
18c Ar = 4-cyanophenyl

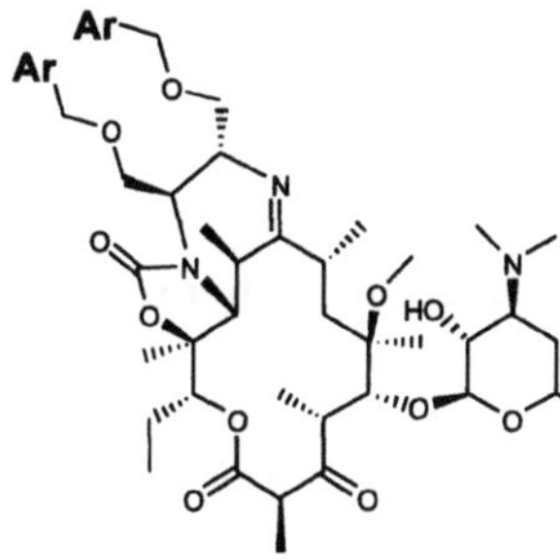

19a Ar = 4-chlorophenyl
19b Ar = phenyl

Figure 7.

(MIC 6.2 µg/ml *versus* > 100 µg/ml for erythromycin). The presence of a chlorine substituent on the aromatic ring was found to be important for the activity against MLS_B constitutively resistant *S. aureus*. A significant loss in activity was observed when the chlorine atoms were removed (**19b**, MIC 50 µg/ml). In addition, the incorporation of two aromatic groups improved the activity against MLS_B-resistant streptococci.

A novel series of tetracyclic ketolide also was prepared [18] that incorporated fused carbocycles and heterocycles to the diazapene ring of TE-802. Heterocycles such as pyrrolidine (**23a,b**) provided an additional site for derivatization (**24a,b**). During the synthesis, *meso*-cis-diamines were employed in the cyclization, which generated both isomers of the cis-fused tetracyclic ring structure. Compounds **20a-24a** were the major isomers.

All unsubstituted tetracyclic compounds were less active against *H. influenzae* and similar in activity against *S. aureus* and streptococci as compared with TE-802. However, the *in vivo* efficacy for the cyclohexane (**20a-b**) and tetrahydrofuran (**22a**) derivatives was comparable to TE-802 and superior to clarithromycin. The pyrrolidine compounds (**23a-b**) exhibited poor oral efficacy. However, subcutaneous efficacy for **23a-b** was improved two-fold against *S. pneumoniae* and was similar against *S. aureus* relative to TE-802. N-Substituted pyrrolidine

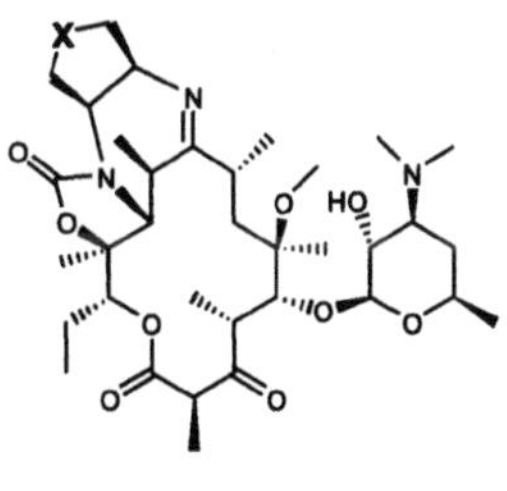

20a X = $-CH_2CH_2-$
21a X = $-CH_2-$
22a X = -O-
23a X = -NH-
24a X = -NR-

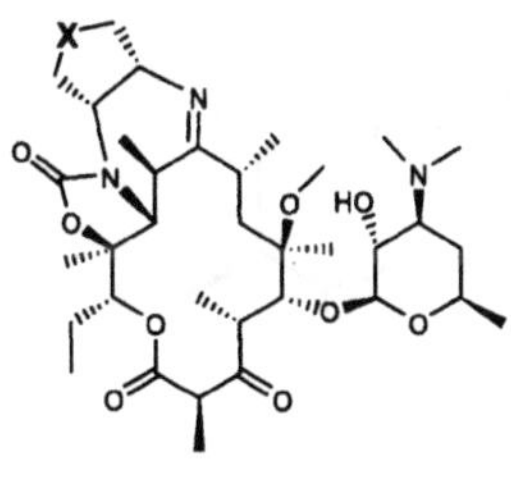

20b X = $-CH_2CH_2-$
21b X = $-CH_2-$
22b X = -O-
23b X = -NH-
24b X = -NR-

Figure 8.

derivatives (**24a-b**), prepared *via* direct N-alkylation, did not provide compounds more active than TE-802.

2-F-tricyclic ketolides

The C-2 position in the ketolide series provided an important site for synthetic modifications. The introduction of a non-sterically demanding group such as fluorine at C-2 had significant effects on the overall biological profile and pharmacokinetic properties of this class of macrolide [19].

2-Fluoro-TE-802 (**25**) improved the overall activity of TE-802 by one dilution but, more significantly, enhanced its *in vivo* efficacy particularly against *H. influenzae* in the rat lung infection model (Tab. 1). Furthermore, the introduction of 2-fluoro increased the $\log P_{(octanol/water)}$ of TE-802 (1.47 *versus* 0.96). Interestingly, replacing the C-2 hydrogen with fluorine altered the solid-state conforma-

Table 1. Comparison of *in vivo* efficacy of 2-F-TE-802 with other macrolides (ED_{50}, mg/kg).

Compound	*S. aureus* 10649[a] ED_{50}[1]	*S. pneumoniae* 6303[a] ED_{50}[1]	*H. influenzae* 1435 ED_{50}[2]
25 (2-F-TE-802)	9.4	7.2	36
TE-802	13	10	> 60
HMR3647	13	34	58
Azithromycin	25	39	35

[a] *S. aureus* 10649 and *S. pneumoniae* 6303 are erythromycin-susceptible strains.
1. ED50 (mg/kg) – mouse protection model.
2. ED50 (mg/kg/day) – 2 log reduction of bacterial burden in rat lung infection model.

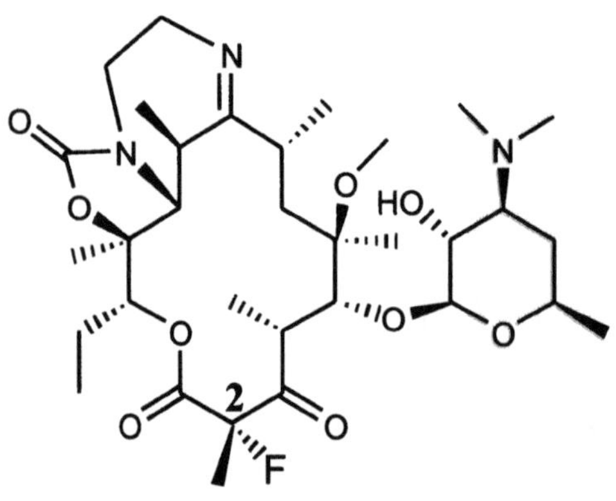

25

Figure 9.

tion around C-1 to C-5 region of the macrocycle including the desosamine sugar as observed in an X-ray crystal structure. All other substituents examined at C-2, including hydroxy, chlorine, bromine, and alkyl, displayed decreased activity.

6-O-substituted erythromycin derivatives

Modification at the C-6 position of erythromycin represented a logical extension to the success of clarithromycin. The major challenge posed by this strategy was the selective introduction of an alkyl group to the sterically hindered C-6 hydroxyl position, which required extensive protection and deprotection. Previous efforts resulted in limited success with a small number of lower alkyl derivatives being prepared [20]. The introduction of higher alkyl groups was sluggish and was complicated by dramatic losses in selectivity for the C-6 position [3, 21]. A general strategy has been developed at Abbott for the introduction of substituents to the C-6 position [22], which involved selective alkylation of the C-6 hydroxyl group with activated alkylating agents such as allylic, propargylic, and benzylic halides. Further elaboration of these intermediates resulted in an array of 6-O-alkyl erythromycin derivatives.

Although the 6-O-propyl erythromycin (**26a**) was several-fold less active than clarithromycin, the 6-O-allyl and 6-O-propargyl analogs (**26b** and **26c**) showed similar activity to clarithromycin. The benzylic analogs (**26d** and **26e**) were less active than clarithromycin against erythromycin-susceptible organisms, but they exhibited improved activity against MLS_B-resistant *S. pyogenes* and *S. pneumoniae*, with MICs at 8 to 64 μg/ml as compared with > 128 μg/ml for clarithromycin.

Further derivatization of 6-O-allyl erythromycin (**26b**) by Heck coupling reaction provided a series of analogs **27a-c**. Theses compounds were as active as clarithromycin against erythromycin-susceptible organisms and were more active than clarithromycin against MLS_B-resistant strains with MICs at 8 to 64 μg/ml.

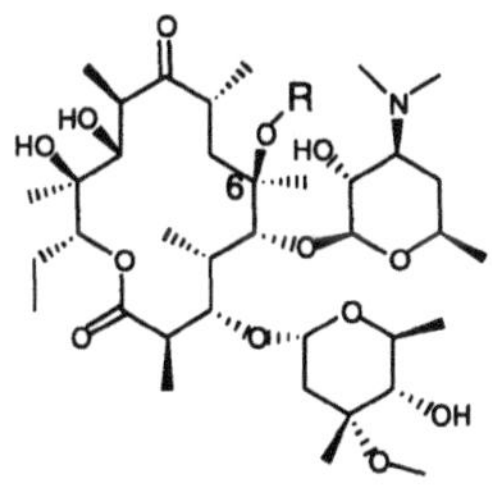

26a R = propyl
26b R = allyl
26c R = propargyl
26d R = benzyl
26e R = 4-fluorobenzyl

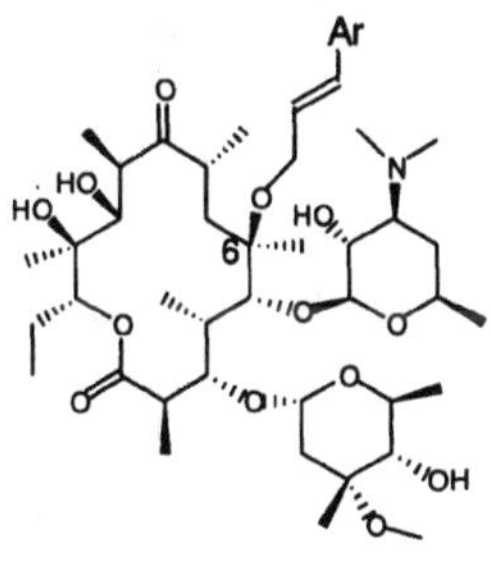

27a Ar = phenyl
27b Ar = (1-naphthyl)
27c Ar = (3-quinolyl)

Figure 10.

Figure 11.

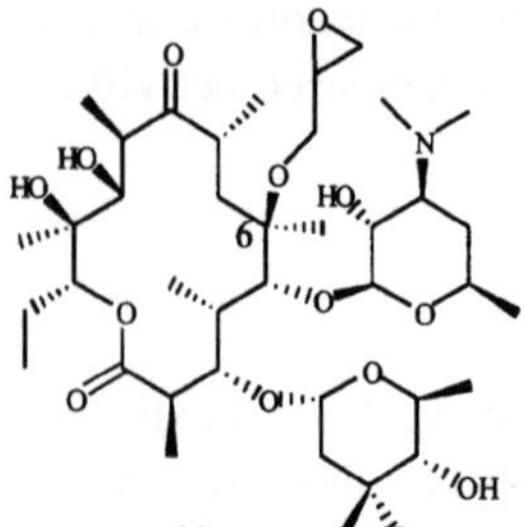

28

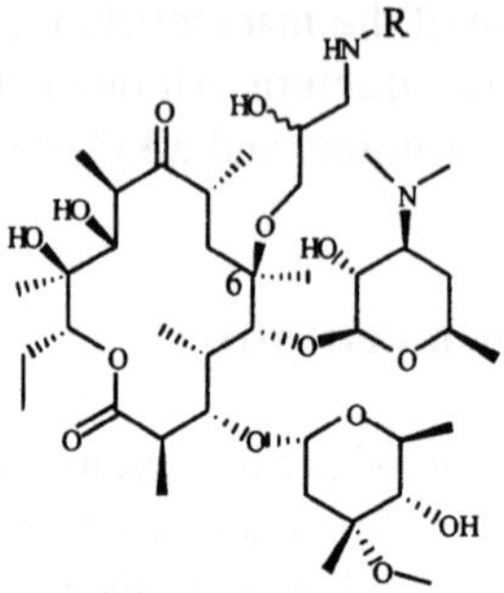

29a R = benzyl
29b R = phenethyl

Compound **26b** also was converted to the corresponding epoxide (**28**), which was further derivatized to a series of aminol analogs (**29a-b**). Although the benzyl analog (**29a**) was less active than clarithromycin, the phenethyl analog (**29b**) was as active as clarithromycin against erythromycin-susceptible strains and more active against MLS_B-resistant bacteria with MIC at 32 μg/ml.

As a versatile intermediate, **26b** was also converted to the corresponding aldehyde (**30**) by ozonolysis. Oximation of **30** provided a series of oximes (**31a-c**), and reactions of **30** with hydrazines provided a series of hydrazones (**32a-b**). All the oxime and hydrazone analogs showed similar or weaker activity than clarithromycin with the exception of compound **31c**, which was as active as

Figure 12.

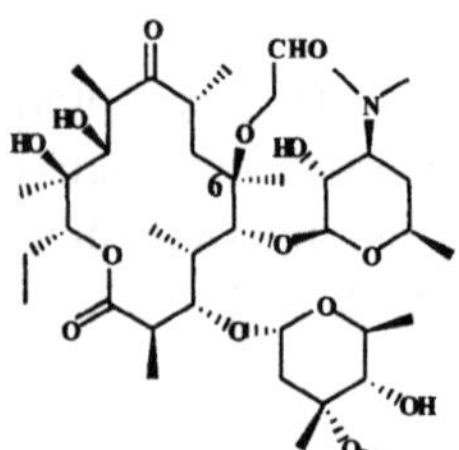

30

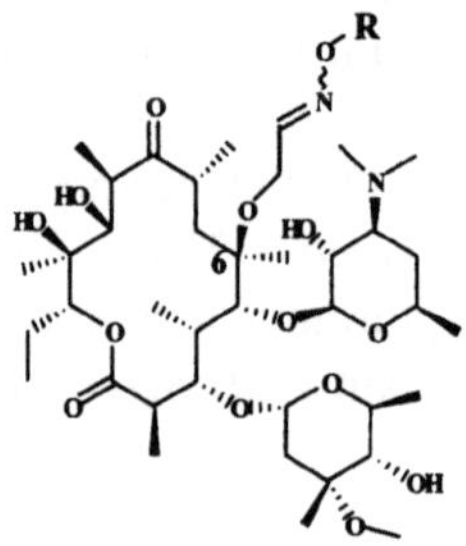

31a R = hydrogen
31b R = methyl
31c R = phenyl

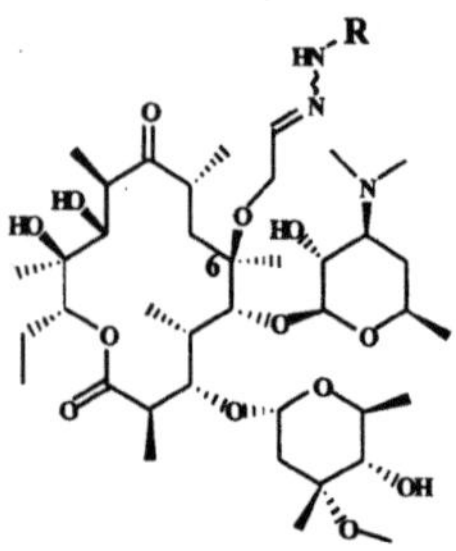

32a R = methyl
32b R = (2-pyridyl)

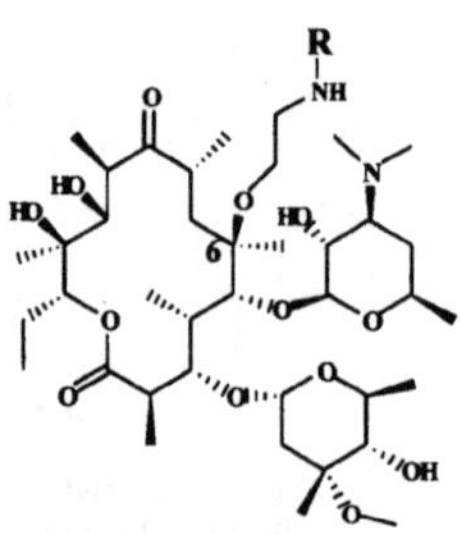

33a R = benzyl
33b R = phenethyl
33c R = 3-phenylpropyl

clarithromycin against susceptible strains and weakly active against MLS_B-resistant strains (MIC 128 μg/ml). Reductive amination of **30** provided a series of amines (**33a-c**) with various chain lengths. Analogs with two and three carbon spacers (**33b** and **33c**) between the phenyl and the amino groups exhibited the best activity against susceptible strains. Among these analogs, compound **33b** gave the best activity against MLS_B-resistant organisms (MIC 64 μg/ml).

6-O-substituted ketolides

To address the increasing antibiotic resistance problem, a novel series of ketolides currently is being developed at Abbott [23]. Based on structure-activity relationship studies, three structural features were identified as key elements for overcoming MLS_B and efflux resistance, which included an aryl group appropriately attached to the lactone ring, a keto group at C-3 position, and an appropriately constrained macrolide conformation.

A series of 6-O-substituted ketolides first was reported in 1998 [24], which included some of the above features. Ketolide **34** first was prepared as a key intermediate for preparing other analogs. Heck coupling reactions of **34** with aryl halides provided a series of (3-aryl)prop-2-enyl analogs (**35a-e**). Conversion of the allyl group to aldehyde **36** followed by reductive amination provided a series of amino analogs (**37a-e**). Compared with the corresponding 6-O-substituted erythromycin analogs, these ketolides were generally less active against erythromycin-susceptible strains except for the (3-quinolyl)prop-2-enyl analog (**35e**), which possessed activity similar to its full macrolide counterpart (**27c**). However, these ketolide analogs showed improved activity against various erythromycin-resistant bacteria. As with the 6-O-substituted erythromycin derivatives, ketolide analogs with an aryl group attached to the C-6 position also showed improved activity against MLS_B-resistant strains. In addition, these analogs exhibited improved activity against inducibly MLS_B-resistant *S. aureus* and efflux resistance. The most active compound of this group, **35e**, gave MICs of 0.2 and 0.25 μg/ml against inducibly MLS_B-resistant *S. aureus* and efflux resistant *S. pneumoniae,* respectively, as compared with 6.2 and 16 μg/ml for erythromycin.

The antibacterial activity of the 6-O-substituted ketolides was greatly enhanced when a 11,12-cyclic carbamate group was introduced [23]. The 6-O-(3-quinolyl)prop-2-enyl-11,12-carbamate ketolide (**38**, ABT-773) showed excellent, well-balanced antibacterial profiles against both susceptible and resistant organisms. ABT-773 provided further improved activity against erythromycin-susceptible *S. aureus*, *S. pyogenes,* and *S. pneumoniae* with MICs at 0.05, < 0.004, and < 0.004 μg/ml, respectively, as compared with 0.2, 0.2, and 0.03 μg/ml for compound **35e**. Furthermore, ABT-773 exhibited remarkably enhanced activity against MLS_B-resistant *S. pyogenes* and *S. pneumoniae,* with MICs at 1 and 0.25 μg/ml as compare with 100 and 128 μg/ml for **35e**. The corresponding carbazate (**39**) and tricyclic (**40**) analogs were very potent against susceptible strains but were less active against MLS_B-resistant strains, with MICs at 16 to 64 μg/ml. All the

Figure 13.

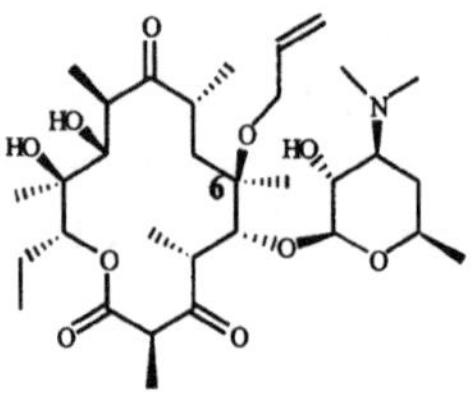

34

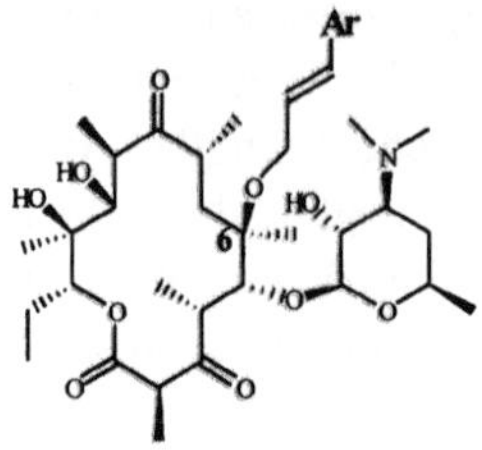

35a Ar = phenyl
35b Ar = 4-fluorophenyl
35c Ar = 4-chlorophenyl
35d Ar = 4-methoxylphenyl
35e Ar = 3-quinolyl

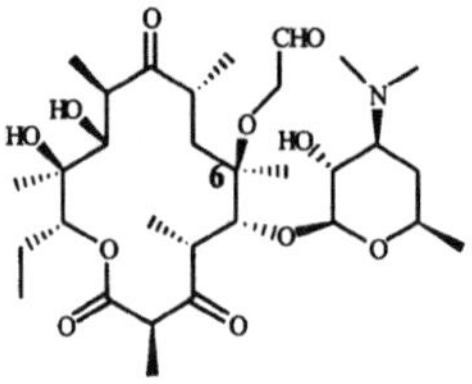

36

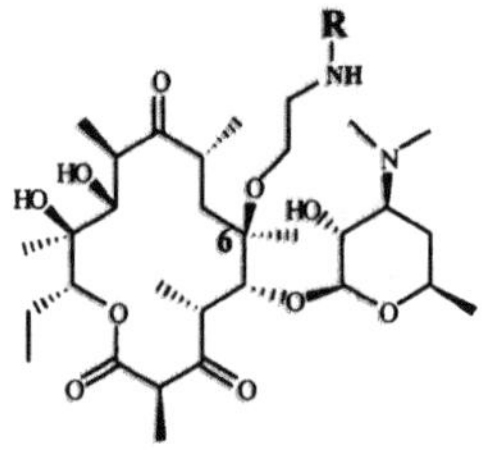

37a Ar = hydrogen
37b Ar = benzyl
37c Ar = phenethyl
37d Ar = (4-pyridyl)methyl
37e Ar = (4-quinolyl)methyl

possible quinolyl regioisomers of **38** were prepared (**41a-f**). The connecting position on quinoline was found to be very important for optimal antibacterial activity, especially against MLS_B-resistant organisms. In addition to the 3-quinolyl analog (**38**), the 6-quinolyl isomer (**41d**) also demonstrated excellent overall antibacterial activity.

The above results indicated that an aryl group linked to the C-6 position was the key element for overcoming MLS_B-resistance, while the 3-keto group provided activity against inducible and efflux resistance. These structural features in combination with a 11,12-carbamate group provided a series of potent analogs highly active against both erythromycin-susceptible and -resistant bacteria.

Profiles of ABT-773

ABT-773 is currently under clinical development for the treatment of respiratory tract infections. Preclinical studies indicated that ABT-773 was superior to all reference macrolides and ketolides against variety of susceptible and resistant respiratory pathogens [25]. As indicated in Table 2, both ABT-773 and telithromycin (HMR-3647) showed significantly improved activity as compared with erythromycin. Furthermore, ABT-773 exhibited better activity than telithromycin against resistant *S. pnuemoniae* and *S. pyogenes*, two key respiratory pathogens.

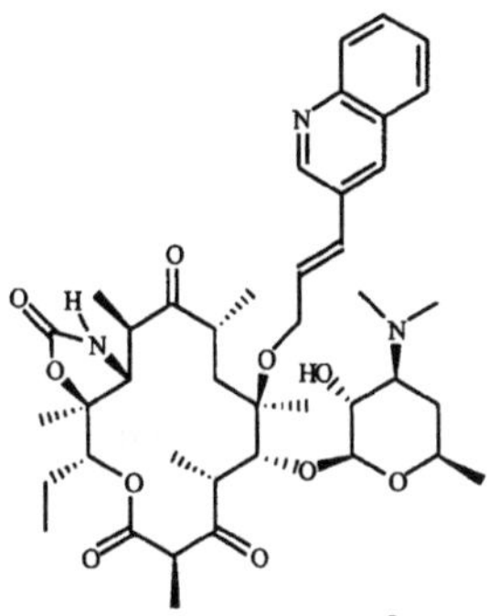

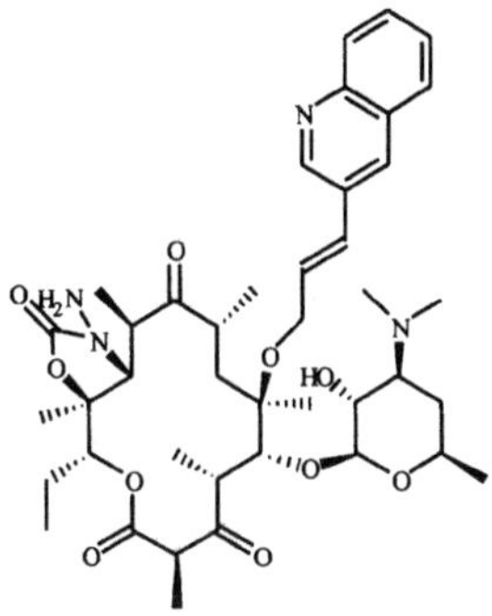

Figure 14.

38 (ABT-773)

39

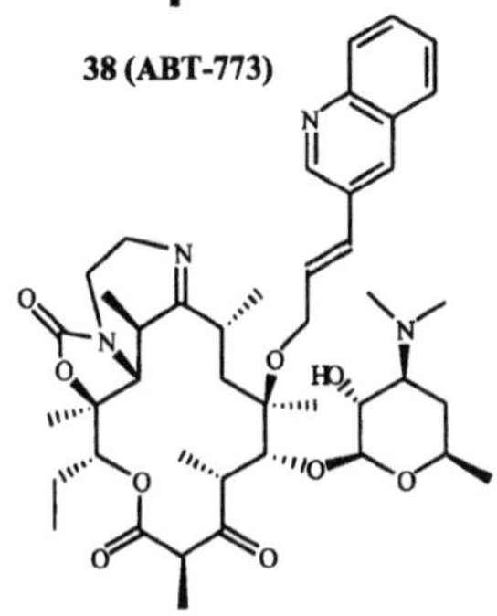

40

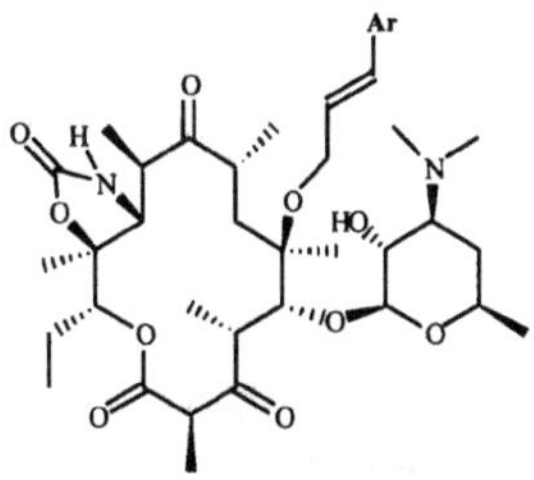

41a Ar = 2-quinolyl
41b Ar = 4-quinolyl
41c Ar = 5-quinolyl
41d Ar = 6-quinolyl
41e Ar = 7-quinolyl
41f Ar = 8-quinolyl

Table 2. Comparison of *in vitro* antibacterial activity (MIC_{90} in µg/ml).

Organism			Compound		
			ABT-773	HMR-3647	Erythromycin
S. pneumoniae	Susceptible	(N = 94)	0.002	0.008	0.06
S. pnuemoniae	Resistant-*mef*	(N = 100)	0.12	1.0	8.0
S. pnuemoniae	Resistant-*erm*	(N = 104)	0.015	0.12	> 32.0
S. pyogenes	Resistant-*mef*	(N = 60)	0.12	1.0	8.0
S. pyogenes	Resistant-*erm*	(N = 30)	0.5	> 8.0	> 32.0
M. catarrhalis		(N = 94)	0.25	0.25	0.5
H. influenzae		(N = 94)	2.0	2.0	8.0
S. aureus	Susceptible	(N = 60)	0.03	0.06	1.0
S. aureus	Resistant-MLS_B-c	(N = 37)	> 128.0	> 128.0	> 128.0

Interestingly, none of the ketolides was active against constitutively MLS_B-resistant *S. aureus*.

ABT-773 demonstrated excellent *in vivo* efficacy in mouse protection test and rat lung infection model [26]. In mouse protection tests, ABT-773 demonstrated improved efficacy against macrolide-susceptible strains as compared with azithromycin and telithromycin (Tab. 3). In rat lung infection models, ABT-773

Table 3. Comparison of *in vivo* efficacy-mouse protection test (ED_{50}, mg/kg).

Compound	*S. aureus* 10649[a] ED_{50}	*S. pneumoniae* 6303[a] ED_{50}	*S. pyogenes* C203[a] ED_{50}
ABT-773	10.4	12.5	2.5
HMR3647	12.5	34.1	
Azithromycin	24.8	18.8	6.1

[a]*S. aureus* 10649, *S. pyogenes* C203, and *S. pneumoniae* 6303 are erythromycin-susceptible strains.

Table 4. Comparison of *in vivo* efficacy in rat lung infection models (ED_{50}, mg/kg/d).

Compound	*S. pneumoniae* 6303[a] ED_{50}	*S. pneumoniae* 5649[a] ED_{50}	*S. pneumoniae* 6396[a] ED_{50}
ABT-773	< 0.63	7.0	1.6
HMR3647	2.3	25.8	26.7
Azithromycin	6.0	78.7	> 100.0

[a]*S. pneumoniae* 6303 is an erythromycin-susceptible strain, *S. pneumoniae* 5649 is an efflux-resistant strain, and *S. pneumoniae* 6396 is a MLS_B-resistant strain.

showed substantially better efficacy than both telithromycin and azithromycin against a macrolide-susceptible strain, *S. pneumoniae* 6303 (Tab. 4). Against infections caused by an efflux resistant strain, *S. pneumoniae* 5649, ABT-773 exhibited a 3-fold improvement in efficacy over telithromycin and a 10-fold improvement over azithromycin. Against infections caused by an MLS_B-resistant strain, *S. pneumoniae* 6396, ABT-773 demonstrated excellent efficacy, while telithromycin showed weaker efficacy and azithromycin showed no efficacy under 100 mg/kg/d dose.

The pharmacokinetic profile of ABT-773 was evaluated in cynomolgus monkey, beagle dog, sprague-dawley rat, and CD-1 mouse [27]. ABT-773 distributed rapidly after intravenous dosing with terminal elimination half lives at 1.6, 4.5, 3.0, and 5.9 h in mouse, rat, monkey, and dog, respectively. Volume of distribution values ranged from 2.5 L/kg in dog to 9.2 L/kg in rat. After oral dosing, ABT-773 was slowly absorbed. Peak plasma concentration averaged at 1.47, 0.52, 0.56, and 0.84 mg/ml with oral bioavailabilities of 49.5%, 60.0%, 35.8%, and 44.1% in mouse, rat, monkey, and dog, respectively. ABT-773 was highly concentrated in lung tissue with over 25-fold higher lung concentrations than plasma concentrations after oral dosing in rat.

Conclusion

Current macrolide research has been focused on the development of novel derivatives that are active against resistant bacteria. The new-generation macrolides, particularly the ketolide derivatives, have been found to be successful against most resistant strains with the exception of MLS_B-resistant *S. aureus*. Future research in this area will be directed at the discovery of new macrolides with potent activity against MLS_B-resistant *S. aureus* and *H. influenzae* and improved pharmacokinetic/pharmacodynamic profiles.

References

1 a) Kurath P, Jones P, Egan R, Perun T (1971) Acid degradation of erythromycin A and erythromycin B. *Experienta* 27: 362. (b) Krowicki K, Zamojski A (1974) Chemical modifications of erythromycins I. 8,9-anhydro-6,9-hemiketal of erythromycin A. *J Antibiotics* 26: 569–574

2 Itoh Z, Nakaya K, Suzuki H, Arai H, Wakabayashi K (1984) Erythromycin mimics exogenous motilin in gastrointestinal contractile activity in the dog. *Am J Physiol* 247: G688–G694

3 Morimoto S, Takahashi Y, Wantanabe Y, Omura S (1984) Chemical modification of erythromycins I. Synthesis and antibacterial activity of 6-O-methylerythromycin A. *J Antibiotics* 37: 187–189

4 Bright GM, Nagel AA, Bordner J, Desai KA, Dibrino JN, Nowakowska J, Vincent L, Watrous RM, Sciavolino FC, English AR et al (1988) Synthesis, *in vitro* and *in vivo* activity of novel 9-deoxo-9a-aza-9a-homoerythromycin A derivatives; a new class of macrolides antibiotics. *J Antibiotics* 41: 1029–1047

5 a) Chantot JF, Bryskier A, Gasc JC (1986) Antibacterial activity of roxithromycin: a laboratory evaluation. *J. Antibiotics* 39: 660–668 (b) Gasc JC, Gouin d'Ambrieres S, Lutz A, Chantot JF (1991) New ether oxime of erythromycin A; a structure activity relationship study. *J Antibiotics* 44: 313–330

6 Kirst HA, Wind JA, Leeds JP, Willard KE, Debono M, Bonjouklian R, Greene JM, Sullivan KA, Paschal JW, Deeter JB et al (1990) Synthesis and structure-activity relationships of new 9-N-alkyl derivatives of 9(S)-erythromycylamine. *J Med Chem* 33: 3086–3094

7 For recent reviews, see: (a) Chu DTW (1999) Recent progress in novel macrolides, quinolones, and 2-pyridones to overcome bacterial resistance. *Med Res Rev* 19(6): 497–520 (b) Bryskier A (1999) New research in macrolides and ketolides since 1997. *Exp Opin Invest Drugs* 8(8): 1171–1194 (c) Bryskier A (1997) Novelties in the field of macrolides. *Exp Opin Invest Drugs* 6: 1697–1709 (d) Chu DTW (1995) Recent developments in 14- and 15-membered macrolides. *Exp Opin Invest Drugs 4(2)*: 65–94

8 a) Baker WR, Clark JD, Stephens RL, Kim KH (1988) Modification of macrolide antibiotics. Synthesis of 11-deoxy-11-(carboxyamino)-6-O-methylerythromycin A 11,12-(cyclic ester) *via* an intramolecular Michael reaction of O-carbamates with an α,β-unsaturated ketone. *J Org Chem 53*: 2340–2345 (b) Fernandes PB, Baker WR, Freiberg LA, Hardy DJ, McDonald ED (1989) New macrolides active against *Streptococcus pyogenes* with inducible or constitutive type of macrolide-lincosamide-streptogramin B resistance. *Antimicrob Agents Chemother* 33: 78–81

9 Neszmelyi A, Bojanska-Dahlig H (1978) A carbon-13 relaxation studies of erythromycin A cyclic 11,12-carbonate. *J Antibiotics* 31: 478

10 Agouridas C, Denis A, Auger JM, Benedetti Y, Bonnefoy A, Bretin F, Chantot JF, Dussarat A, Fromentin C, et al. (1998) Synthesis and antibacterial activity of ketolides (6-O-methyl-3-oxoerythromycin derivatives): A new class of antibacterials highly potent against macrolide-resistant and -susceptible respiratory pathogens. *J Med Chem* 41: 4080–4100

11 For earlier works, see: Daniel T. W. Chu , reference 7 d.

12 Elliott RL, Pireh D, Nilius AM, Johnson PM, Flamm RK, Chu DTW, Plattner JJ, Or YS (1997) Novel 3-deoxy-3-descladinosyl-6-O-methyl erythromycin A analogues. Synthesis and *in vitro* activity. *Bioorg & Med Chem Lett* 7(5): 641–646

13 Elliott RL, Pireh D, Griesgraber G, Nilius AM, Ewing PJ, Bui MH, Raney PM, Flamm RK, Kim K, Henry RF, Chu DTW, Plattner JJ, Or YS (1998) Anhydrolide Macrolides. 1. Synthesis and antibacterial activity of 2,3-anhydro-6-O-methyl 11,12-carbamate erythromycin A analogues. *J Med Chem* 41: 1651

14 Griesgraber G, Kramer MJ, Elliott RL, Nilius AM, Ewing PJ, Raney PM, Bui MH, Flamm RK, Chu DTW, Plattner JJ, Or YS (1998) Anhydrolide Macrolides. 2. Synthesis and antibacterial activity of 2,3-anhydro-6-O-methyl 11,12-carbazate erythromycin A analogues. *J Med Chem* 41:1660

15 The C-10 epimers of the carbazate ketolide series were also inactive. Griesgraber G, Or YS, Chu DTW, Nilius AM, Johnson PM, Flamm RK, Henry RF, Plattner JJ (1996) 3-Keto-11,12-cabazate derivatives of 6-O-methylerythromycin A. Synthesis and *in-vitro* activity. *J Antibiotic* 49: 465

16 Asaka T, Kashimura M, Misawa Y, Ono T, Suzuki K, Yoshida H, Yoshida T, Akashi T, Yokoo C, Nagate T, Morimoto S (1995) A New Macrolide Antibiotic, TE-802; Synthesis and Biological Properties. 35th Interscience Conference on Antimicrobial Agents and Chemotherapy, abstract No. F176

17 Phan LT, Or YS, Spina KP, Chen Y, Tufano M, Chu DTW, Nilius AM, Bui MH, Plattner JJ (1997) Tricyclic Ketolides: Mono-substitution on the Imine Ring. Synthesis and *in-Vitro* Activity. 37th Interscience Conference on Antimicrobial Agents and Chemotherapy, abstract No. F-263

18 Phan LT, Or YS, Spina KP, Chen Y, Tufano M, Chu DTW, Nilius AM, Bui MH, Plattner JJ (1997) Tetracyclic Ketolides: A New Antibacterial Macrolides. Synthesis and *in-Vitro* Activity. 37th Interscience Conference on Antimicrobial Agents and Chemotherapy, abstract No. F-264

19 Phan LT, Or YS, Chen Y, Chu DTW, Nilius AM, Bui MH, Patti R, Hensey-Rudloff D, Henry RF, Mitten M, Plattner JJ (1998) 2-Substituted Tricyclic Ketolides: New Antibacterial Macrolides. Synthesis and Biological Activity. 38th Interscience Conference on Antimicrobial Agents and Chemotherapy, abstract No. F-127

20 Morimoto S, Misawa Y, Adachi T, Nagate T, Watanabe Y, Omura S (1990) Chemical Modification of Erythromycin II. Synthesis and antibacterial activity of *O*-alkyl derivative of erythromycin A. *J Antibiotics* 43: 286–305

21 Watanabe Y, Morimoto S, Adachi S, Kashimura M, Asaka T (1993) Chemical modification of erythromycins. IX. Selective methylation at the C-6 hydroxyl group of erythromycin A oxime derivatives and preparation of clarithromycin. *J Antibiotics* 46: 647–660

22 Clark RF, Ma Z, Wang S, Griesgraber G, Tufano M, Yong H, Li L, Zhang X, Nilius A, Chu DTW, Or YS (2000) Synthesis and antibacterial activity of novel 6-O-substituted erythromycin A derivatives. *Bioorg Med Chem Lett* 10:815–819

23 a) Ma Z, Clark RF, Wang S, Nilius AM, Flamm RK, Or YS (1999) Design, synthesis and characterization of ABT-773: A novel ketolide highly active against multidrug resistant Pathogens. 39th Interscience Conference on Antimicrobial Agents and Chemotherapy, abstract No. 2133 (b) Or YS, Clark RF, Wang S, Chu DTW, Nilius AM, Flamm RK, Mitten M, Ewing P, Ma Z (2000) Design, synthesis and antimicrobial activity of 6-O-substituted ketolides active against resistant respiratory tract pathogens. *J Med Chem* 43: 1045–1049

24 Ma Z, Or YS, Clark RF, Wang S, Brazzale A, Yong H, Tufano M, Nilius AM, Bui MH, Raney P, Flamm RK, Chu DTW, Plattner JJ (1998) Synthesis and antibacterial activity of 6-O-substituted ketolides. 38th Interscience Conference on Antimicrobial Agents and Chemotherapy, abstract No. F126

25 Shortridge D, Ramer NC, Beyer J, Ma Z, Or Y, Flamm RK (1999) The *in vitro* activity of ABT-773 against gram-positive and gram-negative pathogens. 39th Interscience Conference on Antimicrobial Agents and Chemotherapy, abstract No. 2136

26 a) Mitten M, Meulbroek J, Paige L, Alder J, Ewing P, Molison KW, Nilius AM, Flamm RK, Ma Z, Or YS (1999) Efficacies of ABT-773 and HMR-3647 against respiratory pathogens causing acute systemic infections in mice and lung infections in rats. 39th Interscience Conference on Antimicrobial Agents and Chemotherapy, abstract No. 2150 (b) Meulbroek J, Mitten M, Molison KW, Ewing P, Alder J, Nilius AM, Flamm RK, Ma Z, Or YS (1999) Efficacies of ABT-773 and

azithromycin against experimental rat lung infections caused by *Streptococcus pneumoniae*. 39th Interscience Conference on Antimicrobial Agents and Chemotherapy, abstract No. 2151
27 Hernandez L, Sadrzadeh N, Krill S, Ma Z, Marsh K (1999) Preclinical pharmacokinetic profile of ABT-773 in mouse, rat, monkey and dog. 39th Interscience Conference on Antimicrobial Agents and Chemotherapy, abstract No. 2148

Macrolide Antibiotics
ed. by W. Schönfeld and H. A. Kirst

Polyketide diversity

Leonard Katz

Kosan Biosciences Inc., 3832 Bay Center Place, Hayward, CA 94611, USA

Polyketides are natural products made by bacteria, fungi and plants, that have gained widespread use in human medicine (antibacterials, antifungals, anticancers, immunosuppressants), veterinary medicine (anthelmintics), and agriculture (insecticides). The term was coined by Collie in 1907 to describe compounds that were composed of units containing multiple "ketide" (-CH_2-CO-) groups which, as building blocks, either could persist in the final structure or be modified during their biosynthesis [1]. The modification of either carbon center of the ketide unit is the basis for the large and structurally diverse array of compounds that are classified as polyketides.

Polyketides in general can be separated into two groups. The aromatic polyketides contain two or more aromatic rings that are formed through internal aldol condensations of the folded polyketide chain. For this event to occur, the polyketide chain is largely unreduced and can be thought of as a polyketone. Compounds of this type include the tetracycline class of antibiotics, the antitumor agent doxorubicin, and the mycotoxins. Structural diversity of this group is generated through differences in chain length (and hence the number of aromatic rings), folding patterns leading to aromatization, reductions (although only a modest number of reductions per molecule are seen), and post-polyketide modifications including oxidation, methylation, and glycosidation. This chapter does not deal with the aromatic polyketides, but they have been the subject of numerous reviews [2–4].

The second and much larger group generally is called the complex or reduced polyketides, wherein the ketide units are largely in reduced form. Reduction prevents internal aldol condensations, yielding long acyl chains that often are cyclized through the formation of ester linkages. In contrast to the aromatic polyketides, which largely are built on acetyl units, the ketide units in the complex polyketides are not restricted to two-carbon compounds but include three- and four-carbon compounds, as well as a three-carbon unit that contains a hydroxyl function. As will be described in the next section, each unit contributes two carbons to the chain, leaving the remaining moieties as methyl, ethyl, or hydroxymethyl side chains. The selected employment of the various ketide units, along with the stereochemistry imparted to the side chains, contributes to structural diversity. Polyketide synthesis also employs a starter ketide unit that can be selected from a large number of carboxylic acids. Finally, the complex polyketides can undergo various modifications including, as noted above for the aromatics, oxidation, methylation, and glycosidation, as well as decarboxylation, reduction, and dehydration. Some polyketides have peptide units contained within. The structures of representative complex polyketides, underscoring the extensive diversity of the class, are shown in Figure 1. This chapter will be concerned in large part with the structural diversity produced from manipulation of the polyketide backbone. Diversity also can be achieved by manipulation of the various glycosidations that take place on a number of polyketide cores [5, 6].

Though polyketides have been described for over a century and continue to be

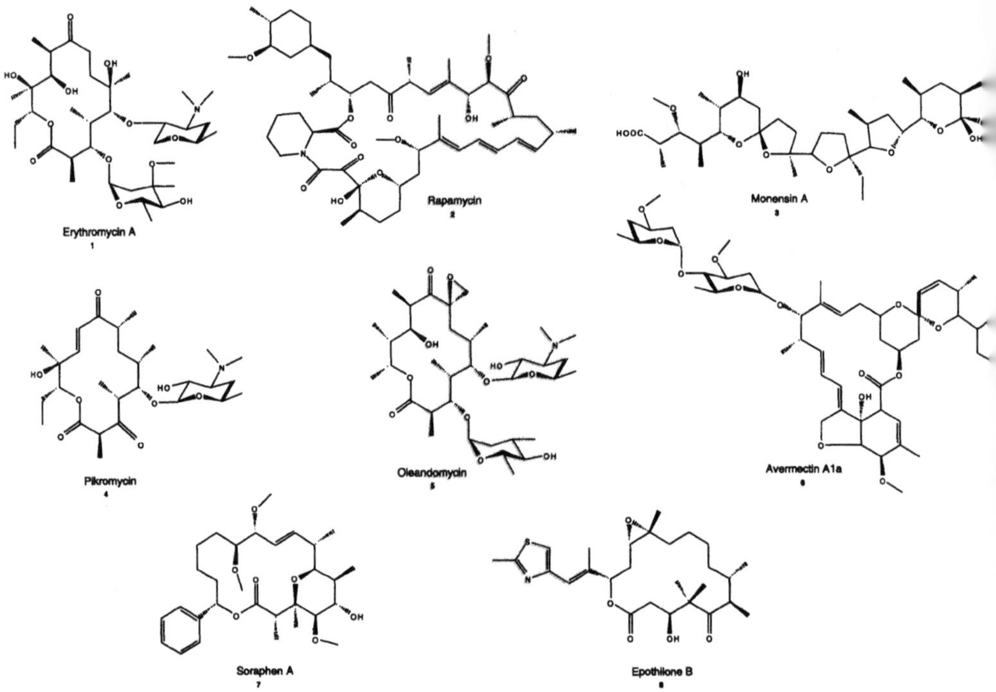

Figure 1. Structures of various complex polyketides..

discovered, it is only in the past 10 years that an understanding of the biochemical basis for diversity has been gained. This understanding has been achieved largely through efforts to determine the nucleotide sequences of the genes controlling the biosynthesis of these compounds. At present, the biosynthesis genes of close to two dozen compounds of this class, including all the molecules shown in Figure 1 (except **3**), have been sequenced in whole or in part. What has emerged is that complex polyketides share a remarkably common mechanism of synthesis, which permits the diversity of structures seen. The chemical, genetic and biochemical basis of complex polyketide synthesis is described in the next section. The understanding of the genetics and biochemistry of polyketide synthesis, along with the advancements of genetic technology in the organisms that produce polyketides, mainly bacteria belonging the actinomycetes family, also has permitted manipulation of polyketide structure by genetic intervention in the laboratory. The succeeding sections of this chapter deal with these approaches, first as single changes and then in combinatorial fashion.

Synthesis of complex polyketides

Polyketides are synthesized in an iterative manner as described in Figure 2. Chain growth is initiated through the condensation of a starter unit with an extender unit. Since the entire process takes place on the enzyme system termed a polyketide synthase (PKS), the units are shown in the enzyme-bound state, but the nature of their interaction with the PKS will be described below. The starter (with few exceptions) and extender units (with no exceptions) are present in the host as Coenzyme A thioesters. In the scheme shown in Figure 2, the starter is the C_3 unit propionyl-CoA (**9**), but acetyl-CoA, 2-methylbutyryl-CoA, and 3,4-dihydroxycyclohexane carboxylic acid (**18–20**) are used as starters in **5**, **6** and **2** (Fig. 1), respectively. **20** is not thought to be in the CoA form when loaded on the rapamycin PKS [7]. 3-Amino-5-hydroxybenzoyl-CoA (**21**) is the starter for rifamycin biosynthesis [8, 9], and benzoyl-CoA (**22**) is used to start synthesis of **7** [10]. In Figure 2, 2-methylmalonyl-CoA (**10**) is the extender used, but malonyl-

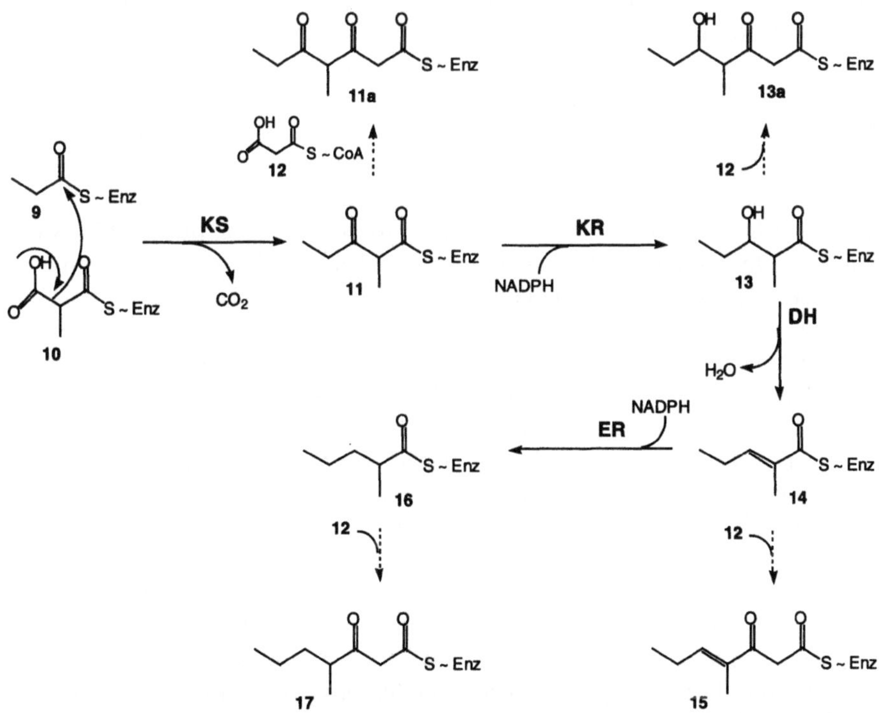

Figure 2. Chemical scheme for synthesis of complex polyketides. Abbreviations as in Figure 4.

CoA (**12**; Figure 2) is commonly used in many polyketides, and 2-ethylmalonyl-CoA (**23**) is seen in **3** and many 16-membered ring polyketides. **7** (Fig. 1) employs 2-hydroxymalonyl-CoA (**24**) [or 2-methoxymalonyl-CoA (**25**)] in 2 places, **10** in 3 places, and **12** in 2 places of the polyketide chain. Though **10**, **23**, **24**, and **25** can exist in the 2-*S* and 2-*R* forms, it has been established only for the synthesis of **1** that only the 2-*S* form of **10** is employed in each of the six condensations [11].

The condensation between **9** and **10** is driven by decarboxylation of **10** and breakage of the thioester linkage of **9** to the enzyme. The enzymatic component of the PKS that conducts the condensation and the decarboxylation is the β-acyl ACP synthase [12, 13], abbreviated ketosynthase or KS. At the start of the reaction, **9** is attached to a cysteine residue in the KS through a thioester linkage. The extender unit is attached to an acyl carrier protein (ACP) domain of the PKS through a thioester linkage to a phosphopantetheine moiety attached to a serine residue. Other than carrying the extender unit and the subsequent diketide, the ACP has not been shown to possess any enzymatic function. The decarboxylative condensation resembles the Claisen condensation employed in the synthesis of fatty acids by the analogous enzyme, fatty acid synthase. Thus, the resulting diketide, **11**, has been formed through extension of the extender unit that stays attached to the ACP.

A choice of two fates awaits **11**. It can undergo β-ketoreduction to yield **13**, which contains a β-hydroxyl group. This is dependent upon the presence of a β-ketoreductase function (KR) that can act upon **11** at the time of its synthesis. If a functional KR is not present, **11** will then undergo a new round of condensation employing a new extender (shown in Figure 2 as malonyl-CoA; **12**). Mechanistically, this resembles the condensation between **9** and **10** except that **11** replaces **9** as the "starter". The triketide formed, **11a**, therefore, contains a δ-ketone, which will persist throughout the succeeding rounds of synthesis and be present in the final product. If **13** is produced, it again is faced with two pathways. If a dehydratase (DH) function capable of acting on **13** is present, it will produce **14**. If the particular DH function is not present in the PKS, **13** will undergo a new round of condensation, yielding **13a**, which carries a δ-hydroxyl group that will be maintained throughout the succeeding rounds of polyketide chain growth. Similarly, if **14** is produced, it will undergo the next step in the reduction cycle, enoylreduction, if the required enoylreductase (ER) function is present to yield **16**, which contains a fully reduced β-carbon. If not, **14** will undergo a new round of condensation resulting in **15**, which will carry the γ,δ-double bond through to the end of the synthesis. If **16** is formed, its only fate is to enter a new round of synthesis. The δ-methylene group will appear at the corresponding position in the final compound. The compound formed from the second condensation, either **11a**, **13a**, **15**, or **17**, will be subject to its degree of reduction dependent upon the presence of the KR, DH, and ER activities that act on the triketide. The reductive fate of the triketide, be it full, partial, or no reduction, does not depend upon the reductive fate of the diketide formed in the prior round of condensation or what will happen to the tetra-, penta-, and hexaketides formed in subsequent condensations. Furthermore, the use of a given extender unit for a given condensation is determined by the specificity of the acyltransferase (AT) function for that condensation cycle only.

The wide latitude in the starters and extenders that can be used by the various PKSs enables the variety of structures that can be made. However, because a PKS only makes a single molecule (in a specific instance, two molecules), in order to ensure fidelity of synthesis, a specific extender is employed and the fate of the resulting β-carbonyl is fixed for each cycle. The polyketide synthase, therefore, must be able to distinguish one condensation/reduction cycle from another and to determine the correct number of cycles to take place. Thus, PKSs are programmed to act faithfully and uniquely at each cycle of synthesis.

Modular polyketide synthases

Information on the nature of PKSs has come mainly from nucleotide sequencing of the corresponding genes. Sequencing of a number of PKS genes has shown that they are large (5 kilobases and up), that the genes contain a number of segments that appear to be repeated (*i. e.,* encode similar functions), and that the number of repeated segments corresponds overall to the number of condensation cycles required to build the molecule. The repeated segments have been termed modules [14]. Each module contains the functional domains responsible for 1) selection of the correct extender unit (AT), 2) the decarboxylative condensation event (KS, ACP), and 3) the reduction of the β-carbonyl formed from the condensation (KR/DH/ER). The first and best-studied example of a modular PKS is 6-deoxyerythronolide B synthase (DEBS) that assembles the polyketide component of **1**. As shown in Figure 4, DEBS is composed of 6 modules, each responsible for the condensation and β-carbonyl processing of a single cycle of 6-deoxyerythronolide B (**31**) synthesis. The PKS is divided into three polypeptide subunits [15, 16]. Each subunit carries two modules; DEBS 1 has an additional loading module. Since each protein, therefore, carries a number of functional domains, DEBS is

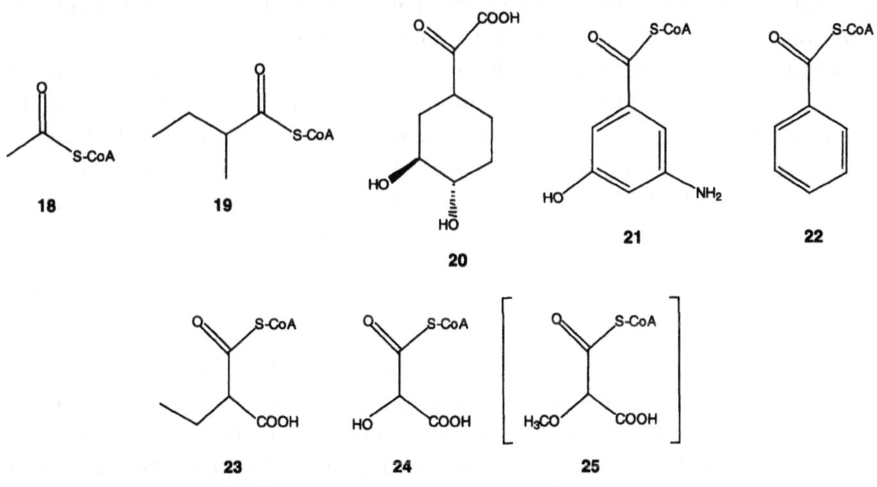

Figure 3. Structures of compounds commonly used to start (**18–22**) and extend (**23 – 25**) the synthesis of complex polyketides.

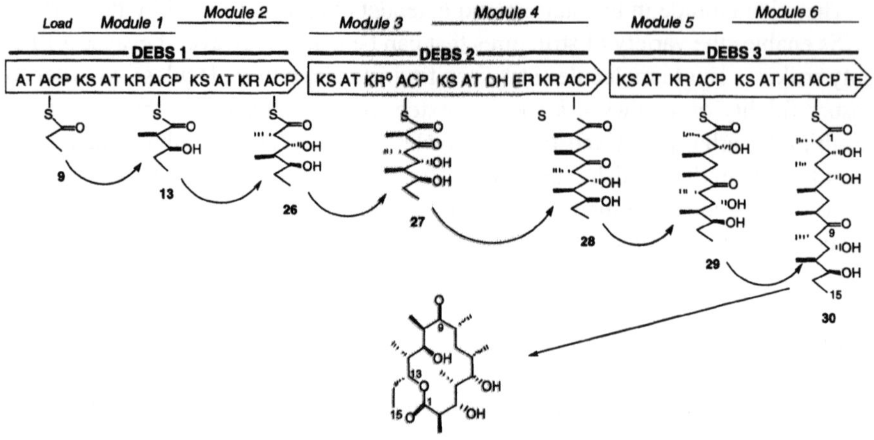

Figure 4. Modular organization of the deoxyerythronolide B synthase (DEBS). Structures attached to the ACP domains are shown to illustrate the pathway of synthesis. Completion of synthesis produces **31**. Abbreviations: KS – β-ketoacyl ACP synthase (ketosynthase); AT – acyltransferase; DH – dehydratase; ER – enoylreductase; KR – ketoreductase; KR° – inactive ketoreductase; TE – thioesterase..

classified as a type I PKS. In DEBS, each of the 6 AT domains binds 2-*S*-methylmalonyl CoA (**10**); the loading module AT binds propionyl-CoA (**9**) normally [17] but also can bind butyryl-CoA and to a lesser extent acetyl-CoA [18, 19]. Synthesis of **31** occurs with the loading of **9** and **10** to the AT domains of the loading module and module 1, respectively, and their subsequent transacylation to the cognate ACP domains. The propionyl thioester is then transacylated to KS1 where it undergoes decarboxylative condensation with **10** attached to the ACP of module 1 (ACP1) to yield a diketide. The β-carbonyl of the diketide then undergoes reduction carried out by the KR1 domain to form **13**. Because no additional functions exist in module 1, **13** represents the end of the first cycle. It is then transferred to KS2, which undergoes condensation with another molecule of **10** attached to ACP2 through attachment and transacylation by AT2. Again, because only a KR domain is present in module 2, β-ketoreduction of the triketide takes place to form **26**. The next step involves transfer to KS3, which requires movement from DEBS/1 to DEBS/2. How the PKS moves the acyl chain to the correct domain is not understood, but it must be based on the correct juxtapositioning of the ACP and KS domains. Once the tetraketide is formed, the β-carbonyl does not undergo reduction because of the absence of a functional KR domain in module 3. Thus, the β-keto group in **27** persists through the subsequent rounds of condensation and appears at C_9 of the product **31**. Module 4 contains a full set of reduction domains; the β-carbonyl of the pentaketide formed from the fourth condensation undergoes β-ketoreduction, dehydration, and enoylreduction to yield **28**. The β-methylene group persists through subsequent chain growth to end as the C_7 methylene in **31**. In modules 5 and 6, only β-ketoreduction takes place after each condensation. A thioesterase (TE) domain resides at the end of module 6 that releases the acyl chain from the enzyme and probably is responsible for the subsequent cyclization to form the macrolactone **31**. The stereochemistry of the hydroxyl groups is determined by the cognate KR domains [20, 21]. What determines the stereochemistry of the methyl side chains in **31** is not fully understood, but this function is believed to reside in the presence (or absence) of an epimerase function that lies within or adjacent to the KS domains [22].

Although the general scheme of the modular PKS architecture and function shown in Figure 4 is maintained in all of the more than 20 modular PKSs examined, some variations have been found and are summarized here. First, though not shown, the linear order of the utilization of the modules is matched at the gene level for DEBS. Co-linearity of modules between the genes and biochemical order does not hold in a number of PKSs, although all PKSs have a loading module and most have a thioesterase. Secondly, the loading domain of the rapamycin (rap) PKS does not contain an AT domain but has a segment that corresponds to an adenosylmonophosphate (AMP)-ligase. It is thought that the starter, 20 – a cyclohexenyl derivative of a carboxylic acid, is converted into an adenylate by the ligase domain and then transferred to the ACP domain of the loading module to initiate polyketide synthesis [7]. Finally, a significant difference among the various PKSs lies in the number of modules carried by a given polypeptide subunit; there are as few as one in the tylosin and niddamycin PKSs [23, 24] and as many as six in the rap PKS. Each PKS is programmed to introduce the correct starter and extender, carry out the appropriate reductions, and ensure the correct stereochemistry.

Manipulation of PKSs

The ability to manipulate PKS genes arose in the late 1970s and was enhanced in subsequent years with the discoveries and improvements in the ability to introduce DNA into actinomycetes and the development of a series of vectors for cloning and expression of the large PKS genes. Much of this work originated in the laboratory of Sir David Hopwood in Norwich, UK; expression of the DEBS genes and production of **31** in a heterologous host was carried out first in Chaitan Khosla's laboratory at Stanford University. The latter employed an autonomously replicating plasmid, into which the *ery* PKS genes were inserted, and the host *Streptomyces coelicolor* CH999, which was depleted of its resident actinorhodin PKS genes [25]. Expression of the DEBS genes in *S. coelicolor* also resulted in production of **32** (Fig. 5), which employed **18** rather than **9** as the starter. Changes to the DEBS genes also have been performed in the erythromycin-producing host *Saccharopolyspora erythraea* by altering the genes either in their natural location in the chromosome [14] or on vectors, which could be subsequently re-introduced in the host [26, 27].

The changes introduced in the DEBS genes can be characterized in one of the following paradigms and are described in schematic outline in Table 1. The corresponding compounds produced are shown in Figure 5. Loss of (enzymatic)

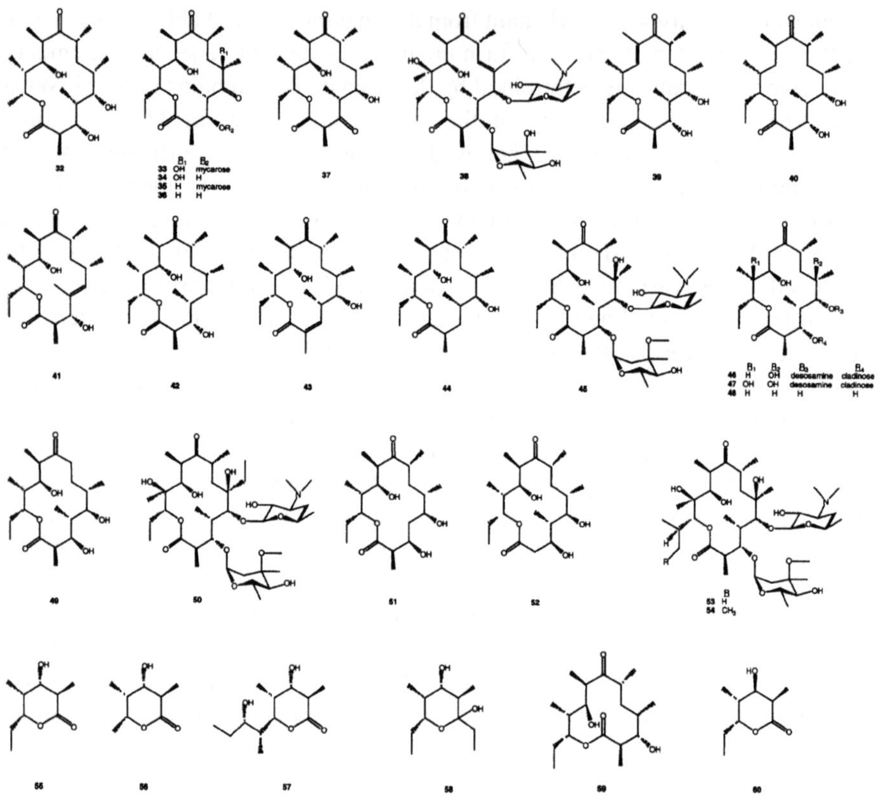

Figure 5. Compounds produced from genetic manipulation of DEBS.

function, through inactivation of one of the domains associated with reduction, results in the production of compounds that are less reduced than their corresponding parent molecules (**33–38**). Gain of function increases the degree of reduction. This is achieved by addition of a reduction domain not present in the native module. The examples described in Table 1 (**39–44**) employ a DH domain from the fourth module of the rap PKS or a DH + ER domain from the first module of the rap PKS. It was found, however, that in order for compounds to be produced, the cognate KR domain from the rap PKS was required, necessitating a replacement of the DEBS KR domain with rap DH/KR or DH/ER/KR encoding sequences [28]. The basis for this requirement is not understood. Gain of function replacements were done only in the *S. coelicolor* host, which resulted only in the production of non-hydroxylated, non-glycosidated macrolactones. Loss of function mutations in *S. erythraea* DEBS produced compounds that could be hydroxylated and glycosidated under some conditions.

Substitution of the AT domain has been achieved in each of the six modules of DEBS. In each case, except module 4, the AT employed specified the incorporation of malonyl-CoA, resulting in the loss of a methyl side chain from the corresponding position of the completed molecule (**45–49, 51, 52**). A number of

Table 1. Genetically engineered changes to DEBS and compounds produced.

N-o.	Change in DEBS	Host	Pro-duced	Ref
1	Loss of function: inactivation of KR5	A/B	33, 34, 35, 36	[14,28]
2	Loss of function: inactivation of KR6	B	37	[28]
3	Loss of function: inactivation of ER4	A	38	[41]
4	Gain of function: addition of rap DH4 (KR4) to module 2	B	39	[28]
5	Gain of function: addition of rap DH4/ER4 (KR4) to module 2	B	40	[28]
6	Gain of function: addition of rap DH4 (KR4) to module 5	B	41	[28]
7	Gain of function: addition of rap DH4/ER4 (KR4) to module 5	B	42	[28]
8	Gain of function: addition of rap DH4 (KR4) to module 6	B	43	[28]
9	Gain of function: addition of rap DH4/ER4 (KR4) to module 6	B	44	[28]
10	Side chain replacement: substitition of AT1 with malonyl AT	A	45	[42]
11	Side chain replacement: substitition of AT2 with malonyl AT	A/B	46, 47, 48	[28,42]
12	Side chain replacement: substitution of AT3 with malonyl AT	B	49	[28]
13	Side chain replacement: substitution of AT4 with ethylmalonyl AT	A	50	[43]
14	Side chain replacement: substitution of AT5 with malonyl AT	B	51	[28]
15	Side chain replacement: substitution of AT6 with malonyl AT	B	52	[28]
16	Loading module (starter) replacement: ave PKS	A	53, 54	[44]
17	Change of length: placement of TE6 at end of module 2	A/B	55, 56	[26, 45]
18	Change of length: placement of TE6 at end of module 3	B	57, 58	[46]
19	Change of length: placement of TE6 at end of module 5	B	59	[47]
20	Change of sterochemistry: exhange of AT2 with AT5	B	60	[20]

AT domains were used: rap PKS; modules 2, 12, or 14; an uncharacterized PKS from the same *Streptomyces hygroscopicus* strain that produces rapamycin; and an uncharacterized PKS from a strain of *Streptomyces venezuelae* that produces pikromycin. An AT exchange in module 4 also was performed using the AT domain from the PKS that specifies the ethyl side chain (oxidized in the final product) at C_6 of the 16-membered macrolide niddamycin. The 6a-methylerythromycin (**50**) produced in *S. erythraea* was shown to have antibacterial activity, but initial tests indicated that it was not as potent as erythromycin. Replacement of the loading module of DEBS with the corresponding module for avermectin, which initiates synthesis with 2-methylbutyryl-CoA (and, rarely, isopropionyl-CoA), yielded the corresponding erythromycin analogs (**53, 54**). Loading module exchanges between the tylosin (propionyl-CoA starter) and spiramycin (acetyl-CoA starter) PKSs resulted in the production of 15-methylspiramycin [29]. Changes at C_{13} and C_{12} also can be introduced by the process termed "chemobiosynthesis", or precursor-directed biosynthesis, which is discussed in a subsequent section of this chapter.

The length of the erythromycin polyketide also could be shortened by re-engineering the DEBS genes so that premature termination of polyketide synthesis took place. This change was accomplished by repositioning the TE domain from the end of module 6 to the end of upstream modules. Placement of the TE domain after ACP2 in both *S. coelicolor* and *S. erythraea* resulted in the production of the predicted triketide (**55**) as well as the 8-desmethyl derivative (**56**), formed through use of acetyl-CoA as the starter. Placement of the TE domain after module 3 resulted in the synthesis of the predicted tetraketide **57** as well as **58,** which arises from decarboxylation and a variation of the cyclization process. Finally, the 12-membered macrolactone **59** with the predicted structure is formed when the TE domain is repositioned after module 5. The stereochemistry of the ring hydroxyl function in the triketide lactone (**60**) was altered by substitution of the KR domain in module 2 with the KR from module 5, suggesting that the chirality of the hydroxyl groups is determined at the time of ketoreduction rather than by epimerization.

Combinatorial PKS manipulations

When using unaltered PKS genes to introduce mutations, exchanges, *etc*., it is rare to find convenient restriction sites that will allow surgical removal of a particular domain for replacement with another. Hence, most of the changes of PKSs employ an *in vivo* process of double reciprocal (homologous) recombination that requires an extensive amount of gene cloning and vector preparation and can take several weeks to months to accomplish because of the slow nature of growth and sporulation of the microorganisms involved. A significant advance in the technology of PKS manipulation was achieved by McDaniel and colleagues at Kosan Biosciences, Inc. [28]. First, the restriction sites for *Pac*I, *Spe*I, *Bgl*II and *EcoR*I were introduced in the DEBS-encoding *eryA* genes as shown in Figure 6, such that all or most of each gene could be removed from the autonomously replicating plasmid that carried the *eryA* genes, engineered, and then returned to the plasmid, which could then be reintroduced to the host. Next, on the separated fragments containing each gene, *BamH*I and *Pst*I restriction sites were introduced upstream and downstream, respectively, of either of the two AT domains, and an *Xho*I site was placed at the end of either KR domain. Placement of the sites was performed without interrupting the reading frame or the function of any domain. Each gene, therefore, was prepared in three versions: unmodified and modified to permit manipulation in either of the two modules. As shown in Figure 6, fragment 1 enabled manipulation of module 1, fragment 2 enabled manipulation of module 2, *etc*. The heterologous PKS segments used for replacement also were prepared with the corresponding restriction sites: the rapAT2 domain (specifying malonyl-CoA) on a *BamH*I-*Pst*I fragment, and a KR, KR+DH, KR+DH+ER, or inactivated KR domain from various rap PKS modules on a *Pst*I-*Xho*I segment (Fig. 6). Replacement of the AT domain in module 3 could be accomplished by cutting fragment 3 with *BamH*I and *Pst*I, isolating the *Spe*I-*BamH*I and *Pst*I-*Bgl*II fragments generated, ligating them with the cassette-carrying rapAT2, and, finally, sub-cloning the reconstructed *Spe*I-*Bgl*II fragment in the host vector that was cut with the same two enzymes and isolated from the segment carrying

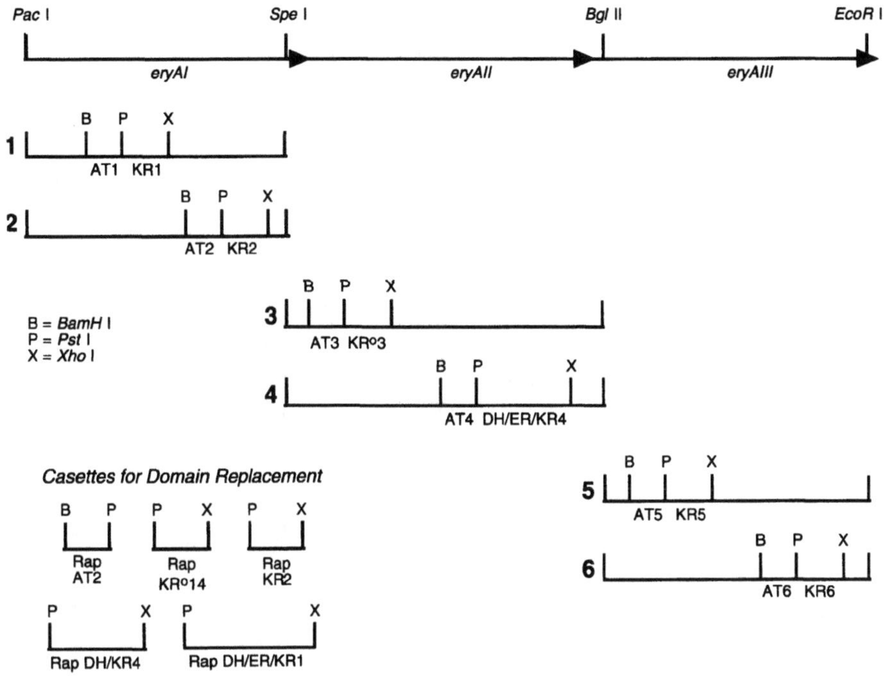

Figure 6. Scheme for re-engineering DEBS. Genes are designated *eryAI, eryAII* and *eryAIII.* DNA shown as bold lines. Segments 1–6 correspond to segment of *eryA* gene shown at top. Selected restriction sites are shown. Abbreviations are as in Figure 4; rap – rapamycin PKS. Numbers beside abbreviations indicate DEBS module..

the unchanged *eryAII.* Similar strategies were used to introduce AT replacements or loss or gain of functions in the reduction domains (KR°, KR, DH/KR or DH/ER/KR-containing cassettes) at other modules. Finally, multiple changes could be introduced simultaneously by combining the manipulations performed at two different modules. However, since only one of each cognate pair of sub-fragments could be manipulated at any given time, only a total of three modules could be changed simultaneously.

A further advance in the technology of combinatorial manipulation of DEBS also was achieved at Kosan by Xue and colleagues [30]. In place of employing the three *eryA* genes on a single plasmid, each gene was cloned on a single plasmid carrying a specific and unique resistance marker for selection in *Streptomyces.* The plasmids either could replicate autonomously or could integrate in the chromosome of several streptomycetes through site-specific recombination directed by segments cloned in the plasmids from genetic elements that normally integrate in the chromosome, either the plasmid pSAM2 [31] or the bacteriophage ϕC31 [32]. In head-to-head comparisons, the strains of *Streptomyces lividans* carrying the three plasmid system produced the same level of **31** as the same host carrying a single plasmid that contained the three *eryA* genes [30]. The *eryA* genes carried the unique *BamH*I, *Pst*I, and *Xho*I sites in either of the two modules to enable direct cloning of the replacement cassettes, as described by McDaniel and colleagues [28]. Although the same number of combinations of "mutant" DEBS proteins could be produced by employing the single- or triple-plasmid systems, high numbers of mutant DEBSs could be generated much more rapidly by employing the three-plasmid system.

The novel analogs of **31**, generated by introducing changes in two or three modules of DEBS employing the single- or three-plasmid system, are shown in Figure 7 (2 changes: **61–87**; 3 changes: **88–92**). All changes in DEBS yielded the predicted compounds, although the yields of the compounds produced varied radically from one "mutant" to another. In general, as the number of changes introduced in DEBS went up, the level of corresponding analog produced decreased. Nevertheless, many compounds were produced at levels sufficient for isolation and testing for enhanced or novel properties. The basis for the effect of changes in DEBS structure on rates of polyketide produced remains to be understood.

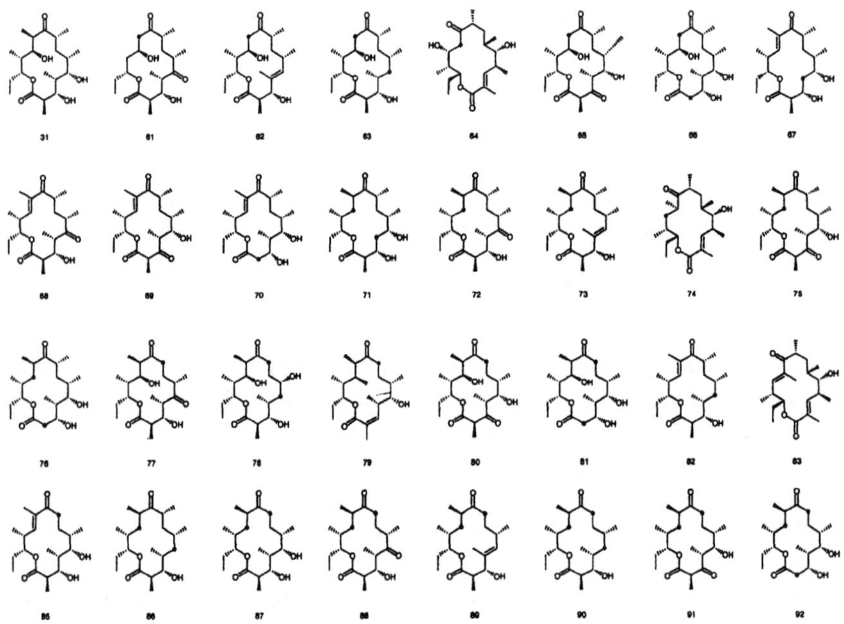

Figure 7. Compounds produced from multiple genetic alterations of DEBS. The wild-type compound, **31**, is shown for comparison..

Hybrid PKSs

The mixed plasmid system to produce a polyketide from its natural PKS components also could be adapted to employ the subunits from different PKS systems. Erythromycin, pikromycin, and oleandomycin, **1**, **4**, and **5**, respectively (Fig. 1), are macrolide antibiotics composed of 14-membered macrolactone (polyketide) rings that are modified by hydroxylation and glycosidation. The aglycones of **1** and **5**, which are **31** and **32**, respectively, differ by the substitution of the C_{13}-ethyl side chain in **31** for the C_{13}-methyl side chain in **32**; this result arises from the synthesis of the polyketide employing acetyl-CoA rather than propionyl-CoA as the starter. **93** (Fig. 8) differs from **31** at C_{10} (H instead of methyl side chain; 10,11-anhydro) and C_3 (3-keto), the result of the use of malonyl-CoA rather than methylmalonyl-CoA as the extender in the second condensation cycle, the dehydration event in the second reduction cycle, and the failure of ketoreduction in the sixth reduction cycle. The PKSs for **93** and **32** have been cloned and sequenced, and the schematic representation of each is shown in Figure 8, along with DEBS for comparison [33, 34]. All are organized similarly: 3 polypeptides, 2 modules per polypeptide, and co-linearity between order of use and linear sequence (at the gene level). In addition, modules 5 and 6 of the Pik PKS are separated on two proteins. The Pik PKS produces **93** as well as the 12-membered macrolactone **94**, which is produced from termination of polyketide synthesis after 5 condensations followed by cyclization. The basis for the apparent premature termination has been explained recently [35].

A number of DEBS – Pik and Pik – Ole hybrid PKSs have recently been constructed recently in *S. lividans*, leading to the synthesis of the predicted "hybrid" compounds, shown in Figure 8 [36]. Compound **37**, made previously by inactivation of the KR domain from module 6 of DEBS, could be made by combining modules 1 through 5(AT) of DEBS with 5(KR) and 6 of Pik. Similarly, by employing the DEBS mutant that carries the DH domain in module 2 in the same DEBS-Pik fusion, the 10,11-anhydro- analog of **37**, **69**, was formed. Exchange of Pik AIII and Pik AIV for EryAIII or Ole AIII resulted in the production of the hybrid compound **95** wherein C_2–C_4 were directed into the polyketide by the Ery or Ole PKS and the remaining atoms of the ring from the Pik PKS. Modified EryAIII, carrying DH or DH+ER domains in modules 5 or 6, in combination with Pik AI and PiKAII, also gave the predicted hybrid compounds. Interestingly, 5-keto (**96**) or 3-keto (**93**) derivatives also were found in extracts that produced reduced C_5 or C_3 derivatives. This unanticipated result could be explained by the failure of the hybrid PKS to carry out the expected β-ketoreduction at steps 5 or 6 of the synthesis on some of the nascent acyl chains produced during synthesis. The hybrid PKSs were made by placing the *eryAIII* (native or altered) or *oleAIII* gene on a plasmid that integrates in the chromosome and the *pikAI*+ *pikAII* genes on a vector that replicates autonomously in the cytoplasm of *S. lividans*.

Chemobiosynthesis

An important methodology has been reported recently by Jacobsen and colleagues [37] that allows incorporation of novel structures into the C_{12} and C_{13} positions of **31**. In this approach, the DEBS was mutated to prevent the synthesis of the initial diketide through the introduction of a cysteine to alanine substitution in the active site of the KS domain of module 1 (the KS1 null mutant cannot form the thioester with the

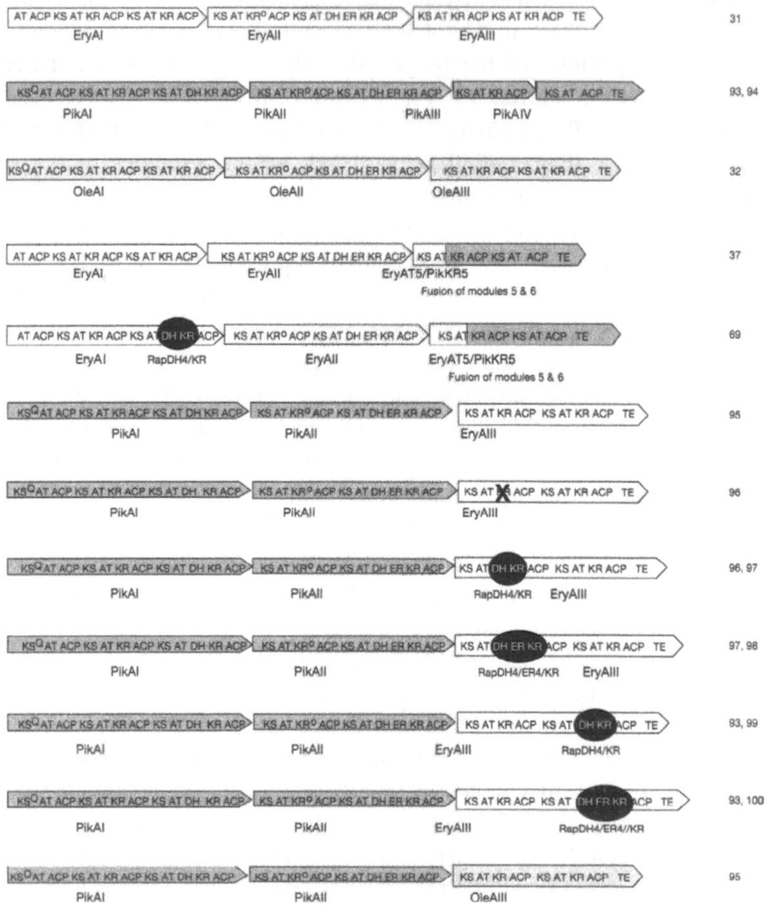

Figure 8a. Compounds produced from hybrid PKSs. Abbreviations: KS^Q – KS domain with active site cysteine replaced by glutamine; Pik – pikromycin PKS; Ole – oleandomycin PKS; all other as in Figs. 4 and 6. PKSs are labeled as shown.

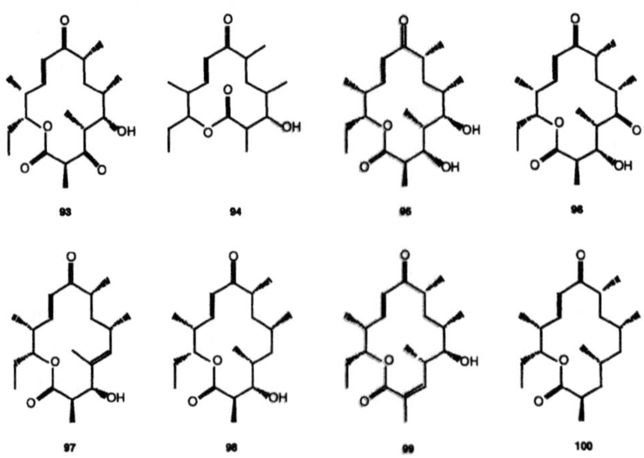

Figure 8b.

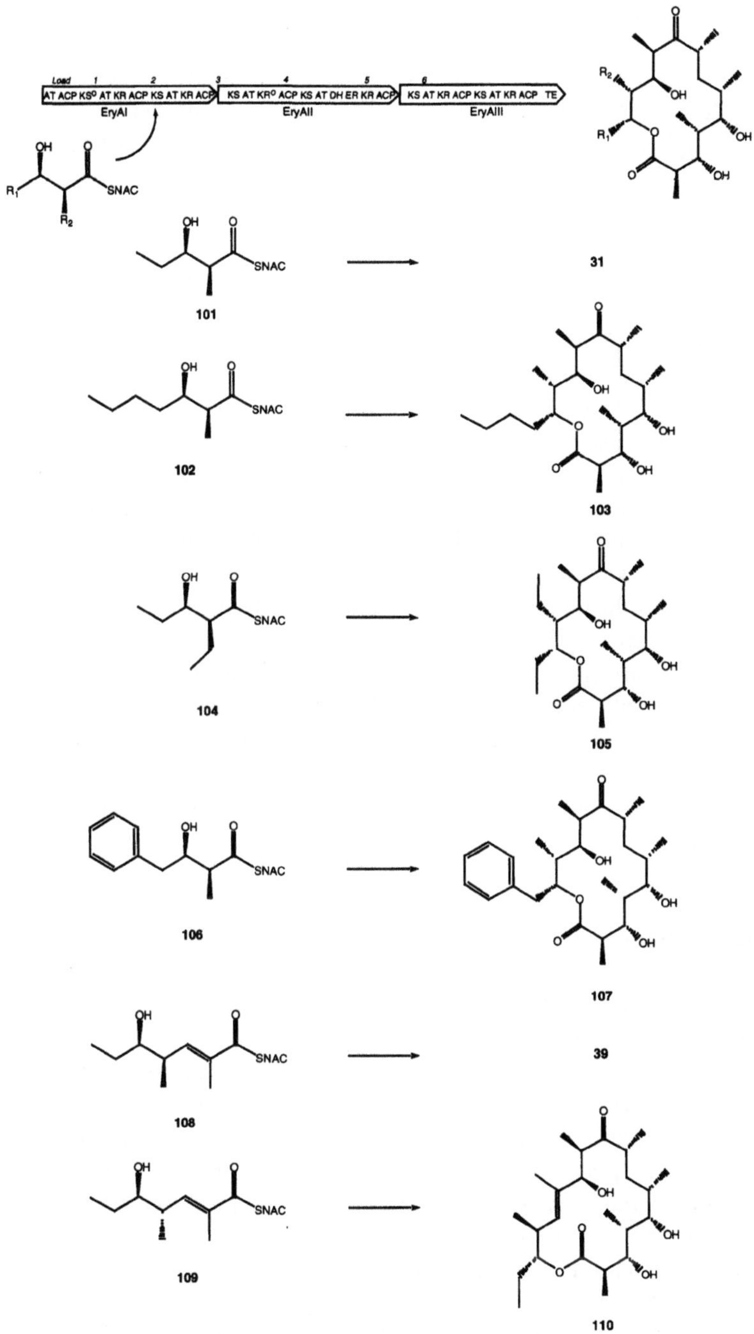

Figure 9. Precursor-directed biosynthesis synthesis of polyketides. Abbreviations: SNAC – *N*-acetylcysteamine thioester; KS° – inactivated KS domain; all other abbreviations as in Figs. 4 and 6. Compounds on left were fed to KS1°-containing strain, leading to production of compounds on right.

propionyl- starter unit). *S. coelicolor* strains carrying the DEBS genes containing the KS1° mutation, however, could incorporate a variety of di- and triketides, fed to cells as *N*-acetylcysteamine (SNAC) thioesters, presumably through thioester exchange at the KS2 domain and subsequent processing through the DEBS in the normal fashion. Thus, through feeding of diketide **101**, (2*S*)-methyl-(3*R*)-hydroxypentanoate N-acetylcysteamine thioester, to the KS1° mutant in DEBS or in the bimodular variant DEBS1-TE, either **31** or **55**, respectively, could be produced [37,38]. However, thioesters carrying (2*R*)-methyl or (3*S*)-hydroxy- substituents did not get processed into **31** or **55** or their corresponding epimeric analogs. Nevertheless, by employing the (2*S*,3*R*)- thioesters, a wide variety of structures could be incorporated successfully to produce 6dEB analogs including those shown in Figure 9 carrying C_{13}-butyryl (**103**) or C_{13}-benzyl (**107**) side chains. An ethyl side chain could be placed at C_{12} (**105**) by feeding the (2*R*)-ethyl substituted diketide SNAC thioester **104** [39]. Feeding of the triketide **108** resulted in the production of **39** [40] through incorporation of the precursor at the KS3 domain, thereby placing the hydroxyl group at C_5 of the precursor at the correct C_{13} position of the completed chain to allow lactonization to yield the 14-membered ring with the correct stereochemistry of the C_{12} methyl side chain. However, when the C_4 enantiomer of the precursor (**109**) was fed, only the 16-membered macrolactone **110** was produced [37] through incorporation at KS2, placing the C_5-hydroxyl group of the precursor at C_{15} of the completed chain and the ene function at $C_{12,13}$. The stereochemistry of the methyl side chain at C_{14} is similar to that found on all 16-membered macrolides that possess a C_{14} methyl side chain (tylosin, rosaramicin, *etc.*). Incorporation of **109** at KS3 would have yielded the C_{12} epimer of **39** if it were allowed to be processed by DEBS. These findings indicate that the stereochemistry of the growing molecule is tightly regulated in the PKS, but the precise elements that control this effect have not yet been rigorously established.

Closing comments

The understanding of the molecular basis for the biosynthesis of complex polyketides has been gained only over the past decade and has provided an explanation for the basis of the extensive structural diversity seen among this class of naturally occurring molecules. In simplified terms, diversity is generated during synthesis by variations in 1) use of different starter and extender units, 2) degrees of reduction, 3) polyketide length, and 4) post-polyketide modification (*e. g.*, glycosidations, methylations, *etc.*). Thus, the structural differences between any two complex polyketides can be explained by employing one or more of these variables. The four types of variations also are explained at the biochemical level: 1–3 in the PKS and 4 in enzymes that modify the completed (or partially completed) polyketide chain or ring. Because the modular architecture of the PKS is common to all complex polyketides, it has been argued (but not proven) that more complicated structures arise from simpler ones through duplication, mutation, and transfer (mixing) of modules. Certainly, in the laboratory, through advances in genetic technology, novel polyketides can be generated by mutation (single or multiple), addition, deletion, and manipulation of modules (from single domains to the full module level) or by assembling functional PKSs from modules originating from two different sources. Manipulations can now be done combinatorially. Thus, our ability to create diversity of polyketides in the laboratory now outpaces our ability to discover novel polyketides from natural sources. Therefore, it is not unreasonable to project that the next generation of polyketides developed as drugs or agricultural or veterinary products could be "designed" and produced from the engineering of a modular polyketide synthase.

Acknowledgement

The author thanks Kevin Kaster for helpful comments on the manuscript.

References

1 Collie JN (1907) Derivatives of the multiple ketene group. *Proc Chem Soc* 23: 230–231

2 Hutchinson CR (1995) Anthracyclines. *Biotechnology* 28: 331–357

3 Hutchinson CR (1998) Combinatorial biosynthesis for new drug discovery. *Curr Opin Microbiol* 1: 319–329

4 Tsoi CJ, Khosla C (1995) Combinatorial biosynthesis of 'unnatural' natural products: the polyketide example. *Chem Biol* 2: 355–362

5 Xue Y, Wilson D, Zhao L, Liu H-w, Sherman DH (1998) Hydroxylation of macrolactones YC-17 and narbomycin is mediated by the pikC-encoded cytochrome P450 in *Streptomyces venezuelae*. *Chem Biol* 5: 661–667

6 Salah-Bey K, Doumith M, Michel JM, Haydock S, Cortes J, Leadlay PF, Raynal MC (1998) Targeted gene inactivation for the elucidation of deoxysugar biosynthesis in the erythromycin producer *Saccharopolyspora erythraea*. *Mol Gen Genet* 257: 542–553

7 Schwecke T, Aparicio JF, Molnar I, Konig A, Khaw LE, Haydock SF, Oliynyk M, Caffrey P, Cortes J, Lester JB et al (1995) The biosynthetic gene cluster for the polyketide immunosuppressant rapamycin. *Proc Natl Acad Sci U S A* 92: 7839–7843

8 Schupp T, Toupet C, Engel N, Goff S (1998) Cloning and sequence analysis of the putative rifamycin polyketide synthase gene cluster from *Amycolatopsis mediterranei*. *FEMS Microbiol Lett* 159: 201–207

9 August PR, Tang L, Yoon YJ, Ning S, Muller R, Yu TW, Taylor M, Hoffmann D, Kim CG, Zhang X et al (1998) Biosynthesis of the ansamycin antibiotic rifamycin: deductions from the molecular analysis of the rif biosynthetic gene cluster of *Amycolatopsis mediterranei* S699. *Chem Biol* 5: 69–79

10 Schupp T, Toupet C, Cluzel B, Neff S, Hill S, Beck JJ, Ligon JM (1995) A *Sorangium cellulosum* (myxobacterium) gene cluster for the biosynthesis of the macrolide antibiotic soraphen A: cloning, characterization, and homology to polyketide synthase genes from actinomycetes. *J Bacteriol* 177: 3673–3679

11 Haydock SF, Aparicio JF, Molnar I, Schwecke T, Khaw LE, Konig AF, Marsden AF, Galloway IS, Staunton J, Leadlay PF (1995) Divergent sequence motifs correlated with the substrate specificity of (methyl)malonyl-CoA: acyl carrier protein transacylase domains in modular polyketide synthases. *FEBS Lett.* 374: 246–248

12 Bisang C, Long PF, Cortes J, Westcott J, Crosby J, Matharu AL, Cox RJ, Simpson TJ, Staunton J, Leadlay PF (1999) A chain initiation factor common to both modular and aromatic polyketide synthases. *Nature* 401: 502–505

13 Witkowski A, Joshik AK, Lindqvist Y, Smith S (1999) Conversion of a β-ketoacyl synthase to a malonyl decarboxylase by replacement of the active-site cysteine with glutamine. *Biochemistry* 38: 11643–11650
14 Donadio S, Staver MJ, McAlpine JB, Swanson SJ, Katz L (1991) Modular organization of genes required for complex polyketide biosynthesis. *Science* 252: 675–679
15 Kao CM, Pieper R, Cane DE, Khosla C (1996) Evidence for two catalytically independent clusters of active sites in a functional modular polyketide synthase. *Biochemistry* 35: 12363–12368
16 Staunton J, Caffrey P, Aparicio JF, Roberts GA, Bethell SS, Leadlay PF (1996) Evidence for a double-helical structure for modular polyketide synthases. *Nature Struct Biol* 3: 188–192
17 Aparicio JF, Caffrey P, Marsden AF, Staunton J, Leadlay PF (1994) Limited proteolysis and active-site studies of the first multienzyme component of the erythromycin-producing polyketide synthase. *J Biol Chem* 269: 8524–8528
18 Pieper R, Luo G, Cane DE, Khosla C (1995) Remarkably broad substrate specificity of a modular polyketide synthase in a cell-free system. *J Am Chem Soc* 117: 11373–11374
19 Wiesmann KE, Cortes J, Brown MJ, Cutter AL, Staunton J, Leadlay PF (1995) Polyketide synthesis in vitro on a modular polyketide synthase. *Chem Biol* 2: 583–589
20 Kao CM, McPherson M, McDaniel R, Fu H, Cane D, Khosla C (1998) Alcohol stereochemistry in polyketide backbones is controlled by the ß-ketoreductase domains of modular polyketide synthases. *J Am Chem Soc* 120: 2478–2479
21 Holzbaur IE, Harris RC, Bycroft M, Cortes J, Bisang C, Staunton J, Rudd BA, Leadlay PF (1999) Molecular basis of Celmer's rules: the role of two ketoreductase domains in the control of chirality by the erythromycin modular polyketide synthase. *Chem Biol* 6: 189–195
22 Weissman KJ, Timoney M, Bycroft M, Grice P, Hanefeld U, Staunton J, Leadlay PF (1997) The molecular basis of Celmer's rules: the stereochemistry of the condensation step in chain extension on the erythromycin polyketide synthase. *Biochemistry* 36: 13849–13855
23 DeHoff BS, Sutton KL, Rosteck Jr. PR. (Eli Lilly & Co., 1997).
24 Kakavas SJ, Katz L, Stassi D (1997) Identification and characterization of the niddamycin polyketide synthase genes from *Streptomyces caelestis*. *J Bacteriol* 179: 7515–7522
25 Kao CM, Luo G, Katz L, Cane DE, Khosla C (1994) Engineered biosynthesis of a triketide lactone from an incomplete modular polyketide synthase. *J Am Chem Soc* 116: 11612–11613
26 Cortes J, Wiesmann KE, Roberts GA, Brown MJ, Staunton J, Leadlay PF (1995) Repositioning of a domain in a modular polyketide synthase to promote specific chain cleavage. *Science* 268: 1487–1489
27 Rowe CJ, Cortes J, Gaisser S, Staunton J, Leadlay PF (1998) Construction of new vectors for high-level expression in actinomycetes. *Gene* 216: 215–223
28 McDaniel R, Thamchaipenet A, Gustafsson C, Fu H, Betlach M, Ashley G (1999) Multiple genetic modifications of the erythromycin polyketide synthase to produce a library of novel "unnatural" natural products. *Proc Natl Acad Sci USA* 96: 1846–1851
29 Kuhstoss S, Huber M, Turner JR, Paschal JW, Rao RN (1996) Production of a novel polyketide through the construction of a hybrid polyketide synthase. *Gene* 183: 231–236
30 Xue Q, Ashley G, Hutchinson CR, Santi DV (1999) A multiplasmid approach to preparing large libraries of polyketides. *Proc Natl Acad Sci USA* 96: 11740–11745
31 Mazodier P, Thompson C, Boccard F (1990) The chromosomal integration site of the Streptomyces element pSAM2 overlaps a putative tRNA gene conserved among actinomycetes. *Mol Gen Genet* 222: 431–434
32 Bierman M, Logan R, O'Brien K, Seno ET, Nagaraja R, Schoner BE (1992) Plasmid cloning vectors for the conjugal transfer of DNA from *Escherichia coli* to *Streptomyces* spp. *Gene* 116: 43–49
33 Xue Y, Zhao L, Liu HW, Sherman DH (1998) A gene cluster for macrolide antibiotic biosynthesis in *Streptomyces venezuelae*: architecture of metabolic diversity. *Proc Natl Acad Sci USA* 95: 12111–12116
34 Shah S, Xue Q, Tang L, Carney JR, Betlach M, McDaniel R (2000) Cloning, characterization and heterologous expression of a PK gene cluster involved in the biosynthesis of the antibiotic, oleandomycin. *J Antibiot* 53: 502–508
35 Xue Y, Sherman DH (2000) Alternative modular polyketide synthase expression controls macrolactone structure. *Nature* 403: 571–575

36 Tang L, Fu H, McDaniel R (2000) Formation of functional heterologous complexes using subunits from the picromycin, erythromycin and oleandomycin polyketide synthases. *Chem Biol* 7: 77–84
37 Jacobsen JR, Hutchinson CR, Cane DE, Khosla C (1997) Precursor-directed biosynthesis of erythromycin analogs by an engineered polyketide synthase. *Science* 277: 367–369
38 Weissman KJ, Bycroft M, Cutter AL, Hanefeld U, Frost EJ, Timoney MC, Harris R, Handa S, Roddis M, Staunton J et al (1998) Evaluating precursor-directed biosynthesis towards novel erythromycins through in vitro studies on a bimodular polyketide synthase. *Chem Biol* 5: 743–754
39 Jacobsen JR, Keatinge-Clay AT, Cane DE, Khosla C (1998) Precursor-directed biosynthesis of 12-ethyl erythromycin. *Bioorg Med Chem* 6: 1171–1177
40 Jacobsen JR, Cane DE, Khosla C (1998) Dissecting the evolutionary relationship between 14-membered and 16-membered macrolides. *J Am Chem Soc* 120: 9096–9097
41 Donadio S, Staver MJ, McAlpine JB, Swanson SJ, Katz L (1992) Biosynthesis of the erythromycin macrolactone and a rational approach for producing hybrid macrolides. *Gene* 115: 97–103
42 Donadio S, McAlpine JB, Sheldon PJ, Jackson M, Katz L (1993) An erythromycin analog produced by reprogramming of polyketide synthesis. *Proc Natl Acad Sci USA* 90: 7119–7123
43 Ruan X, Pereda A, Stassi DL, Zeidner D, Summers RG, Jackson M, Shivakumar A, Kakavas S, Staver MJ, Donadio S et al (1997) Acyltransferase domain substitutions in erythromycin polyketide synthase yield novel erythromycin derivatives. *J Bacteriol* 179: 6416–6425
44 Stassi D, Post D, Satter M, Jackson M, Maine G (1998) A genetically engineered strain of *Saccharopolyspora erythraea* that produces 6,12-dideoxyerythromycin A as the major fermentation product. *Appl Microbiol Biotechnol* 49: 725–731
45 Marsden AF, Wilkinson B, Cortes J, Dunster NJ, Staunton J, Leadlay PF (1998) Engineering broader specificity into an antibiotic-producing polyketide synthase. *Science* 279: 199–202
46 Kao CM, Luo G, Katz L, Cane DE, Khosla C (1996) Engineered biosynthesis of structurally diverse tetraketides by a trimodular polyketide synthase. *J Am Chem Soc* 118: 9184–9185
47 Kao CM, Luo G, Katz L, Cane DE, Khosla C (1995) Manipulation of macrolide ring size by directed mutagenesis of a modular polyketide synthase. *J Am Chem Soc* 117: 9105–9106

Macrolide Antibiotics
ed. by W. Schönfeld and H. A. Kirst

Biosynthesis of the macrolide antibiotic, tylosin

Eric Cundliffe

Department of Biochemistry, University of Leicester, Adrian Bldg., University Road, Leicester LE1 7RH, United Kingdom

Tylosin is produced by *Streptomyces fradiae via* a combination of polyketide and deoxyhexose metabolism. Elucidation of the biosynthetic route to tylosin involved tracer incorporation studies and bioconversion analysis, with heavy reliance on the use of mutants of *S. fradiae* blocked in tylosin production [1–5]. The primary product of the TylG polyketide synthase is a 16-atom lactone (protylonolide, synonym tylactone) that subsequently acquires three deoxyhexose substituents (D-mycaminose, 6-deoxy-D-allose and L-mycarose) in a preferred but not obligatory order, although mycaminose is always added first. Thereafter, the deoxyallose moiety is converted to D-mycinose *via* bis-*O*-methylation. The polyketide lactone is also hydroxylated following attachment of the first sugar. This occurs at C-20 and C-23, the latter being the site at which deoxyallose subsequently is added (Fig. 1). Complementation of blocked mutants with cloned DNA fragments [6, 7] allowed the mapping of 13 *tyl* loci within the *S. fradiae* genome, alongside other attempts to identify the tylosin-production genes. Success in this regard eventually resulted from two convergent approaches instigated at Lilly Research Laboratories, Indianapolis.

Following purification of macrocin *O*-methyltransferase (MOMT; the enzyme that catalyses the terminal step in tylosin biosynthesis), deoxyoligonucleotide probes ostensibly specific for the MOMT-encoding gene were designed based on the N-terminal amino-acid sequence of the protein. Those probes found hybridisation targets in a library of *S. fradiae* DNA [6], including a 2.3 kb fragment that expressed MOMT activity when cloned in *S. lividans*. That same DNA fragment also restored tylosin production in a *tylF* mutant of *S. fradiae* that otherwise

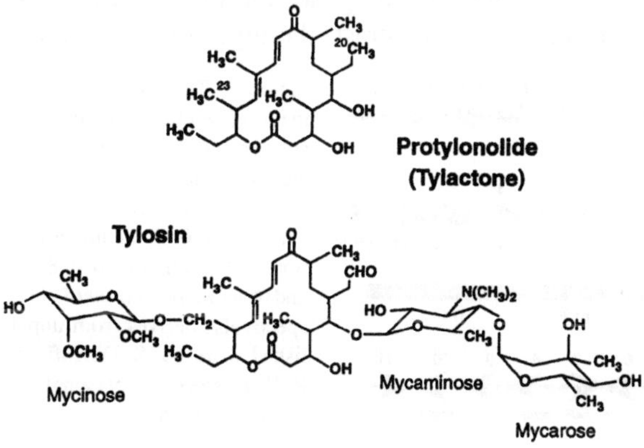

Figure 1. Structures of tylosin and the aglycone.

accumulated macrocin (3"-*O*-demethyl-tylosin). In parallel studies, three tylosin-resistance determinants were isolated from *S. fradiae* [8, 9], and one of them, *tlrB*, was shown to hybridise with DNA fragments that contained *tylF*. By hybridization analysis with overlapping cosmid inserts, another resistance gene (*tlrC*) was shown to be about 85 kb distant from *tlrB* and, significantly, all of the *tyl* loci lay between *tlrB* and *tlrC*. It therefore seemed plausible that many or all of the tylosin-biosynthetic genes might be clustered within that region of the *S. fradiae* genome [9]. That notion has since been confirmed by sequence analysis.

Although not all of the data were made public, DNA adjacent to *tlrB* and *tlrC* was sequenced at Lilly in the late 1980s [10, 11; B. S. DeHoff and P. R. Rosteck Jr., personal communication] together with a contiguous piece of DNA (about 41 kb: accession number U78289) located between *tlrB* and *tlrC* (but separate from both) that encodes the TylG polyketide synthase complex. More recently, the rest of the DNA between *tlrB* and *tlrC* has been sequenced in this laboratory [12–17], and functions have been assigned to specific gene products by a combination of database comparisons, enzymic analysis, complementation of *tyl* mutants, and targeted gene disruptions.

Structural genes in the *tyl cluster*

Between *tlrB* and *tlrC*, occupying about 1% (i. e., 85 kb) of the *S. fradiae* genome, are 43 contiguous open reading frames (orfs) that apparently include the full complement of structural genes needed for tylosin production, together with three resistance determinants, at least five regulatory genes, and a small number of unassigned orfs (Fig. 2). The TylG polyketide synthase (PKS) complex is encoded by 5 giant orfs (*tylGI-GV*) that span about 41 kb, upstream of which are 12 genes (orfs 1, 1a-11) including *tlrC*, while a further 26 genes (orfs 1* through 26*) lie downstream of *tylG* culminating in *tlrB*. Structural genes for production of the tylosin sugars (Fig. 3) are arranged in discrete blocks, although two of these are incomplete. Thus, *tylB* (orf2; involved in mycaminose biosynthesis) and *tylCVI* (orf6; required for mycarose production) are located upstream of *tylG* among a miscellaneous collection of orfs, whereas the other (*tylM*) mycaminose genes (orfs 1*–3*; [14]) and the (*tylC*) mycarose-biosynthetic genes (orfs 6*–10*; [17]) are over 50 kb distant, downstream of *tylG*. In contrast, the mycinose-biosynthetic

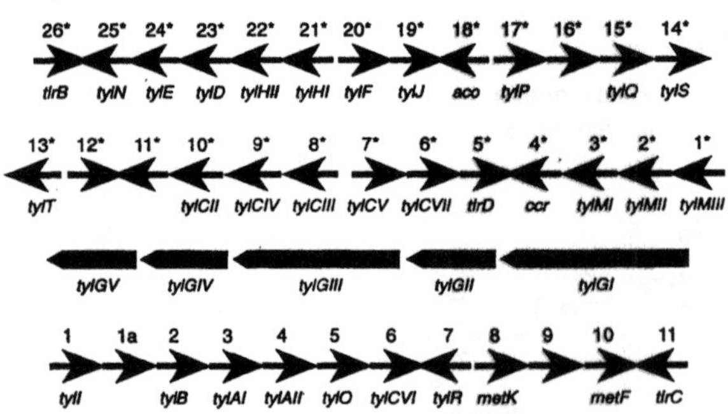

Figure 2. The tylosin-biosynthetic gene cluster. Five orfs are currently unassigned although one of these, orf16*, is deduced to encode a cytochrome P450 of unknown function. Designation of orfs 8 and10 as *metK* and *metF*, respectively, derives from unpublished work (B. S. DeHoff and P. R. Rosteck Jr., personal communication).

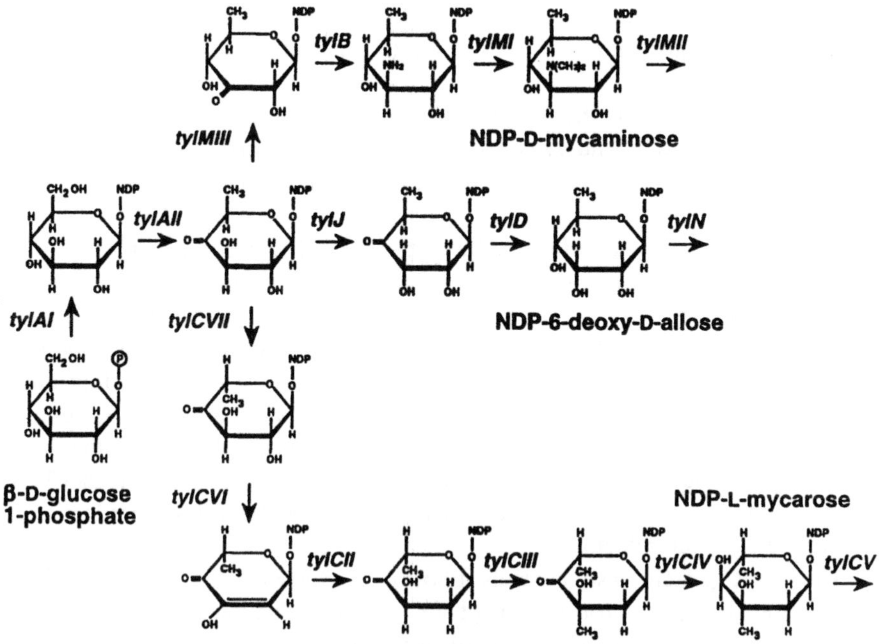

Figure 3. Synthesis of the tylosin sugars. Deoxyallose is converted to mycinose by the products of *tylE* and *tylF* sequentially after addition to the polyketide ring.

genes (orfs 19*–25*; [16]) form a complete cassette that also includes *tylHI*, the product of which is a cytochrome P450 that hydroxylates the polyketide lactone at C-23, and a ferredoxin gene, *tylHII*. Bacterial cytochromes P450 typically receive electrons from ferredoxins. It will therefore be interesting to determine the specificity of TylHII ("tylodoxin"), since *tylHII* is the only ferredoxin gene in the *tyl* cluster.

Regulatory genes in the *tyl cluster*

Antibiotic-biosynthetic gene clusters in actinomycetes typically contain pathway-specific regulators that are, in turn, controlled in "cascade" fashion by additional regulators [18]. The latter may control morphological differentiation in addition to secondary metabolism and are not commonly present in antibiotic-biosynthetic gene clusters. Elsewhere, only two candidate regulatory genes have been identified in macrolide-producing organisms, namely, *srmR* [19] and *acyB2* [20], and their impact on the production of spiramycin and carbomycin, respectively, remains to be studied in detail. It is therefore particularly interesting that the *tyl* cluster contains at least five such genes, four of which (*tylP,Q,T,S*) are tightly bunched, while the fifth, *tylR*, is almost 60 kb away on the other side of *tylG*. Two of the putative regulatory genes (*tylS* and *tylT*) are of a type commonly found in antibiotic-biosynthetic clusters, although the presence of two such genes in the same cluster is unprecedented. These encode proteins of the Streptomyces Antibiotic Regulatory Protein (SARP) family that are typically transcriptional activators [21].

Equally remarkable is the presence in the *tyl* cluster of candidate pleiotropic regulatory genes, *tylP* and *tylQ*. Among the actinomycetes, diffusible signal molecules of the γ-butyrolactone family, sometimes referred to as microbial "hormones", are probably ubiquitous. These currently are believed to be inducers in the classical sense that influence the expression of regulatory genes. Thus, in *Streptomyces virginiae*, the transcriptional repressor BarA (closely related to the product of *tylP*) binds to the promoter of a downstream gene *barB* (an apparent orthologue of *tylQ*) and controls virginiamycin production plus sporulation [22, 23]. Release of BarA from the target DNA is triggered by γ-butyrolactones that bind directly to BarA [22]. Similarly in *S. griseus*, A-factor causes dissociation of a repressor, ArpA, from its target *adpA* and turns on sporulation together with streptomycin production [24,25]. Arguing by analogy, it seems plausible that TylP might be a repressor with *tylQ* as its possible target and that tylosin production is controlled by γ-butyrolactone(s).

The TylR protein also controls tylosin biosynthesis but does not affect sporulation. Thus, most (or all) aspects of tylosin production were shut down in *S. fradiae* when *tylR* (orf7) was specifically disrupted [15]. The resultant strain, which sporulated normally, was unable to bioconvert exogenously added precursors of tylosin and appeared defective in polyketide metabolism, synthesis or addition of all three sugars, and terminal methylation of the deoxyallose moiety. The TylR protein is similar to AcyB2 from the carbomycin producer, *Streptomyces thermotolerans,* which was first suggested to be a positive regulator [20]

Feedback control of tylosin production

While confirming the role of the *tylMII* product as the mycaminosyltransferase involved in tylosin biosynthesis, it was observed that disruption of this gene reduced tylactone production to undetectable levels in *S. fradiae* [26]. This was an unexpected result, prior to which it was anticipated that such strains would accumulate the aglycone. However, when tylosin (or any of its glycosylated precursors) was added to the fermentation medium, polyketide metabolism was restored in the *tylMII*-disrupted strain and tylactone accumulated. In contrast, when genes involved in the biosynthesis of mycarose or mycinose were disrupted, polyketide metabolism was not obviously affected and the expected macrolide intermediates accumulated ([17]; A.R. Butler, unpublished data, this laboratory). Since mycaminose is the first sugar added to tylactone during tylosin production, it is proposed that polyketide metabolism can occur only at minimal levels unless the product gets glycosylated. The mechanism of such regulation is not known. Do glycosylated macrolides relieve negative control of *tylG* by acting as inducers, or do they function as transcriptional co-activators?

Polyketide editing

The PKS enzymes that produce macrolide aglycones are complexes of giant multifunctional proteins, within which discrete catalytic domains sequentially manipulate the nascent polyketide. The TylG PKS produces an octaketide (16-atom ring) and consists of five proteins, each of which contains one or two complete sets (modules) of chain extension domains [27, 28]. Each module selects the incoming acyl extender unit, catalyses decarboxylative condensation, and determines the reductive state of the newly incorporated unit. Nascent polyketides are attached to the PKS as thioesters, and TylGV possesses a carboxy-terminal thioesterase (TE-I) domain that terminates chain extension and cyclises the product. Transplantation of such TE-I domains onto other PKS components results in truncated products and allows the synthesis of novel polyketides with elective ring size [29, 30]. However, additional thioesterase genes (encoding so-called TE-II enzymes) commonly are found adjacent to the PKS-encoding genes in macrolide producers, for example, *tylO* in *S. fradiae* [12]. Disruption of *tylO* greatly reduces antibiotic production (*i. e.,* by at least 85%) and its product is proposed to serve an editing function by removing aberrant material(s) that would otherwise block the TylG enzymes [31]. A similar role has been proposed for "free" thioesterase activity during non-ribosomal peptide synthesis in *Bacillus subtilis* [32].

Resistance genes in the *tyl cluster*

Antibiotic-producing organisms must be able to tolerate their products and typically contain one or more resistance determinants (for a review, see [33]). These are commonly clustered together with antibiotic-biosynthetic genes, as in the genome of *S. fradiae* from which four genes have been isolated that confer resistance when cloned and expressed elsewhere. Three of these genes (*tlrB*, *tlrC*, and *tlrD*) are present in the *tyl* cluster (Fig. 2), whereas the fourth, *tlrA*, occupies an undetermined location elsewhere in the genome. The TlrD protein (encoded by orf5*) is produced constitutively and monomethylates 23S rRNA, thereby rendering the ribosomes moderately resistant to macrolides [34]. In the presence of tylosin or its glycosylated precursors, expression of *tlrA* is induced, leading to further methylation of 23S rRNA at the same target nucleotide and increased levels of tylosin resistance [35]. In addition, *tlrB* encodes a methyltransferase that confers resistance to tylosin in an ill-defined manner [36], whereas *tlrC* encodes an ATP-binding protein with a presumed role in tylosin-efflux [11].

Concluding comments

The *tyl* cluster of *S. fradiae* apparently contains the full complement of structural genes required for tylosin production, together with resistance determinants and an unexpected congregation of regulatory genes. The clear implication is that tylosin production is controlled at the genetic level in a multifactorial manner by pathway-specific and pleiotropic regulators, also involving γ-butyrolactone signalling factors. Polyketide synthesis is subject to feedback control (presumably at the transcriptional level) by glycosylated macrolides, and activity of the PKS enzyme complex depends heavily on the editing activity of a TE-II thioesterase. These controls operate alongside the time-honoured (but still poorly understood) physiological influence of carbon and nitrogen sources on tylosin production and repression of antibiotic biosynthesis by inorganic phosphate.

Acknowledgements

This work was supported by Lilly Research Laboratories, Indianapolis, Indiana, and by project grant 91/T08195 from BBSRC. Contributions to this work were made by colleagues in Leicester (especially Neil Bate, Andrew Butler, Steven Fish, Atul Gandecha, and Louise Merson-Davies) and at Lilly Research Laboratories (too numerous to mention, but including Richard Baltz, Charles Hershberger, Herbert Kirst, Paul Rosteck, Jr., and Eugene Seno).

References

1 Ōmura S, Takeshima H, Nakagawa A, Miyazawa J, Piriou F, Lukacs G (1977) Studies on the biosynthesis of 16-membered macrolide antibiotics using carbon-13 nuclear magnetic resonance spectroscopy. *Biochemistry* 16: 2860–2866

2 Baltz RH, Seno ET (1981) Properties of *Streptomyces fradiae* mutants blocked in biosynthesis of the macrolide antibiotic tylosin. *Antimicrob Agents Chemother* 20: 214–225

3 Ōmura S, Sadakane N, Matsubara H (1982) Bioconversion and biosynthesis of 16-membered macrolide antibiotics. XXII. Biosynthesis of tylosin after protylonolide formation. *Chem Pharm Bull* 30: 223–229

4 Ōmura S, Tanaka H, Tsukui M (1982) Biosynthesis of tylosin: oxidations of 5-*O*-mycaminosyl-protylonolide at C-20 and C-23 with a cell-free extract of *Streptomyces fradiae*. *Biochem Biophys Res Comm* 107: 554–560

5 Baltz RH, Seno ET, Stonesifer J, Wild GM (1983) Biosynthesis of the macrolide antibiotic tylosin. A preferred pathway from tylactone to tylosin. *J Antibiot* 36: 131–141

6 Fishman SE, Cox K, Larson JL, Reynolds PA, Seno ET, Yeh W-K, Van Frank R, Hershberger CL (1987) Cloning genes for the biosynthesis of a macrolide antibiotic. *Proc Natl Acad Sci USA* 84: 8248–8252

7 Beckmann RJ, Cox K, Seno ET (1989) A cluster of tylosin biosynthetic genes is interrupted by a structurally unstable segment containing four repeated sequences. In: CL Hershberger, SW Queener, G Hegeman (eds): *Genetics and molecular biology of industrial microorganisms*. American Society for Microbiology, Washington DC, 176–186

8 Birmingham VA, Cox KL, Larson JL, Fishman SE, Hershberger CL, Seno ET (1986) Cloning and expression of a tylosin resistance gene from a tylosin-producing strain of *Streptomyces fradiae*. *Mol Gen Genet* 204: 532–539

9 Baltz RH, Seno ET (1988) Genetics of *Streptomyces fradiae* and tylosin biosynthesis. *Annu Rev Microbiol* 42: 547–574

10 Szoke PA, Reynolds PA, Rosteck Jr PR, Kreuzman AJ, Yeh W-K, Becker GW, Hershberger CL (1989) Sequence analysis of tylosin biosynthetic genes. Abstracts of Posters of Annual Meeting of American Society for Microbiology, New Orleans, abstract # H-76
11 Rosteck Jr, PR, Reynolds PA, Hershberger CL (1991) Homology between proteins controlling *Streptomyces fradiae* tylosin resistance and ATP-binding transport. *Gene* 102: 27–32
12 Merson-Davies LA, Cundliffe E (1994) Analysis of five tylosin biosynthetic genes from the *tylIBA* region of the *Streptomyces fradiae* genome. *Mol Microbiol* 13: 349–355
13 Gandecha AR, Cundliffe E (1996) Molecular analysis of *tlrD*, an MLS resistance determinant from the tylosin producer, *Streptomyces fradiae*. *Gene* 180: 173–176
14 Gandecha AR, Large SL, Cundliffe E (1997) Analysis of four tylosin biosynthetic genes from the *tylLM* region of the *Streptomyces fradiae* genome. *Gene* 184: 197–203
15 Bate N, Butler AR, Gandecha AR, Cundliffe E (1999) Multiple regulatory genes in the tylosin-biosynthetic cluster of *Streptomyces fradiae*. *Chem Biol* 6: 617–624
16 Bate N, Cundliffe E (1999) The mycinose-biosynthetic genes of *Streptomyces fradiae*, producer of tylosin. *J Ind Microbiol Biotechnol* 23: 118–122
17 Bate N, Butler AR, Smith IP, Cundliffe E (2000) The mycarose-biosynthetic genes of *Streptomyces fradiae*, producer of tylosin. *Microbiology* 146: 139–146
18 Chater KF, Bibb MJ (1997) Regulation of bacterial antibiotic production. In: H Kleinkauf, H von Dören (eds): *Biotechnology, vol. 7; Products of secondary metabolism*. VCH, Weinheim, Germany, 59–105
19 Geistlich M, Losick R, Turner JR, Rao RN (1992) Characterization of a novel regulatory gene governing the expression of a polyketide synthase gene in *Streptomyces ambofaciens*. *Mol Microbiol* 6: 2019–2029
20 Arisawa A, Kawamura N, Tsunekawa H, Okamura K, Tone H, Okamoto R (1993) Cloning and nucleotide sequences of two genes involved in the 4"-*O*-acylation of macrolide antibiotics from *Streptomyces thermotolerans*. *Biosci Biotech Biochem* 57: 2020–2025
21 Wietzorrek A, Bibb M (1997) A novel family of proteins that regulates antibiotic production in streptomycetes appears to contain an OmpR-like DNA-binding fold. *Mol Microbiol* 25: 1177–1184
22 Kinoshita H, Ipposhi H, Okamoto S, Nakano H, Nihira T, Yamada Y (1997) Butyrolactone autoregulator receptor protein (BarA) as a transcriptional regulator in *Streptomyces virginiae*. *J Bacteriol* 179: 6986–6993
23 Nakano H, Takehara E, Nihira T, Yamada Y (1998) Gene replacement analysis of the *Streptomyces virginiae barA* gene encoding the butyrolactone autoregulator receptor reveals that BarA acts as a repressor in virginiamycin biosynthesis. *J Bacteriol* 180: 3317–3322
24 Horinouchi S, Beppu T (1994) A-factor as a microbial hormone that controls cellular differentiation and secondary metabolism in *Streptomyces griseus*. *Mol Microbiol* 12: 859–864
25 Ohnishi Y, Kameyama S, Onaka H, Horinouchi S (1999) The A-factor regulatory cascade leading to streptomycin biosynthesis in *Streptomyces griseus*: identification of a target gene of the A-factor receptor. *Mol Microbiol* 34: 102–111
26 Fish SA, Cundliffe E (1997) Stimulation of polyketide metabolism in *Streptomyces fradiae* by tylosin and its glycosylated precursors. *Microbiology* 143: 3871–3876
27 Bevitt DJ, Cortés J, Haydock SF, Leadlay PF (1992) 6-Deoxyerythronolide B synthase from *Saccharopolyspora erythraea*. Cloning of the structural gene, sequence analysis and inferred domain structure of the multifunctional enzyme. *Eur J Biochem* 204: 39–49
28 Donadio S, Katz L (1992) Organization of the enzymatic domains in the multifunctional polyketide synthase involved in erythromycin biosynthesis in *Saccharopolyspora erythraea*. *Gene* 111: 51–60
29 Cortés J, Wiesmann KEH, Roberts GA, Brown MJB, Staunton J, Leadlay PF (1995) Repositioning of a domain in a modular polyketide synthase to promote specific chain cleavage. *Science* 268: 1487–1489
30 Kao CM, Luo G, Katz L, Cane DE, Khosla C (1995) Manipulation of macrolide ring size by directed mutagenesis of a modular polyketide synthase. *J Am Chem Soc* 117: 9105–9106
31 Butler AR, Bate N, Cundliffe E (1999) Impact of thioesterase activity on tylosin biosynthesis in *Streptomyces fradiae*. *Chem Biol* 6: 287–292

32 Schneider A, Marahiel MA (1998) Genetic evidence for a role of thioesterase domains, integrated in or associated with peptide synthetases, in non-ribosomal peptide biosynthesis in *Bacillus subtilis. Arch Microbiol* 169: 404–410
33 Cundliffe E (1989) How antibiotic-producing organisms avoid suicide. *Annu Rev Microbiol* 43: 207–233
34 Zalacain M, Cundliffe E (1991) Cloning of *tlrD,* a fourth resistance gene, from the tylosin producer, *Streptomyces fradiae. Gene* 97: 137–142
35 Kelemen GH, Zalacain M, Culebras E, Seno ET, Cundliffe E (1994) Transcriptional attenuation control of the tylosin resistance gene, *tlrA,* in *Streptomyces fradiae. Mol Microbiol* 14: 833–842
36 Wilson VTW, Cundliffe E (1999) Molecular analysis of *tlrB*, an antibiotic-resistance gene from tylosin-producing *Streptomyces fradiae*, and discovery of a novel resistance mechanism. *J Antibiot* 52: 288–296

In vitro activity of macrolides against traditional susceptible bacteria

Adel Ben Ali, Fred W. Goldstein and Jacques F. Acar

Hôpital Saint Joseph, Laboratoire de Microbiologie Médicale, 185 rue Raymond Losserand, 75674 Paris Cedex 14, France

Antibiotics belonging to the macrolide class have been in use for almost 40 years and are considered to be among the best-tolerated antibiotics.

They are indicated principally for the treatment of upper and lower respiratory tract and skin structure infections, mainly in children and adults allergic to beta-lactam antibiotics, or infections due to intracellular microorganisms and atypical pathogens such as *Mycoplasma* or *Chlamydia* and *Legionella* spp.

This review gives ranges of MIC, MIC_{50} and/or MIC_{90} values of three subclasses: 14-, 15-, or 16-membered macrolides; streptogramins (RP 59500 [Synercid]); and ketolides.

Ketolides are new semi-synthetic 14-membered-ring macrolides derived from erythromycin. This group is represented by Ketek (Telithromycin, HMR 3647). These compounds have been demonstrated to be more active than existing macrolides against erythromycin-resistant, gram-positive cocci and have improved anti-anaerobic activity.

The increased use of macrolides has been accompanied by increased prevalence of macrolide-resistant strains of staphylococci, streptococci, and pneumococci [1–4]. Resistant strains that have been classified showed either constitutive resistance or inducible resistance as a result of methylation of 23S rRNA. Another mechanism of resistance, involving efflux, also has been reported. It is characterized by the presence of efflux genes, such as the *mefE* gene (see Chapter 17). This review summarizes the susceptibility to macrolides and ketolides of different species and their phenotypes.

A number of precautions must be taken in evaluating the data presented. In particular, not all the compounds have been compared directly against the same groups of bacteria (Tabs. 5, 11, 15, 17, 20).

In addition, methodological differences can affect significantly the activity of a given macrolide against a given organism *in vitro*; these include the type of medium used, inoculum size, and the pH of the medium. For example, most of the studies on anaerobes resulted in higher MICs to macrolides, since the incubation with CO_2 lowers the pH on the agar and decreases the activity of the compounds.

Table 1. MICs for *Staphylococcus aureus* [1–3, 5–7]

	Susceptible	Inducible	Constitutive
Erythromycin	0.06–0.25	4.0– > 128.0	> 128.0
Roxithromycin	0.06–0.25	4.0– > 128.0	> 128.0
Clarithromycin	0.03–0.25	4.0–> 128.0	> 128.0
Dirithromycin	0.06–0.50	4.0– > 128.0	> 128.0
Azithromycin	0.06–0.50	4.0– > 128.0	> 128.0
Josamycin	0.5–1.0	0.5–2.0	> 64.0
Spiramycin	1–4	1.0–4.0	> 64.0
Rokitamycin	0.25–1.0	0.25–1.0	> 64.0
Miocamycin	0.5–2.0	0.5–4.0	> 64.0
Midecamycin	0.25–4.0	0.25–4.0	> 64.0
Quinipristin (Q)	0.5–4.0	1.0–8.0	> 64.0
Dalfopristin (D)	2–4.0	2.0–4.0	2.0–4.0
Q/D	0.06–1.0	0.2–1.0	0.2–2.0
HMR 3647	0.01–0.06	0.01–0.12	> 128.0
ABT 773	0.01–0.06	0.01–0.12	32.0– > 128.0

The 16-membered macrolides inhibit inducible erythromycin-resistant strains, but not those expressing a constitutive phenotype.
Only the combination Q/D is active against a Staphylococci with MLS_Bconstitutive phenotype.

Table 2. Staphylococci phenotypes

Types	14-Memb	15-Memb	16-Memb	Quinupristin	Dalfopristine	Q/D	Ketolides
1	S	S	S	S	S	S	S
2[a]	R	R	S	S	S	S	S
3[b]	R	R	R	R	S	S	R

a: Inducible type
b: Constitutive type

Table 3. MICs for Streptococci [1–3, 5, 6, 8–18]

	S,pneumoniae			*S. pyogenes*				*S. agalactiae*		
	Susceptible	Inducible	Constitutive	Susceptible	Inducible	Constitutive	mefA (MIC90)	Susceptible	Inducible	Constitutive
Erythromycin	0.01–0.06	4.0–16.0	> 128.0	0.015–0.06	4.0–16.0	> 128.0	8.0	0.01–0.06	2.0–16.0	> 128.0
Roxithromycin	0.03–0.06	4.0–16.0	> 128.0	0.03–0.06			16.0	0.03–0.1.0		> 128.0
Clarithomycin	< 0.01–0.03	4.0–16.0	> 128.0	< 0.01–0.03			4.0	0.01–0.03		> 128.0
Dirithromycin	0.01–0.06	4.0–16.0	> 128.0	0.01–0.06				0.06–0.12		> 128.0
Azithromycin	0.03–0.12	2.0–8.0	> 128.0	0.03–0.12	8.0–16.0	> 128.0	8.0	0.06–0.12	4.0–128.0	> 128.0
Josamycin	0.06–0.25	0.5–1.0	4.0– > 128.0	0.06–0.25	0.5	> 128.0	0.25	0.12–1.0		
Spiramycin	0.06–0.12	16.0– > 128.0	32.– > 128.0	0.06–0.25	1.0–4.0	64.0– > 128.0		0.12–0.5		
Rokitamycin	0.12–0.25			0.12–0.25			0.12	0.12–0.5		
Miocamycin	0.06–1.0			0.03–1.0				0.25–1.0		
Midecamycin	0.12–1.0			0.2–2.0						
Quinipristin/ Dalfopristin	0.06–0.5	0.06–0.5	0.06–0.5	0.03–0.06	0.06	0.06–1.0	1.0	0.03–0.06	0.03–0.06	0.06
HMR 3647	0.015–0.06	0.03–0.06	0.06–0.5	0.015–0.06	0.125–0.25	0.125–32.0	0.12	0.03–0.06	0.06–0.25	0.06–0.5
ABT 773	0.0078–0.15	0.015–0.03	0.015–2.0	0.0078–0.15	0.03–0.15	0.015–8.0	0.12	0.0078–0.03	0.015–0.03	0.03–8
Clindamycin	0.03–0.125	0.03–0.125	> 64.0	0.03–0.125	0.03–0.125	> 64.0	0.064			

Resistant strains to erythromycin with MLS_B constitutive phenotype are resistant to C14-, C15- and C16-membered macrolides.
Only Josamycin, Rokitamycin and ketolides are active against *S. pyogenes* with the efflux phenotype (*mefA*).
For resistant strains of *Streptococcus pneumoniae* with MLS_B or mefA phenotype, ketolides and Q/D remain active with low MIC levels.

Table 4. MICS for *H. influenzae* and *M. catarrhalis* [1, 2, 6, 8, 9, 13, 15, 16, 18, 19]

	Haemophilus influenzae			*Moraxella catarrhalis*	
	MIC_{50}	MIC_{90}	MIC range	MIC_{50}	MIC range
Erythromycin	2.0	4.0	0,12– > 8.0	< 0,12	< 0,12–0,5
Roxythromycin	16.0	16.0	0,25– > 32.0	0.25	< 0,03–2.0
Clarithromycin	8.0	16.0	0,25–32.0	0.06	< 0,016–0,25
Dirithromycin	16.0	32.0	0,25– > 32.0	0.5	0,12–1.0
Azithromycin	1.0	2.0	0,25–8.0	< 0,06	< 0,06
Josamycin	8.0	16.0	4–32.0	1.0	0,25–1.0
Spiramycin	8.0	16.0	4–32.0	1.0	1.0–4.0
Rokitamycin	8.0	16.0	4–32.0	0.12	0,12–0,25
Miocamycin				2.0	1.0–4.0
Q/D	4.0	8.0	< 0,12–16.0	0.5	0,12–1.0
ABT 773	1.0	2.0	0,06–4.0	0.12	0,008–0,12
HMR 3647	2.0	4.0	0,125–8.0	0.03	0,015–4.0

The most active macrolides against *H. influenzae are* azithromycin and the ketolide ABT-773. *Moraxella catarrhalis* is extremely susceptible to all macrolides and ketolides.

Table 5. MICS for *B. pertussis, B.parapertussis and B. bronchiseptica* [20–22]

	B. pertussis			***B. parapertussis***			***B. bronchiseptica***
	MIC_{50}	MIC_{90}	MIC range	MIC_{50}	MIC_{90}	MIC range	MIC range
Erythromycin	0.03	0.06	0.03–0.06	0.5	0.5	0.5	8.0–32.0
Roxithromycin	0.06	0.125	0.03–0.25	0.5	0.5	0.5–1.0	4.0–8.0
Clarithromycin	0.06	0.06	0.015–0.125	0.5	0.5	0.25–2.0	
Dirithromycin	0.03	0.03	0.03–0.12		0.125	0.125	
Azithromycin	0.03	0.06	0.008–0.06	0.06	0.06	0.06–0.25	1.0–16.0
Josamycin	< 0.015	0.06	< 0.015–05		1	1	
Spiramycin	0.12	0.25	0.12–05				
Rokitamycin	0.03	0.12	0.03–0.25				
Miokamycin	0.06	0.12	0.03–0.25				
HMR 3647	0.015	0.03	0.004–0.06	0.125	0.25	0.125–0.5	

B. pertussis and *B. parapertussis* are highly susceptible to macrolides and ketolides.
B. brochiseptica is resistant to erythromycin, but susceptibilities of only a few strains are reported.

Table 6. MICs for *N. gonorrheae* and *N. meningitidis*. [23]

	N.gonorrheae			*N.meningitidis*		
	MIC_{50}	MIC_{90}	MIC range	MIC_{50}	MIC_{90}	MIC range
Erythromycin	0.25	2.0	0.03–1.0	0.12	0.25	0.12–0.5
Roxithromycin	0.25	0.5	0.03–1.0	0.12	0.25	0.03–1.0
Clarithromycin	0.06	0.12	0.03–0.25	0.03	0.06	0.03–0.5
Dirithromycin	2.0		0.5–4.0			
Azithromycin	0.125	0.25	0.03–0.5	0.015		
Josamycin	0.25		0.25–2.0	0.12		0.12–0.5
Spiramycin	1.0		0.25–2.0	1		0.25–2.0
Rokitamycin	0.5		0.12–1.0	0.5		0.12–1.0
Miocamycin	0.12		0.12–4.0	0.12		0.12–4.0
RP59500	4.0		2.0–4.0	4.0		2.0–4.0
HMR 3647	0.03	0.03	0.002–0.12	0.015	0.03	0.008–0.25

Neisseria species are highly susceptible to most macrolides: Clarithromycin, azithromycin, and ketolide HMR 3647 are the most active agents.

Table 7. MICs for *Campylobacter jejuni* and *Helicobacte pylori*. [24–27]

	C. jejuni		*H.pylori*	
	MIC_{50}	MIC range	MIC_{50}	MIC range
Erythromycin	0.12	0.06–1.0	0.12	0.12–0.25
Roxithromycin	1.0	0.25–8.0	0.12	0.12–0.25
Clarithromycin	0.25	0.12–2.0	0.03	0.03–0.06
Dirithromycin	0.25	0.06–0.5	0.5	0.25–0.5
Azithromycin	0.06	0.03–0.12	0.25	0.25
Josamycin	0.25	< 0.03–2.0	1.0	0.5–1.0
Spiramycin	0.5	0.25–2.0	0.5	0.25–2.0
Miocamycin	2.0	0.5– > 4.0	0.5	0.5–1.0
Rokitamycin	1.0	0.12–2.0	0.5	0.5–1.0
HMR 3647			0.25	
ABT-773			0.12	

In vitro, macrolides have excellent activity against *C. jejuni* and *H.pylori*. However, *in vivo* efficacy is different (see Chapter 13 authored by Francis Megraud).

Table 8. MICs for *Listeria monocytogenes, Rhodococcus equi*, and *Erysopelothrix rhusiopathiae* [27, 28]

	L. monocytogenes			*Rhodococcus equi*			*Erysopelothrix rhusiopathiae*		
	MIC_{50}	MIC_{90}	MICs	MIC_{50}	MIC_{90}	MICs	MIC_{50}	MIC_{90}	MICs
Erythromycin	0.125	0.25	0.25–1.0	0.25	0.25	< 0.015–0.25	0.03	0.03	0.03
Roxithromycin	0.5	0.5	0.5–1.0	0.125	0.25	< 0.015–0.5	0.06	0.12	0.06–0.12
Clarithomycin	0.06	0.125	0.25–1.0	0.06	0.125	< 0.015–0.125	0.06	0.06	0.06
Dirithromycin			1.0–2.0						
Azithromycin	1.0	1.0	1.0–2.0	1.0	1.0	0.03–2.0	0.03	0.03	0.03
Josamycin	1.0	1.0	2.0–4.0	2.0	4.0	0.03–2.0	0.05	0.05	0.05
Spiramycin			4.0–4.0			4.0–32.0			
Rokitamycin			2.0–2.0						
Miocamycin			2.0–2.0						
Quinipristin/ Dalfopristin	4.0	4.0	2.0–16.0	8.0	8.0	0.12–8.0	2.0	2.0	1.0–2.0
HMR 3647	0.03	0.03	0.03–0.06	0.125	0.25	< 0.015–0.25	< 0.05	< 0.05	< 0.05
ABT 773		0.06							
Clindamycin	8.0	16.0	2.0– > 128.0	16.0	16.0	0.25–16.0	0.06	1.0	0.06–1.0

Table 9. MICs for *Corynebacterium species* [28]

	C. diphteriae		C. minutissimum		C. striatum		C. jeikeium		*C. urealyticum*	
	MIC_{50}	MIC range	MIC_{50}	MIC range	MIC_{50}	MIC range	MIC_{50}	MIC range	MIC_{50}	MIC range
Erythromycin	0.008	0.002–0.125	1.0	< 0.015–8.0	> 128.0	< 0.015– > 128.0	> 128.0	< 0.015– > 128.0	1.0	< 0.015– > 128.0
Roxithromycin	0.008	0.016–2.0	2.0	0.03–32	> 128.0	< 0.015– > 128.0	> 128.0	< 0.015– > 128.0	4.0	< 0.015–128.0
Clarithomycin	0.004	0.004–0.5	0.25	0.015–8.0	> 128.0	< 0.015– > 128.0	> 128.0	< 0.015– > 128.0	0.5	< 0.015–128.0
Azithromycin	0.015	0.031–4.0	2.0	0.12– > 128.0	> 128.0	< 0.015– > 128.0	> 128.0	0.06– > 128.0	1.0	< 0.015– > 128.0
Josamycin	0.5	0.03–32.0	16.0	0.5–64.0	> 128.0	0.06– > 128.0	> 128.0	0.25– > 128.0	32.0	0.03– > 128.0
Spiramycin	0.5	0.06–64.0								
Quinipristin/ Dalfopristin	0.25	0.03–2.0	0.5	0.25–2.0	2.0	0.12–12.0	0.5	0.25–2.0	0.5	0.12–0.5
HMR 3647	0.004	0.002–0.125	0.03	< 0.015–0.06	16.0	< 0.015–64.0	0.12	< 0.015– > 128.0	0.25	< 0.015–4.0
ABT 773	0.015									
Clindamycin	> 128	0.25– > 128.0	2.0	0.5– > 128	> 128.0	0.25– > 128.0	> 128.0	0.25– > 128.0	> 128.0	0.06– > 128.0

C. diphteriae is highly susceptible to erythromycin and to the other macrolides and ketolides.
The other corynebacterium species have macrolide MICs ranging from 0.03 to 128 mg/l with 25% to 30% resistant isolates.

Table 10. MICs for *Lactobacillus spp*, *Leuconostoc*, and *Pediococcus spp.* [24–26]

	Leuconostoc			*Pediococcus*			*Lactobacillus*		
	MIC_{50}	MIC_{90}	MIC range	MIC_{50}	MIC_{90}	MIC range	MIC_{50}	MIC_{90}	MIC range
Erythromycin	0.03	0.06	0.015–0.06	0.03	0.06	> 128.0	0.06	0.06	0.03–0.06
Roxithromycin	0.12	0.12	0.06–0.25	< 0.06	0.12	< 0.06– > 16.0	< 0.06	0.12	> 0.06–0.12
Clarithromycin	0.03	0.03	0.007–0.03	0.06	0.06	0.007–128.0	0.015	0.03	0.015–128.0
Azithromycin	0.125			0.125			0.06		
Josamycin	0.12	0.25	< 0.06–0.25	0.25	0.25	< 0.06–0.25	0.12	0.12	< 0.06–0.25
Spiramycin	0.25	0.5	0.25–0.5	0.5	1.0	0.25– > 64.0	0.25	0.5	0.06–16.0
HMR 3647	0.007	0.015	< 0.007–0.015	0.007	0.015	< 0.0007–4.0	0.007	0.015	0.0007–0.5

Table 11. MICs for *Eikenella corrodens, Actinobacillus actinomycetemcomitans, and Pasteurella multocida* [29]

	E. corrodens			*A. actinomycetemcomitans*			*P. multocida*		
	MIC_{50}	MIC_{90}	MIC range	MIC_{50}	MIC_{90}	MIC range	MIC_{50}	MIC_{90}	MIC range
Erythromycin	1.5	1.0	0.25–16.0	2.0	16.0	0.5–32.0	2.0	2.0	0.25–2.0
Roxithromycin	8.0	16.0	2.0–16.0	1.0	16.0	< 0.016–32.0	4.0	8.0	0.5–8.0
Clarithromycin	4.0	4.0	0.25–8.0	0.5	2.0	0.12–8.0	4.0	8.0	0.5–4.0
Azithromycin	1.0	4.0	0.25–8.0	0.25		< 0.016–8.0	1.0	1.0	0.25–1.0
HMR 3647	0.5	1.0	0.03–1.0	0.25		< 0.016–8.0	1.0	1.0	0.25–1.0
ABT 773	0.5	1.0	0.25–1.0				1.0	1.0	0.125–1.0
Q/D							2.0	4.0	0.125–8.0

Table 12. MICs for *Haemophilus ducreyi, Gardnerella vaginalis, and Mobiluncus* [30]

	H. ducreyi			*G. vaginalis*	*Mobiluncus*
	MIC_{50}	MIC_{90}	MIC range	MIC_{50}	MIC range
Erythromycin	0.008	0.125	0.002–4.0	0.06	0.002–0.2
Roxithromycin	0.03	0.06	0.008–0.06	0.03	0.004–0.25
Clarithromycin	0.008	0.06	0.004–0.006	0.008	0.002–0 006
Azithromycin	0.004	0.03	0.002–0.06	0.06	0.12–1.0
Josamycin	0.12	0.12	0.008–0.12	0.03	0.008–0.4
Miokamycin	0.06	0.12	0.008–0.12	0.03	
HMR 3647	0.004	0.008		< 0.002	

This group is extremely susceptible to macrolides and ketolides.

Table 13. MICS and MIC_{50} for *B. fragilis, Prevotella bivia, Fusobacterium spp., and Porphyromonas spp.* [29, 31–36]

	B. fragilis		*P. bivia*		*Fusobacterium.spp*		*Porphyromonas. spp*	
	MIC_{50}	MIC range	MIC_{50}	MIC range	MIC_{50}	MIC range	MIC_{50}	MIC range
Erythromycin	16.0	2.0–64	2.0	1.0–16.0	4.0	< 0.016– > 32.0	0.25	0.06–0.25
Roxithromycin	32.0	1.0–64.0	1.0	0.5–4.0	8.0	< 0.016– > 32.0	0.25	0.125–0.25
Clarithromycin	4.0	1.0–64.0	0.25	< 0.25–1.0	2.0	0.06–32.0	0.06	0.03–0.125
Dirithromycin	128.0	128.0						
Azithromycin	16.0	4.0–64.0	1.0	0.25–4.0	0.5	0.125–8.0	0.5	0.25–1.0
Josamycin	1.0	0.25–128.0						
Spiramycin	8.0	4.0–128.0						
Rokitamycin	0.25	0.25–128.0						
Miocamycin	2.0	1.0–128.0						
Q/D	4.0	2.0–4.0						
HMR 3647	0.5	0.25–1.0	0.25	< 0.016–1.0	1.0	< 0.016–8.0	0.06	0.03–0.125
ABT 773	4.0		0.06	0.06–0.125	1.0	0.015–8.0	< 0.015	0.015–0.25
Clindamycin	1.0	< 0.006–> 6.0	< 0.06	< 0.06–0.5	0.06	< 0.06–0.25	< 0.016	0.016

Except for *B. fragilis* and *Porphyromonas* spp, MIC_{50} of azithromycin is generally one dilution lower than that of other macrolides.
The MIC_{50} of ketolides is generally one log2 lower than that of erythromycin.

Table 14. MICs and MIC_{50} for *C. perfringens, C. difficile, Peptostreptococcus spp, Propionibacterium acnes*, and *Actinomyces* spp [29, 31–36]

	C. perfringens		*C. difficile*		*Peptostreptococcus spp*		*Propionibacterium acnes*		*Actinomyces spp.*	
	MIC_{50}	MIC range	MIC_{50}	MIC range	MIC_{50}	MIC range	MIC_{50}	MIC range	MIC_{50}	MIC range
Erythromycin	1.0	0.5–1.0	0.25.0	0.25– > 128.0	0.5	0.015– > 128.0	0.03	0.03–128.0	0.03	< 0.015–0.06
Roxithromycin	2.0	1.0–2.0	0.5	0.5– > 128.0	1.0	0.03– > 128.0	0.125	0.03–64.0	0.06	0.03–0.06.0
Clarithromycin	0.25	0.12–0.5	0.12	0.12– > 128.0	0.12	0.015– > 128.0	0.016	0.03–64.0	< 0.015	
Dirithromycin	4.0	2.0–4.0						0.25–1.0		
Azithromycin							0.06	0.004–4.0	0.03	0.015–0.06
Josamycin	1.0	1.0–1.0					0.12	0.06–8.0		
Spiramycin	2.0	2.0–2.0					0.12	0.12–4.0		
Rokitamycin	0.12	0.12–0.12					0.06	0.03–2.0		
Miocamycin	0.5	0.5–1.0					0.12	0.12–8.0		
Q/D	0.12	0.12–0.25								
HMR 3647	0.06	0.03–0.12.0	0.06	0.03– > 128.0	0.004	0.002–0.25	0.004		0.015	0.015
ABT 773	0.03		0.12.0		0.03	0.015–0.25	0.016		<0.015	<0.015–4.0

C. difficile, *Peptostreptococcus* spp, and *Propionibacterium acnes* strains fall into two groups based on their MIC levels: a sensitive group (MIC < 2 mg/l) and a highly resistant group (MIC > 64 mg/l).

Table 15. MICs for *Legionella pneumophila*. [37, 38]

	MIC_{90}	MIC range
Erythromycin	0.12	0.008–0.25
Roxithromycin	0.03	0.004–0.06
Clarithromycin	< 0.004	0.03–0.06
Dirithromycin		1.0–16.0
Azithromycin	0.03	0.004–0.06
Josamycin	0.25	
Spiramycin		8.0–64.0
Miocamycin	0.12	
ABT 773		0.03–0.12
HMR 3647	0.03	< 0.004–0.06
Q/D	0.5	0.015–0.5
Clindamycin	8.0	0.008–8.0

Clarithromycin, azithromycin, and ketolides appear to be more active than erythromycin.

Table 16. *Mycoplasma* spp MIC range [39, 40]

	M. pneumoniae	*M. hominis*	*M. genitalium*	*M. fermentans*	*M. penetrans*	*U. urealyticum*
Erythromycin	< 0.015	> 64.0	> 64.0	64.0– > 64.0	2.0	0.12–1.0
Roxithromycin	< 0.015–0.03	> 64.0	> 64.0	32.0–64.0	0.5	0.06–0.5
Clarithromycin	< 0.015	> 64.0	> 64.0	16.0–32.0	0.12	< 0.015–0.03
Dirithromycin	< 0.015–0.06	> 64.0	> 64.0	64.0– > 64.0	16.0	0.25–2.0
Azithromycin	< 0.015	32.0– > 64.0	< 0.015–0.03	2.0–8.0	0.12–0.5	0.06–0.25
Josamycin	< 0.015–0.03	0.06–0.25	0.015–0.03	0.12–0.5	0.12–0.25	0.03–0.12
Spiramycin	< 0.015–0.25	32.0– > 64.0	0.12–1.0	2.0–4.0	16.0	4.0–32.0
Midecamycin	0.004–0.03	0.008–0.12				0.003–0.25
ABT 773	< 0.0005					
HMR 3647	< 0.015	2.0–16.0	< 0.015	0.06–0.25	0.12	< 0.015–0.06
Clindamycin		0.008–0.016	0.25	0.016–0.125	0.008	

14-membered macrolides are inactive against *M. hominis*, *M. genitalium*, and *M. fermentans*.
So far, all clinically isolated strains of *M. pneumoniae* have been found to be clinically susceptible to erythromycin.

Table 17. *Rickettsiae* spp: MIC range [41–43]

	Group 1	Group 2	Group 3	Group 4	Group 5	*Coxiella burnettii*
Erythromycin	2.0–8.0	2.0–8.0	2.0–8.0	1.0–8.0	0.125–1.0	4.0– > 8.0
Clarithromycin	1.0–4.0	0.5–4.0	0.5–4.0	0.5–2.0	0.5–1.0	1.0–4.0
Roxithromycin	8.0–16.0				1.0	
Dirithromycin	16.0				16.0	
Azithromycin	8.0				0.25	
Josamycin	0.5–1.0	0.5–1.0	0.5–1.0	0.5–2.0	0.5–1.0	
Pristinamycin	1.0–4.0	1.0–8.0	2.0–4.0	1.0–4.0	2.0–4.0	
HMR 3647	0.5				0.5	1.0

Group 1: *R. rickettsii; R. conorii* Moroccan, Seven, and Israeli; *R. sibirica; R. australis;* and *R. akari.*
Group 2: *R. japonica, R. honei, R. conorii Astrakhan, R. africae, "R. mongolotimonae"*, strain 13 B, and the human isolate of *R. slovaca.*
Group 3: *R. bellii, R. Canada, R. helvetica, R. conorii, M1, R. parkeri,* and Thai tick typhus rickettsia.
Group 4: *Bar 29, R. massiliae, R. aeschlimanii, R. montana,* and *R. rhipicephali.*
Group 5: *R. typhi and R. prowazekii.*

Table 18. *Bartonella spp* MICs [44, 45]

	B. quintana	*B. henselae*	*B. vinsonii*	*B. elizabethae*	*B. bacilliformis*
Erythromycin	0.06	0.06–0.25	0.25	0.12	0.06
Roxithromycin	0.06	0.015–0.03	0.06	0.06	0.03
Clarithromycin	0.015	0.006–0.03	0.03	0.015	0.015
Azithromycin	0.006	0.006–0.015	0.015	0.006	0.015
Dirithromycin	1.0	0.125		0.1	
HMR3647	0.006	0.003			0.015
Clindamycin	8.0	2.0–4.0	8.0	8.0	

Clarithromycin, azithromycin and HMR 3647 are the most active macroldies against Bartonella.

Table 19. MIC_{90} for some *Enterobacteriacae* and other gram-negative bacteria [11, 46]

	Erythromycin	Roxithromycin	Clarithromycin	Azithromycin	D/Q*	HMR 3647
E.coli	64.0	128.0	128.0	4.0	128.0	16.0
Salmonella enteritidis	128.0		128.0	4.0		32.0
S.typhi	32.0			4.0		
Shigella Spp	128.0	128.0	64.0	8.0	64.0	
Yersinia enterecolitica	128.0	128.0	128.0	64.0		
Y. pestis	16.0	> 16				0.5
V. cholerae	4.0			0.12		
V.parahemolyticus	8.0			0.25		
Physiomonas shigelloïdes	8.0			1.0		
Alcagenes spp	32.0	> 32.0	32.0	4.0		16.0
Arcobacter butzleri	12.5	12.5	12.5	25.0		6.25
Stenotrophomonas maltophilia	128.0		64.0	32.0		16.0

References

1 Felmingham D, Grüneberg RN, and the Alexander Project Group (2000) The Alexander Project 1996–1997: latest susceptibility data from this international study of bacterial pathogens from community-acquired lower respiratory tract infections. *J Antimicrob Chemother* 45: 191–20

2 Schmitz FJ, Verhoef J, Fluit AC, and the Sentry Participants Group (1999) Prevalence of resistance to MLS antibiotics in 20 european university hospitals participating in the european SENTRY surveillance programme. *J Antimicrob Chemother* 43: 783–792

3 Shortridge D, Doern GV, Brueggemann AB, Beyer JM, Flamm RK (1999) Prevalence of macrolide resistance mechanisms in *Streptococcus pneumoniae* isolates from a multicenter antibiotic resistance surveillance study conducted in the United States in 1994–1995. *Clin Infect Dis* 29: 1186–1188

4 Weisblum B (1985) Inducible resistance to macrolides, lincosamides and streptogramin type B antibiotics: the resistance phenotype, its biological diversity, and structural elements that regulate expression. A review. *J Antimicrob Chemother* 16 (*Suppl.* A): 63–90

5 Barry AL, Fuchs PC, Brown SD (1998) Susceptibilities to RPR 106,972, quinupristin/dalfopristin and erythromycin among recent clinical isolates of enterococci, staphylococci and streptococci from north american medical centres. *J Antimicrob Chemother* 42: 651–655

6 Jamjian C, Biedenbach DJ, Jones RN (1997) *In vitro* evaluation of a novel ketolide antimicrobial agent, RU-64004. *Antimicrob Agents Chemother* 41(2): 454–459

7 Schmitz FJ, Sadurski R, Kray A, Boos M, Geisel R, Köhrer K, Verhoef J, Fluit AC (2000) Prevalence of macrolide-resistance genes in *Staphylococcus aureus* and *Enterococcus faecium* isolates from 24 European university hospitals. *J Antimicrob Chemother* 45: 891–894

8 Brueggemann AB, Doern GV, Huynh HK, Wingert EM, Rhomberg PR (2000) *In vitro* activity of ABT-773, a new ketolide, against recent clinical isolates of *Streptococcus pneumoniae, Haemophilus influenzae*, and *Moraxella catarrhalis. Antimicrob Agents Chemother* 44(2): 447–449

9 Boswell FJ, Andrews JM, Ashby JP, Fogarty C, Brenwald NP, Wise R (1998) The *in vitro* activity of HMR 3647, a new ketolide antimicrobial agent. *J Antimicrob Chemother* 42: 703–709

10 Marshall SA, Erwin ME, Jones RN (2000) Determination of MIC quality control ranges for ABT-773, a novel ketolide antimicrobial agent. *J Clin Microbiol* 38(6): 2462–2463

11 Shortridge D, et al (1999) The *In vitro* activity of ABT-773 against gram-positive and gram-negative pathogens. ICAAC, Abstract 2136, p. 346. *In* Abstracts of the 39th ICAAC. American Society for Microbiology, Washington, D.C.

12 Davies TA, Kelly LM, Jacobs M, Appelbaum PC (2000) Antipneumococcal activity of telithromycin by agar dilution, microdilution, E-test, and disk diffusion methodologies. *J Clin Microbiol* 38(4): 1444–1448

13 Jacobs MR, Bajaksouzian S, Zilles A, Lin G, Pankuch GA, Appelbaum PC (1999) Susceptibilities of *Streptococcus pneumoniae* and *Haemophilus influenzae* to 10 oral antimicrobial agents based on pharmacodynamic parameters: 1997 U.S. surveillance study. *Antimicrob Agents Chemother* 43(8): 1901–1908

14 Nishijima T, Saito Y, Aoki A, Toriya M, Toyonaga Y, Fujii R (1999) Distribution of *mefE* and *ermB* genes in macrolide-resistant strains of *Streptococcus pneumoniae* and their variable susceptibility to various antibiotics. *J Antimicrob Chemother* 43: 637–643

15 Thornsberry C, Ogilvie PT, Holley HP, Sahm DF (1999) Survey of susceptibilities *of Streptococcus pneumoniae, Haemophylus influenzae*, and *Moraxella catarrhalis* isolates to 26 antimicrobial .agents: a prospective U.S. study. *Antimicrob Agents Chemother* 43 (11): 2612–2623

16 Thornsberry C, Jones ME, Hickey ML, Mauriz Y, Kahn J, Sahm DF (1999) Resistance surveillance of *Streptococcus pneumoniae*, *Haemophilus influenzae* and *Moraxella catarrhalis* isolated in the United States, 1997–1998. *J Antimicrob Chemother* 44: 749–759

17 Waites K, Johnson C, Gray B, Edwards K, Crain M, Benjamin W (2000) Use of clindamycin disks to detect macrolide resistance mediated by *ermB* and *mefE* in *Streptococcus pneumoniae* isolates from adults and children. *J Clin Microbiol* 38 (5): 1731–1734

18 Wootton M, Bowker KE, Janowska A, Holt HA, MacGowan AP (1999) *In vitro* activity of HMR 3647 against *Streptococcus pneumoniae*, *Haemophilus influenzae* and *Moraxella catarrhalis* and β-haemolytic streptococci. *J Antimicrob Chemother* 44: 445–453

19 Jorgensen JH, McElmeel ML (1997) Activity of quinupristin/dalfopristin and its components against *Haemophilus influenzae*. *J Antimicrob Chemother* 39(*Suppl.* A): 69–73

20 Brett M, Short P, Beatson S (1998) The comparative *in vitro* activity of roxithromycin and other antibiotics against *Bordetella pertussis*. *J Antimicrob Chemother* 41(*Suppl.* B): 23–27

21 Hoppe JE, Bryskier A (1998) *In vitro* susceptibilities of *Bordetella pertussis* and *Bordetella parapertussis* to two ketolides (HMR 3004 and HMR 3647), four macrolides (azithromycin, clarithromycin, erythromycin A, and roxithromycin), and two ansamycins (rifampicin and rifapentine). *Antimicrob Agents Chemother* 42(4): 965–966

22 Korgenski EK, Daly JA (1997) Surveillance and detection of erythromycin resistance in *Bordetella pertussis* isolates recovered from a pediatric population in the intermountain west region of the united states. *J Clin Microbiol* 35(11): 2989–2991

23 Slaney L, Chubb H, Ronald A, Brunham R (1990) *In vitro* activity of azithromycin, erythromycin, ciprofloxacin and norfloxacin against *Neisseria gonorrhoeae*, *Haemophilus ducreyi*, and *Chlamydia trachomatis*. *J Antimicrob Chemother* 25(*Suppl. A*): 1–5

24 Loo VG, et al 1997. *In vitro* susceptibility of *Helicobacter pylori* to six antibiotics. ICAAC, Abstract E 20, p. 117. *In* Abstracts of the 37 th ICAAC. American Society for Microbiology, Washington, D.C.

25 Sanchez R, Fernandez-Baca V, Diaz MD, Munoz P, Rodriguez-Creixems M, Bouza E (1994) Evolution of susceptibilities of *Campylobacter* spp. to quinolones and macrolides. *Antimicrob Agents Chemother* 38(9): 1879–1888

26 Zarazaga M, Saenz Y, Portillo A, Tenorio C, Ruiz-Larrea F, Del Campo R, Baquero F, Torres C (1999) *In vitro* activities of ketolides HMR3647, macrolides, and other antibiotics against *Lactobacillus*, *Leuconostoc*, and *Pediococcus* isolates. *Antimicrob Agents Chemother* 43 (12): 3039–3041

27 Moore LS, Schneider B, Holloway WJ (1997) Minimal inhibitory concentrations of quinupristin/dalfopristin against clinical isolates of *Corynebacterium jeikeium* and *Listeria monocytogenes*. *J Antimicrob Chemother* 39(*Suppl.* A): 67–68

28 Soriano F, Fernandez-Roblas R, Calvo R, Garcia-Calvo G (1998) *In vitro* susceptibilities of aerobic and facultative non-spore-forming gram-positive bacilli to HMR 3647 (RU 66647) and 14 other antimicrobials. *Antimicrob Agents Chemother* 42 (5): 1028–1033
29 Goldstein EJC, Citron DM , Vreni Merriam C (1999) Linezolid activity compared to those of selected macrolides and other agents against aerobic and anaerobic pathogens isolated from soft tissue bite infections in humans. *Antimicrob Agents Chemother* 43(6): 1469–1474
30 Knapp JS, Back AF, Babst AF, Taylor D, Rice R (1993) *In vitro* susceptibility of isolates of *Haemophilus ducreyi* from Thailand and the United States to currently recommended and newer agents for treatment of chancroid. *Antimicrob Agents Chemother* 37 (7): 1552–1555
31 Credito KL, Ednie LM, Jacobs MR, Appelbaum PC (1999) Activity of Telithromycin (HMR 3647) against anaerobic bacteria compared to those of eight other agents by time-kill methodology. *Antimicrob Agents Chemother* 43 (8): 2027–2031
32 Ednie LM, Spangler SK, Jacobs MR, Appelbaum PC (1997) Antianaerobic activity of the ketolide RU 64004 compared to activities of four macrolides, five β-lactams, clindamycin, and metronidazole. *Antimicrob Agents Chemother* 41 (5): 1037–1041
33 Ednie LM, Jacobs MR, Appelbaum PC (1997) Comparative antianaerobic activities of the ketolides HMR 3647 (RU 66647) and HMR 3004 (RU 64004). *Antimicrob Agents Chemother* 41: 2019–2022
34 Goldstein EJC, Citron DM , Gerardo SH, Hudspeth M, Vreni Merriam C (1998) Activities of HMR 3004 (RU 64004) and HMR 3647 (RU 66647) compared to those of erythromycin, azithromycin, clarithromycin, roxithromycin, and eight other antimicrobial agent against unusual aerobic and anaerobic human and animal bite pathogens isolated from skin and soft tissue infections in humans. *Antimicrob Agents Chemother* 42 (5): 1127–1132
35 Goldstein EJC, Citron DM , Vreni Merriam C, Warren Y, Tyrrell K (1999) Activities of Telithromycin (HMR 3647, RU 66647) compared to those of erythromycin, azithromycin, clarithromycin, roxithromycin, and other antimicrobial agents against unusual anaerobes. *Antimicrob Agents Chemother* 43 (11): 2801–2805
36 Goldstein EJC et al (2000) Comparative *In vitro* activity of ABT-773 against aerobic and anaerobic human and animal bite pathogens isolated from skin and soft tissue. Abstract 2.31, p. 29. *In* Abstracts of ICMASKO 5, Wallace Communications, Atlanta GA.
37 Marques T, Piedad J (1997) Susceptibility testing by E-test and agar dilution of 30 strains of *Legionella* spp. isolated in Portugal. *Clin Microb Infect* 3(3): 365–368
38 Schulin T, Wennerstern CB, Ferraro MJ, Moellering RCJ, Eliopoulos GM (1998) Susceptibilities of *legionella* spp. to newer antimicrobials in vitro. *Antimicrob Agents Chemother* 42: 1520–1523
39 Bebear CM, Renaudin H, Bryskier A, Bebear C (2000) Comparative activities of telithromycin (HMR 3647), levofloxacin, and other antimicrobial agents against human mycoplasmas. *Antimicrob Agents Chemother* 44 (7): 1980–1982
40 Bebear CM, Renaudin H, Aydin MD, Chantot JF, Bebear C (1997) *In vitro* activity of ketolides against mycoplasmas. *J Antimicrob Chemother* 39: 669–670
41 Rachek LI, Hines A, Tucker AM, Winkler HH, Wood DO (2000) Transformation of *Rickettsia prowazekii* to erythromycin resistance encoded by the *Escherichia coli ereB* gene. *J Bacteriol* 182 (11): 3289–3291
42 Rolain JM, Maurin M, Vestris G, Raoult D (1998) *In vitro* susceptibility of 27 *Rickettsiae* to 13 antimicrobials. *Antimicrob Agents Chemother* 42 (7): 1537–1541
43 Rolain JM, Maurin M, Bryskier A, Raoult D (2000) *In vitro* activities of telithromycin (HMR 3647) against *Rickettsia rickettsii, Rickettsia conorii, Rickettsia africae, Rickettsia typhi, Rickettsia prowazekii, Coxiella burnetti, Bartonella henselae, Bartonella quintana, Bartonella bacilliformis*, and *Ehrlichia chaffeensis*. *Antimicrob Agents Chemother* 44 (5): 1391–1393
44 Maurin M, Gasquet S, Ducco C, Raoult D (1995) Minimal inhibitory concentrations of 28 antibiotic compounds for 14 *Bartonella* isolates. *Antimicrob Agents Chemother* 39 (11): 2387–91
45 Maurin M, Raoult D (1993) Antibiotic susceptibility of *Rochalimaea quintana, Rochalimaea vinsonii*, and the newly described *Rochalimeae henselae*. *J Antimicrob Chemother* 32: 587–94
46 Stock I, Wiedemann B (1999) An *In vitro* study of the antimicrobial susceptibilities of *Yersinia enterocolitica* and the definition of a database. *J Antimicrob Chemother* 43: 37–45

Macrolide Antibiotics
ed. by W. Schönfeld and H. A. Kirst

Activity of macrolides against mycobacteria

Lowell S. Young and Luiz E. Bermudez

Kuzell Institute for Arthritis and Infectious Diseases, California Pacific Medical Center Research Institute, 2200 Webster Street, Suite 305, San Francisco, CA 94115, USA;

Introduction

The description of human disease caused by mycobacterial pathogens dates back to Biblical times. Presently, mycobacterial diseases account for a large proportion of all serious infectious disorders observed worldwide. Estimates of the numbers of leprosy cases exceed 20 million. Tuberculosis in all of its forms is believed to be the most common of the fatal infections, with total annual mortality figures of three million adult deaths of adults in developing countries (malaria may be numerically even more common but kills fewer patients) [1]. Tuberculosis is a re-emergent problem in many industrialized countries. In the modern world of global interdependency, rapid transportation, expanding trade, and migration, tuberculosis in any country is a threat to people of every country. The current global re-emergence of tuberculosis can be attributed to several factors, among them, the HIV epidemic, social dislocation, poverty, overcrowding, and inadequate investment in public-health measures.

As a result of the AIDS pandemic, non-tuberculous mycobacteria were recognized as important opportunistic pathogens. In hospitals dealing with immune-suppressed patients, or where extensive reconstructive and prosthetic surgery is undertaken, the non-tuberculous mycobacteria account for a small but very challenging number of complicating nosocomial infections [2–4]. Acquired or therapeutically induced immune suppression that results in impairment of TH1-type lymphocyte responses appears to predispose humans to mycobacterial disease. Numerous medications, the best known of which are the glucocorticoids, are recognized to suppress this limb of the human host response. Non-tuberculous mycobacteria, and in particular *M. kansasii* and organisms of the *Mycobacterium avium* complex (MAC), cause pulmonary diseases in patients who may or may not be overtly immune suppressed.

Mycobacteria are largely environmental in origin, and studies of phylogenetic relationships (comparison of nucleic acid pattern), as well as an appreciation of the entire mycobacterial genomes that have recently been decoded, strongly suggest that those pathogens causing human disease were derived from environmental sources and in fairly recent evolutionary time. The adaptation of pathogens such as *M. tuberculosis* to its primary human host is unique. Nonetheless, organisms such as *M. bovis* serve as the basis of the Bacille Calmette-Guerin (BCG) vaccine against tuberculosis, and *M. bovis* has a genome quite similar to *M.*

tuberculosis. The therapeutic use of BCG in oncology also clearly has led to iatrogenic disease when this live-attenuated organism has been used as a component of adjuvant chemotherapy.

The classification of mycobacteria dates back to the work of Runyon and colleagues [5] and is particularly useful from the viewpoint of growth characteristics (Table 1). However, a more clinically oriented classification of the nontuberculous mycobacteria is summarized in Table 2. This table classifies mycobacteria not by their appearance, growth characteristics, or host range, but from the viewpoint of their organ involvement when they cause disease in humans. In AIDS patients many, if not almost all, of the species listed in Table 2 can cause disseminated diseases including some novel, newly described species. Clearly, *M. tuberculosis* is the most important pathogen and can involve virtually every organ site in the body. *M. leprae* is primarily cutaneous in its manifestations, but systemic disease has been noted. As a result of the AIDS pandemic, the nontuberculous organisms such as *M. avium intracellulare* complex, *M. genovense*, and *M. hemophilum* have received clinical attention. What has been known or learned about *M. avium* in terms of chemotherapeutic approaches may be applicable to *M. hemophilum* and *M. genovense*. The rapidly growing mycobacteria *M. fortuitum M. chelonei,* and *M. abscessus* have a number of phenotypic characteristics that distinguish them from other mycobacteria, and, indeed, the general antimicrobial susceptibility patterns may vary significantly [3, 6].

Disease-causing mycobacteria are considered facultative intracellular pathogens. They invade and can multiply within the phagosomes (endosomes) of mononuclear phagocytes. *M. leprae* is known to invade and survive within Schwann cells of the nervous system. Other evidence indicates that organisms of the MAC can replicate within fibroblasts, endothelial cells, intestinal epithelial cells, and dendritic cells. The properties of an effective group of antimicrobial

Table 1. Classification of mycobacteria (Based on work of Runyon, [5])

Group	Representative species of mycobacteria	
Typical, slow-growing, strict pathogens	*M. tuberculosis, M. bovis, M. leprae*	
Photochromogens	*M. kansasii*	
	M. marinum	
Scotochromogens	*M. scrofulaceum*	
	M. szulgai	
	M. xenopi	
Nonphotochromogens	*M. avium*	*Mycobacterium avium*
	M. intracellulare	*Complex*
	M. malmoense	
	M. haemophilum	
Rapidly growing organisms	*M. abscessus*	
	M. fortuitum	
	M. chelonei	

Photochromogen: isolate is buff-colored in the dark but turns yellow with brief exposure to light.
Scotochromogen: isolate is yellow-orange or orange-colored even when grown in the dark.

Table 2. Clinical disease and the nontuberculous mycobacteria recovered from humans

Clinical disease	Common etiologic species	Growth rate	Morphologic growth features	Macrolide susceptible	Ref
Pulmonary	*M. avium* Complex	Slow (> 7 days)	Usually not pigmented	+	[4, 37]
	M. kansasii	Slow	Photochromogen	+	[6]
	M. abscessus	Rapid(< 7days)	Not pigmented	+	[47]
	M. xenopi	Slow	Pigmented, grows at 45°C	?	
	M. terrae	Slow	Not pigmented	+	[41]
Lymphadenitis	*M. avium* complex	Slow	Usually not pigmented	+	[4]
	M. scrofulaceum	Slow	Scotochromogen	+	[42]
Cutaneous	*M. leprae*	V. slow	Not cultureable *ex vivo*	+	[11]
	M. marinum	Rapid	Photochromogen;requires low temp (28–30°C) for	+	[6]
	M. fortuitum	Rapid	isolation	+	[47]
	M. chelonei	Rapid	Not pigmented	+	[47]
	M. ulcerans	Slow	Not pigmented	+	[43]
			Usually a scotochromogen: requires low temp for isolation		
Disseminated	*M. avium* complex	Slow	Isolates from patients with AIDS, often pigmented	+	[27, 28]
	M. genovense	V.slow(< 6wks)	(80%)	+	[45, 46]
	M. kansasii	Slow	Growth better in broth > agar	+	[6]
	M. chelonei	Rapid	Photochromogen	+	[40]
	M. haemophilum	Slow	Not pigmented	+	[45]
	M. simiae	Slow	Not pigmented; requires hemin, often needs low	?	
	M. malmoense	V.slow(> 6wks)	temp and CO_2	+	[46]
			Photochromogen		
			Prefers low pH		

agents against mycobacteria would include stability, ready absorption from gut, excellent tissue distribution, and the ability to penetrate into host defense cells such as mononuclear phagocytes. Since pathogenic mycobacteria appear to prevent acidification of the vacuole and to block phagolysosome fusion, active antimicrobial agents should exert their activity over a broad pH's range. A bactericidal effect clearly would be desirable. Since the organisms replicate slowly and intracellularly, the pharmacology of any potential agent necessarily would require access to intracellular "sanctuaries" as well as activity against organisms that are both replicating and metabolically inactive.

With regard to the desirable properties of antimycobacterial agents, many of them are represented by the new-generation macrolides (azithromycin, clarithromycin, and roxithromycin) and macrolide-related compounds such as the ketolides. However, not all of the newer agents have been studied adequately in mammalian hosts. There is little evidence suggesting that any macrolide or related compound offers reliable activity against organisms of the *M. tuberculosis* complex, and the basis for this difference between *M. tuberculosis* and other mycobacteria remains unclear.

Mycobacterium tuberculosis

Controversy surrounds the potential application of any of the macrolide or related compounds for the treatment of tuberculosis. An initial, encouraging report showed MICs of clarithromycin against *M. tuberculosis* ranging from 4 µg/ml to greater than 16 µg/ml [7]. There was some variability in clarithromycin's potentiation of activity of rifampin and isoniazid when multi-drug combinations were tested. When these investigators evaluated clarithromycin in a macrophage test system, clarithromycin was active and was synergistic with rifampin against some strains of tubercle bacilli. The virulent but drug-susceptible challenge strain, H37Rv, was used in murine challenge experiments, and clarithromycin reduced mortality associated with tuberculosis for up to eight weeks; however, colony counts of lungs and spleens showed that the anti-tuberculosis activity of clarithromycin was inferior to that of isoniazid and streptomycin. These investigators felt that when used as part of a multi-drug combination, clarithromycin's activity was comparable to that of thiacetazone (a widely used anti-tuberculosis agent in Africa, which is considered to be of "second-" or "third-line" efficacy). This relative ranking of activity suggested clarithromycin's potential usefulness as a component of multi-drug therapy for tuberculosis. However, in this study, the mode MICs of wild-type *M. tuberculosis* organisms assayed was 16 µg/ml or greater. Similarly, Cavalieri and colleagues reported on the synergistic activity of clarithromycin and some anti-tuberculous agents against multi-drug resistant *M. tuberculosis* (an approach that has not been investigated further in murine challenge models) [8].

Less encouraging, however, is the experience of Truffot-Pernot and colleagues, who reported at almost the same time that the MIC_{50} and MIC_{90} of 12 strains of *M.*

tuberculosis were 64 μg/ml and greater than 128 μg/ml, respectively [9]. Taking this work further in murine challenge models, four to six weeks of clarithromycin at 250 mg/kg yielded neither a bactericidal or bacteriostatic effect against *M. tuberculosis* H37Rv (the same challenge bacterium employed by Luna-Herrera). This group noted, similar to the experience of Luna-Herrera, that four weeks of clarithromycin did reduce mortality associated with *M. tuberculosis* of infection, but they found no effect on the multiplication of *M. tuberculosis in vivo*. Clearly, more information is needed about the potential of a macrolide, such as clarithromycin, as part of a multi-drug regimen in experimental challenge studies, either as a substitute for a component of a multi-drug regimen or as an added drug. Until then, it would seem prudent to conclude that no macrolide at present can be considered a part of a multi-drug, anti-tuberculosis regimen.

Mycobacterium leprae

Macrolides have been studied to a greater degree against *M. leprae* than against *M. tuberculosis,* despite the fact that the leprosy bacillus has not been cultured for extended passages in *ex vivo* culture. Non-culture systems have been utilized for *in vitro* drug-susceptibility screening, and it was with such a test system that Franzblau reported potent activity of erythromycin against *M. leprae* using an adenosine tri-phosphate (ATP) assay [10]. However, the drug was lacking *in vivo* activity. Similar conclusions were reached by other authors. In contrast, studies with clarithromycin *in vitro* suggested an MIC of 0.1 to 2.0 μg/ml, and the clarithromycin activity was confirmed by murine studies that suggested the presence of bactericidal activity. Comparative studies indicated that orally administered roxithromycin or clarithromycin was bactericidal in murine challenge systems but azithromycin was not [11]. The efficacy in humans of roxithromycin or azithromycin has not been studied.

Confirmation in humans that newer macrolides such as clarithromycin are therapeutically active comes from studies of lepromatous leprosy as reported by Chan and Ji [12–14]. The potency of clarithromycin using skin biopsy material inoculated into mouse footpad test systems approached -4_{10} logarithmic after a month of treatment. This effect was further enhanced with the concomitant use of minocycline, an established agent for treatment of leprosy. Taken together, the experience with the new macrolides offers these agents as another therapeutic alternative besides standard treatment regimens consisting of dapsone, clofazimine, and rifampicin. The limiting factor in the application of such therapy to areas where leprosy remains a serious problem is the cost of the drug in the populations where it is most needed. Still, the potency of these agents is sufficiently great to consider them as components of multi-drug "cocktails" where the frequency of dosing of the more expensive components of the regimen may be reduced (*i. e.,* longer drug-free intervals), thus lowering the total cost of treatment.

Mycobacterium avium complex

The first report of activity of any of the modern macrolides against non-tuberculous mycobacteria was the small study of Casal published in 1987 in which roxithromycin was assessed *in vitro* [15]. When cultured macrophages containing *M. avium* were stimulated with the cytokine TNF-α, bacterial activity of roxithromycin was observed [16]. At approximately that time, the clinical development of azithromycin and clarithromycin began. The organisms of the *Mycobacterim avium* complex were recognized previously to be the cause of serious, chronic, progressive lung disease that could imitate the clinical picture of tuberculosis [17, 18]. Standard therapies often were comprised of some of the mycobacterial agents, and some authorities believed that even isoniazid had activity against the MAC. As pointed out in many reviews, the *Mycobacterium avium* complex consists of two closely related groups of organisms, *Mycobacterium avium*, which consists of serotypes 1 through 12 (with one exception), and the *Mycobacterium intracellulare* species comprising the higher serotypes [19, 20].

Recognition that organisms of the *Mycobacterium avium* complex, almost all of which were *M. avium*, cause serious systemic disease in AIDS patients triggered the search for more effective chemotherapy than what had been employed until the mid-1980s. It is in this area that the modern macrolides have made a significant contribution [21].

The characteristics of non-tuberculous mycobacterial infections include chronicity, persistence, and the ability to survive within the cells of the host. Remarkably, the host cell range would include monocytes, macrophages, dendritic cells, and enterocytes. The organisms persist within intracellular vacuoles, and hence these sites may serve as an intracellular sanctuary where the mycobacteria are relatively protected from host defense. Cytokine-mediated activation of intracellular killing by phagocytes is believed to be the principal mode of elimination of the organism from the host. Nonetheless, with the abundant data that AIDS patients in their advanced clinical stages developed persistent bacteremia due to MAC, a logical hypothesis was that intracellular killing and host recognition of this important pathogen was defective. Information that the newer macrolides achieved high intracellular concentrations and were active at pHs within phagocytic vacuoles seems to explain their *in vitro* activity against the MAC.

Prior to the initiation of human studies, an assessment of the potential of a chemotherapeutic agent is not only desirable but also essential. In this regard, the search for suitable animal models or test systems to assess *in vivo* activity had been prepared by the work of Gangadharam and colleagues. In 1981 these investigators reported the use of the beige mouse as a suitable animal test system [22], and this was confirmed by Bertram and colleagues [23]. The beige mouse is defective in natural killer cell activity, hence mimicking in some respects the characteristics of individuals with acquired immune deficiency (or for that matter impaired lymphocyte function secondary to therapeutic agents such as steroids that can predispose to mycobacterial disease). The subject of animal models has been reviewed extensively [4, 24]. Suffice it to say that the beige mouse is but one of several small animal species that proved to be useful for the assessment of *in vivo* anti-mycobacterial activity. Studies with similar rodents or involving therapeutic immune suppression also yielded results that pointed toward the activity of the modern macrolides.

In 1989 two groups, Fernandes at Abbott Laboratories [25], and ourselves with research support from Pfizer [26], demonstrated in the beige mouse test system that clarithromycin and azithromycin, respectively, were active against disseminated MAC disease. We found that it was important for screening to choose a virulent challenge organism. Beige mice *per se* do not succumb to challenge from routine environmental isolates, but, from a collection of bacteremic isolates from AIDS patients, we have identified a suite of challenge organisms that are animal-virulent in terms of capability of replicating and increasing tissue burden as well as causing mortality at a reasonable interval (four weeks of experimental infection, longer if the challenge is *via* the gastrointestinal route). In this regard, *M. avium* strain 101 (MAC 101) proved to be consistently virulent and is now widely used in studies of MAC pathogenesis and therapy.

The studies carried out in the beige mouse system set the stage for human clinical trials of macrolides for disseminated MAC disease in AIDS patients.. The first report was an intriguing small study of bacteremic AIDS patients in which clarithromycin monotherapy was compared with a multi-drug regimen and a cross-over design [27]. Although the number of patients enrolled was small, quantitative blood cultures were used to demonstrate the conclusive effect of clarithromycin treatment. A similar approach was published using azithromycin monotherapy [28]. The latter study did not employ a cross-over, but the control phase involved allowing patients' bacteremia to rebound, whereupon the resumption of therapy unequivocably demonstrated an *in vivo* effect against mycobacteremia (patient as own comparator). Encouraged by these results, multi-center, clinical trials were carried out for the therapy of MAC bacteremia. These include those organized by the AIDS Clinical Trial Groups [29], a dose-ranging study, and a multi-center Azithromycin Study [30]. One, two, and four grams per day of clarithromycin have been used for treatment, but the one gram total daily dose is recommended because of side-effects at higher doses. The therapeutic azithromycin dose is 0.5 g once daily for an indefinite period or until the CD4 lymphocyte count is above 100 cells/ mm^3 for at least three to six months.

Roxithromycin in certain animal studies appeared to be comparably active against the MAC *in vitro* and in beige mice [31]. However, no large-scale human trial of roxithromycin has been reported using microbiological endpoints that are similar to those employed in the azithromycin and clarithromycin MAC bacteremia treatment studies.

The basis for the improved activity of modern macrolides *versus* MAC has been attributed to high tissue concentration [32] and penetration into phagosomes where the organisms are localized following phagocytosis. Improved drug delivery to active sites of infection has also been postulated [33]. For clarithromycin, a post-antibiotic effect of 5 to 16 h has been reported [34]. Use of drug combinations containing macrolides is discussed later (see resistance, page 209).

The major goal of AIDS treatment has always been effective control of HIV replication. Prior to the successful introduction of multi-drug regimens that accomplished adequate suppression of HIV viremia, the major management approach focused on prevention of life-threatening opportunistic infections. Thus, many studies were undertaken to evaluate the effect of macrolide prophylaxis. These agents have been shown to be conclusively effective in randomized, prospective, double-blind trials [35, 36]. Not only was there an effect in reducing the incidence of MAC bacteremia, but also a concomitant decline in pneumonias, respiratory infections, and other opportunistic processes was observed. In the United States, both azithromycin and clarithromycin are approved for prophylaxis of bacteremic MAC disease. The regimens have differed in that clarithromycin was administered in a dose of 0.5 g twice daily, whereas the azithromycin trials used a 1.2 g weekly dose, the latter being more convenient for long-term prophylaxis. More extensive data has been also obtained with combinations of macrolides with other drugs, but macrolide mono-prophylaxis is simple and effective with fewer overall side effects.

While most of the clinical attention of the last two decades has focused on systemic MAC infections, pulmonary disease has proved to be a particularly nettlesome clinical problem. MAC organisms have long been recognized as the cause of chronic pulmonary disease, particularly in patients who have had a history of smoking or lung damage [5,17,18]. MAC lung disease mimics chronic pulmonary tuberculosis with lung infiltrates, cavitation, fibrotic calcifications, and bronchiectasis. It is not uncommon, however, to diagnose MAC lung disease in patients with no obvious predisposing factors and no evidence of immune suppression has been observed. For these individuals, macrolide use has become a cornerstone of management, but additional drugs are clearly needed [37]. The number of other active agents that should be employed, the duration of therapy, and the endpoints for treatment (*e. g.*, culture negativity, x-ray improvement) are largely unresolved issues that underscore the need for large comparative trials. Based on the AIDS experience, it is clear that agents such as azithromycin and clarithromycin can be tolerated for years without serious sequelae.

Non-tuberculous mycobacteria other than MAC

A tremendous diversity of mycobacterial species exist in nature [3, 38]. Viewed in this light, human disease-causing strains such as *M. leprae, M. tuberculosis,* and *M. avium* have been specially adapted and have followed genetic routes among the environmental, naturally occurring mycobacteria. Large reviews of the non-tuberculous mycobacteria and their treatment have been published [3, 6]. Table 2 is a summary of the non-tuberculous pathogens and clinical syndromes and provides references for macrolide activity. Most of the species listed would be considered susceptible by *in vitro* criteria [3, 6, 37–47]. Nonetheless, caution should be employed in extrapolating from the results of purely laboratory studies to conclusions about clinical utility. These species cause a wide variety of diseases, as reflected by their potential to contaminant aqueous sources. Additionally, organisms other than those belonging to the MAC can cause systemic and pulmonary disease in suitably immune suppressed hosts. The clinical picture has been very difficult to distinguish between *M. avium* complex and system disease caused by *M. malmoense*, *M. hemophilum*, and *M. genovense* – mycobacteria that were not widely appreciated or even described before the onset of the AIDS pandemic.

While some generalizations can be made to the effect that what may be applicable for MAC chemotherapy should at least be considered for the non-tuberculous mycobacteria, *in vitro* susceptibility testing should be performed if available. Only clarithromycin has been studied against the MAC, resulting in observation of a relationship between clinical response and susceptibility (MICs < 8 μg/ml) [19]. This information may be extended to azithromycin, although specific data is lacking.

Macrolide resistance in mycobacteria

There is a limited amount of information about the molecular basis for macrolide resistance [48–50]. In the case of the *M. avium* complex, it appears to be the selection of a small, already-resistant subpopulation that contains 23S ribosomal mutations [48, 50]. Additional ribosomal alterations also have been postulated [49]. What can be said is that organisms of the MAC, if resistant to one agent such as clarithromycin, are usually resistant to the alternative macrolides [51]. The same is probably true for the macrolide-related compounds, such as the ketolides, which are in early laboratory and clinical investigation. The presence of enzymatic inactivation mechanisms and efflux mechanisms have not been adequately studied, and genomic mapping of MAC in comparison with other pathogens is likely to foster information about the potential presence of these resistance mechanisms. Combination therapy with at least one additional agent will reduce the emergence of resistance [51, 52]. The optimum number of agents for a multidrug regimen requires further study in different disease states, *e. g.*, pulmonary MAC [53] and disseminated disease [54].

Ketolides

Ketolide derivatives of macrolides have attracted much attention because of their effect against some macrolide-resistant respiratory pathogens, including *Streptococcus pneumoniae*. However, on a weight basis they are not as potent as clarithromycin *versus* the MAC [55, 56]. *In vivo* activity has been observed with HMR3004 [55], telithromycin [56], and ABT-773 [57], but not to the degree that is seen with azithromycin and clarithromycin. Unfortunately, clarithromycin resistant *M. avium* are also resistant to the ketolides tested thus far. This observation was extended to the non-tuberculous mycobacteria as well.

In contrast to HMR3004, telithromycin and ABT-773 achieve high intracellular concentration. Telithromycin is bactericidal at 400 mg/kg/d treatment against *M. avium in vivo* but is bacteriostatic at lower concentrations [56]. Although telithromycin is not active against clarithromycin-resistant *M. avium*, the use of telithromycin as monotherapy to treat clarithromycin-susceptible *M. avium* resulted in significantly less emergence of resistance than did treatment of beige mice with clarithromycin [56]. The latter observation was made in beige mice infected for up to 12 weeks and harvested to obtain quantitative blood cultures of organs and quantitative plating of tissue homogenates onto macrolide-containing media. The level of resistance of telithromycin after therapy is comparable to what is observed with azithromycin for 12 weeks, suggesting that compounds that achieve very high tissue concentrations select significantly less resistance than those compounds that achieve high blood levels, *e. g.*, clarithromycin, which appears to be less tissue active.

Concluding perspective

Modern macrolides have become a major component of the therapy of non-tuberculous mycobacterial diseases, but not for tuberculosis itself. Optimal human treatment regimens still require drug combinations. As new macrolide derivatives are being studied, exploration of structure-activity relationships against disease-causing mycobacteria may be a fruitful area for future investigation.

References

1 Snider DE, Raviglione M, Kochi A (1994) Global burden of tuberculosis. In: B Bloom (ed): *Tuberculosis Pathogenesis: Protection and Control.* American Society for Microbiology, Washington, D.C., 3–12

2 Wolinsky E (1979) Nontuberculous mycobacteria and associated diseases. *Am Rev Respir Dis* 119:107–159

3 Falkinham JO, 3rd (1996) Epidemiology of infection by nontuberculous mycobacteria. *Clin Microbiol Rev* 9:177–215

4 Korvick JA, Benson CA (eds) (1996) *Mycobacterium avium-complex infection. Progress in research and treatment.* Marcel Dekker, Inc., New York

5 Runyon E (1959) Anonymous mycobacteria in pulmonary disease. *Med Clin North Am* 43: 273–290

6 Wallace RJ, Glassroth J, Griffith DE, Oliver KN, Cook JL, Gordon F (1997) Diagnostic and treatment of disease caused by non tuberculous mycobacteria. *Am J Respir Crit Care Med* 156(2): S1-S25

7 Luna-Herrera J, Reddy VM, Daneluzzi D, Gangadharam PR. (1995) Antituberculosis activity of clarithromycin. *Antimicrob Agents Chemother* 39: 2692–2695

8 Cavalieri SJ, Biehle JR, Sanders WE, Jr. (1995) Synergistic activities of clarithromycin and antituberculous drugs against multidrug-resistant *Mycobacterium tuberculosis. Antimicrob Agents Chemother* 39:1542–1545

9 Truffot-Pernot C, Lounis N, Grosset JH, Ji B. (1995) Clarithromycin is inactive against *Mycobacterium tuberculosis. Antimicrob Agents Chemother* 39: 2827–2878
10 Franzblau SG, Hastings RC. (1988) *In vitro* and *in vivo* activities of macrolides against *Mycobacterium leprae. Antimicrob Agents Chemother* 32:1758–1762
11 Gelber RH (1990) Progress in the chemotherapy of leprosy: status, issues and prospects. *Prog Drug Res* 34: 421–445
12 Chan GP, Garcia-Ignacio BY, Chavez VE, Livelo JB, Jimenez CL, Parrilla ML, Franzblau SG. (1994) Clinical trial of clarithromycin for lepromatous leprosy. *Antimicrob Agents Chemother* 38: 515–517
13 Ji B, Perani EG, Grosset JH (1991) Effectiveness of clarithromycin and minocycline alone and in combination against experimental *Mycobacterium leprae* infection in mice. *Antimicrob Agents Chemother* 35: 579–581
14 Ji B, Jamet P, Perani EG, Bobin P, Grosset JH (1993) Powerful bactericidal activities of clarithromycin and minocycline against *Mycobacterium leprae* in lepromatous leprosy. *J Infect Dis* 168:188–190
15 Casal M, Rodriguez F, Villalba R (1987) *In vitro* susceptibility of *Mycobacterium avium* to a new macrolide (RU- 28965). *Chemotherapy* 33: 255–258
16 Bermudez LE, Young LS (1988) Activities of amikacin, roxithromycin, and azithromycin alone or in combination with tumor necrosis factor against *Mycobacterium avium* complex. *Antimicrob Agents Chemother* 32:1149–1153
17 Prince DS, Peterson DD, Steiner RM *et al.* (1989) Infection with *Mycobacterium avium* complex in patients without predisposing conditions. *N Engl J Med* 321: 863–868
18 Reich JM, Johnson RE (1992) *Mycobacterium avium* complex pulmonary disease presenting as an isolated lingular or middle lobe pattern. The Lady Windermere syndrome. *Chest* 101:1605–1609
19 Inderlied CB, Nash KA (1996) Microbiology and *in vitro* susceptibility testing. In: JA Korvick, CA Benson (eds): *Mycobacterium avium-complex infection: Progress in research and treatment.* Marcel Dekker, Inc., New York, 109–140
20 Inderlied CB (1997) Microbiology and minimum inhibitory concentration testing for *Mycobacterium avium* complex prophylaxis. *Am J Med* 102: 2–10
21 Ives DV, Davis RB, Currier JS (1995) Impact of clarithromycin and azithromycin on patterns of treatment and survival among AIDS patients with disseminated *Mycobacterium avium* complex. *Aids* 9: 261–266
22 Gangadharam PR, Edwards CK, 3rd, Murthy PS, Pratt PF (1983) An acute infection model for *Mycobacterium intracellulare* disease using beige mice: preliminary results. *Am Rev Respir Dis* 127: 648–649
23 Bertram MA, Inderlied CB, Yadegar S, Kolonoski P, Yamada JK, Young LS (1986) Confirmation of the beige mouse model for study of disseminated infection with *Mycobacterium avium* complex [letter]. *J Infect Dis* 154:194–195
24 Young LS, Bermudez LE (1996) Animal models in anti-*Mycobacterium avium*-complex drug development. In: JA Korvick, CA Benson (eds) *Mycobacterium avium complex infection: Progress in research and treatment.* Marcel Dekker, Inc., New York, 141–161
25 Fernandes PB, Hardy DJ, McDaniel D, Hanson CW, Swanson RN (1989) *In vitro* and *in vivo* activities of clarithromycin against *Mycobacterium avium. Antimicrob Agents Chemother* 33: 1531–1534
26 Inderlied CB, Kolonoski PT, Wu M, Young LS (1989) *In vitro* and *in vivo* activity of azithromycin (CP 62,993) against the *Mycobacterium avium* complex. *J Infect Dis* 159: 994–997
27 Dautzenberg B, Truffot C, Legris S, Meyohas MC, Berlie HC, Mercat A, Chevret S, Grosset J (1991) Activity of clarithromycin against *Mycobacterium avium* infection in patients with the acquired immune deficiency syndrome. *Am Rev Respir Dis* 144: 561–569
28 Young LS, Wiviott L, Wu M, Kolonoski P, Bolan R, Inderlied CB (1991) Azithromycin for treatment of *Mycobacterium avium-intracellulare* complex infection in patients with AIDS. *Lancet* 338: 1107–1109
29 Chaisson RE, Benson CA, Dube MP, Heifets LB, Korvick JA, Elkin S, Smith T, Craft JC, Sattler FR (1994) Clarithromycin therapy for bacteremic *Mycobacterium avium* complex disease. A

randomized, double-blind, dose-ranging study in patients with AIDS. AIDS Clinical Trials Group Protocol 157 Study Team. *Ann Intern Med* 121: 905–911
30 Koletar SL (1997) Treatment of *Mycobacterium avium* in human immunodeficiency virus-infected individuals. *Am J Med* 102: 16–21
31 Struillou L, Cohen Y, Lounis N, Bertrand G, Grosset J, Vilde JL, Pocidalo JJ, Perronne C (1995) Activities of roxithromycin against *Mycobacterium avium* infections in human macrophages and C57BL/6 mice. *Antimicrob Agents Chemother* 39: 878–881
32 Killian AD, Kanyok TP, Drusano GL (1996) Pharmacokinetics of drugs used for the therapy of *Mycobacterim avium*-complex infection. In: JA Korvick, CA Benson (eds) *Mycobacterium avium-complex infection: Progress in research and treatment.* Marcel Dekker, Inc., New York, 197–240
33 Gladue RP, Bright GM, Isaacson R., Newborg MF (1989) *In vitro* and *in vivo* uptake of azithromycin (CP-62,993) by phagocytic cells: possible mechanism of delivery and release at sites of infection. *Antimicrob Agents Chemother* 33: 277–282
34 Ellis LC, Benson CA. Koenig GI., Trenholme GM (1995) Postantibiotic effect of clarithromycin alone and combined with ethambutol against *Mycobacterium avium* complex. *Antimicrob Agents Chemother* 39: 2803–2806
35 Havlir DV, Dube MP, Sattler FR, Forthal DN, Kemper CA, Dunne MW, Parenti DM, Lavelle JP, White AC, Jr., Witt MD et al (1996) Prophylaxis against disseminated *Mycobacterium avium* complex with weekly azithromycin, daily rifabutin, or both. California Collaborative Treatment Group. *N Engl J Med* 335: 392–398
36 Benson CA, Williams PL, Cohn DL, Becker S, Hojczyk P, Nevin T, Korvick JA, Heifets L, Child CC, Lederman MM et al (2000) Clarithromycin or rifabutin alone or in combination for primary prophylaxis of *Mycobacterium avium* complex disease in patients with AIDS: A randomized, double-blind, placebo-controlled trial. The AIDS Clinical Trials Group 196/Terry Beirn Community Programs for Clinical Research on AIDS 009 Protocol Team. *J Infect Dis* 181: 1289–1297
37 Wallace RJ Jr., Brown BA, Griffith DE, Girard WM, Murphy DT, Onyi GO, Steingrube VA, Mazurek GH (1994) Initial clarithromycin monotherapy for *Mycobacterium avium- intracellulare* complex lung disease. *Am J Respir Crit Care Med* 149: 1335–1341
38 Wallace RJ Jr. (1994) Recent changes in taxonomy and disease manifestations of the rapidly growing mycobacteria. *Eur J Clin Microbiol Infect Dis* 13: 953–960
39 Brown BA, Wallace RJ Jr., Onyi GO (1992) Activities of clarithromycin against eight slowly growing species of nontuberculous mycobacteria, determined by using a broth microdilution MIC system. *Antimicrob Agents Chemother* 36: 1987–1990
40 Wallace RJ Jr., Tanner D, Brennan PJ, Brown BA (1993) Clinical trial of clarithromycin for cutaneous (disseminated) infection due to *Mycobacterium chelonae. Ann Intern Med* 119: 482–486
41 Carbonara S, Tortoli E, Costa D, Monno L, Fiorentino G, Grimaldi A, Boscia D, Rollo MA, Pastore G, Angarano G (2000) Disseminated *Mycobacterium terrae* infection in a patient with advanced human immunodeficiency virus disease. *Clin Infect Dis* 30: 831–835
42 Sanders JW, Walsh AD, Snider RL, Sahn EE (1995) Disseminated *Mycobacterium scrofulaceum* infection: a potentially treatable complication of AIDS. *Clin Infect Dis* 20: 549
43 Portaels F, Traore H, De Ridder K, Meyers WM (1998) *In vitro* susceptibility of *Mycobacterium ulcerans* to clarithromycin. *Antimicrob Agents Chemother* 42: 2070–2073
44 Matsiota-Bernard P, Thierry D, De Truchis P, Saillour M, Paraire F, Guesdon JL, Nauciel C (1995) *Mycobacterium genovense* infection in a patient with AIDS who was successfully treated with clarithromycin. *Clin Infect Dis* 20:1565–1566
45 Kiehn TE, White M (1994) *Mycobacterium haemophilum*: an emerging pathogen. *Eur J Clin Microbiol Infect Dis* 13: 925–931
46 Buchholz UT, McNeil MM, Keyes LE, Good RC (1998) *Mycobacterium malmoense* infections in the United States, January 1993 through June 1995. *Clin Infect Dis* 27: 551–558
47 Mushatt DM, Witzig RS (1995) Successful treatment of *Mycobacterium abscessus* infections with multidrug regimens containing clarithromycin. *Clin Infect Dis* 20:1441–1442
48 Roberts MC, Sutcliffe J, Courvalin P, Jensen LB, Rood J, Seppala H (1999) Nomenclature for macrolide and macrolide-lincosamide-streptogramin B resistance determinants. *Antimicrob Agents Chemother* 43: 2823–2830

49 Doucet-Populaire F, Truffot-Pernot C, Grosset J, Jarlier V (1995) Acquired resistance in *Mycobacterium avium* complex strains isolated from AIDS patients and beige mice during treatment with clarithromycin. *J Antimicrob Chemother* 36: 129–136

50 Nash KA, Inderlied CB (1996) Rapid detection of mutations associated with macrolide resistance in *Mycobacterium avium* complex. *Antimicrob Agents Chemother* 40: 1748–1750

51 Bermudez LE, Petrofsky M, Kolonoski P, Young LS (1998) Emergence of *Mycobacterium avium* populations resistant to macrolides during experimental chemotherapy. *Antimicrob Agents Chemother* 42: 180–183

52 Bermudez LE, Inderlied CB, Kolonoski P, Petrofsky M, Young LS (1994) Clarithromycin, dapsone, and a combination of both used to treat or prevent disseminated *Mycobacterium avium* infection in beige mice. *Antimicrob Agents Chemother* 38: 2717–2721

53 Griffith DE, Wallace RJ (1997) Treatment of pulmonary *Mycobacterium avium* complex lung disease in non-acquired immunodeficiency syndrome (AIDS) patients in the era of the newer macrolides and rifabutin. *Am J Med* 102: 22–27

54 Shafran SD, Singer J, Zarowny DP, Phillips P, Salit I, Walmsley SL, Fong IW, Gill MJ, Rachlis AR, Lalonde RG, Fanning MM, Tsoukas CM (1996) A comparison of two regimens for the treatment of *Mycobacterium avium* complex bacteremia in AIDS: rifabutin, ethambutol, and clarithromycin versus rifampin, ethambutol, clofazimine, and ciprofloxacin. Canadian HIV Trials Network Protocol 010 Study Group. *N Engl J Med* 335: 377–383

55 Bermudez LE, Inderlied CB, Kolonoski P *et al.* (1998) Activity of HMR3004 against *Mycobacterium avium* complex *in vitro*, in human macrophages and in beige mice. *Clin Microb Infect* 4: 325–331

56 Bermudez LE, Inderlied CB, Kolonoski P, Wu M, Aralar P, Young LS (2001) Telithromycin is active against *Mycobacterim avium* in mice despite lacking significant activity in standard *in vitro* and macrophage assays and is associated to low frequency of resistance during treatment. *Antimicrob Agents Chemother* 45: 2210–2216

57 Cynamon MH, Carter JL, Shoen CM (2000) Activity of ABT-773 against *Mycobacterium avium* complex in the beige mouse model. *Antimicrob Agents Chemother* 44: 2895–2896

Macrolide Antibiotics
ed. by W. Schönfeld and H. A. Kirst

Chlamydia pneumoniae and asthma and atherosclerosis: role of macrolides

Margaret R. Hammerschlag

Division of Infectious Diseases, Department of Pediatrics, SUNY Health Science Center at Brooklyn, 450 Clarkson Ave., Brooklyn, NY 11203–2098, USA

Chlamydia pneumoniae was first described as a respiratory tract pathogen by Grayston and colleagues in 1986 [1]. The genus *Chlamydiae* is a group of obligate intracellular parasites that have a unique developmental cycle with morphologically distinct infectious and reproductive forms. All members of the genus have a gram-negative envelope without peptidoglycan, share a genus-specific lipopolysaccharide (LPS) antigen, and utilize host ATP for the synthesis of chlamydial protein. The genus now contains four species: *Chlamydia psittaci, C. trachomatis, C. pneumoniae,* and *C. pecorum.* Macrolide antibiotics have long been used for treatment of infections due to *C. trachomatis,* and, by extrapolation, they have been used for treatment of *C. pneumoniae* infections. Macrolide antibiotics, especially the newer agents, have a number of properties that make them ideal agents for the treatment of infections due to intracellular pathogens such as *C. pneumoniae.* They achieve high concentrations in tissue and cells, including polymorphonuclear leukocytes and macrophages. These drugs also have long half-lives in tissue, allowing once-daily dosing and shorter duration of therapy. However, data on the treatment of even respiratory infection due to *C. pneumoniae* is limited. Although currently available macrolides have good activity against *C. pneumoniae in vitro*, the majority of published treatment studies have relied on serologic diagnosis, and thus microbiological efficacy has not been assessed [2].

C. pneumoniae appears to be a primary human pathogen, although the organism has been isolated from other species, including koalas [3]. The mode of transmission remains uncertain but is probably *via* infected respiratory secretions. Serologic surveys have documented rising prevalence of antibody to *C. pneumoniae* with increasing age, from 10% of children 5 to 10 years of age, reaching 30% to 45% by adolescence, and often exceeding 80% in the elderly [4]. The proportion of community-acquired pneumonias associated with *C. pneumoniae* infection has ranged from 6% to 22%, varying with geographic location, age group examined, and diagnostic methods used [5–10]. Most of these studies were based on serology alone. *C. pneumoniae* also has been associated with other respiratory infections, including acute exacerbations of chronic bronchitis, otitis media, sinusitis, and reactive airway disease [11–13]. Although initial studies suggested that infection with *C. pneumoniae* was uncommon in young children, subsequent studies, utilizing isolation of the organism in tissue culture, found the prevalence to be similar to that observed in adults [8, 9]. Asymptomatic respiratory infection may occur in 2% to 5% of children and adults [12–14]. Persistent nasopharyngeal infection with *C. pneumoniae* following acute respiratory infection has been documented in adults for periods of months to several years [15, 16].

Recently, *C. pneumoniae* has been implicated with disseminated disease outside the respiratory tract, notably atherosclerosis [17]. Although the organism has been identified in atheromatous tissue, causality has not been directly established. Interpretation of many studies is made more difficult by the lack of standardized serological and non-culture methods for the detection of the organism. These problems also have an impact on efforts to study treatment of *C. pneumoniae* infections.

In vitro activity of macrolides against *C. pneumoniae*

C. pneumoniae is susceptible *in vitro* to agents that affect protein or DNA synthesis; macrolides, tetracyclines and fluoroquinolones (Tab. 1) [2, 18–32]. Unlike *C. trachomatis, C. pneumoniae* is resistant to sulfonamides. The methods used for *in vitro* susceptibility testing of *C. pneumoniae* have been adapted largely from those used for *C. trachomatis*. The methods are not standardized and the results can be influenced by a number of variables including the tissue culture system used, inoculum size, timing of the addition of the antibiotic, and the

Table 1. *In vitro* activity of various antibiotics against *C. pneumoniae*

	MIC (range) (μg/ml)	MIC_{90}	MBC_{90}
Drug			
Erythromycin	0.015–0.25	0.25	0.25
Azithromycin	0.015–0.5	0.25	0.25
Clarithromycin	0.004–0.03	0.03	0.03
Dirithromycin	0.5–4	1	1
Erythromycylamine	0.5–4	1	1
Roxithromycin	0.06–2	0.5	0.5
Telithromycin	0.03–2	0.25	0.25
ABT 773	0.008–0.015	0.015	0.015
Ciprofloxacin	1–2	2	4
Levofloxacin	0.25–1	0.5	0.5
Doxycycline	0.06–0.25	0.25	0.25
Sulfamethoxazole	> 500	–	–

From [2, 18–32]

number and type of isolates used for testing. Many *in vitro* studies reported in the literature have used ≤ 5 isolates of *C. pneumoniae*, and many have used only one, usually laboratory isolates such as TW 183 and IOL 207. There are a limited number of studies that have tested large numbers of recent clinical isolates.

Macrolides (including azalides and ketolides) remain among the most active antibiotics against *C. pneumoniae in vitro*. As shown in Table 1, the most active compounds tested so far are ABT 773, a new ketolide, and clarithromycin, with MIC_{90}s of 0.015 mg/l and 0.03 mg/l, respectively. Erythromycin, azithromycin, and another ketolide, telithromycin (HMR 3647), fall into an intermediate range with MIC_{90}s of 0.25 mg/l. The least active macrolides *in vitro* are dirithromycin and its metabolite, erythromycylamine, and roxithromycin, having MIC_{90}s of 1 mg/l and 0.5 mg/l, respectively. The combination of dirithromycin and erythromycylamine was found to be additive. A recent study from Germany evaluated several antibiotic combinations for synergy against *C. pneumoniae in vitro* [33]. Combinations of azithromycin with either ofloxacin, doxycycline, or rifampin, as well as combinations of these three antibiotics, were found to be synergistic.

Questions have been raised about the relevance of *in vitro* testing of *C. pneumoniae* to treatment *in vivo*, as the methods currently used are not analogous to the infection as it occurs *in vivo*. In most studies, the antibiotic has been added after the cells are inoculated; however, *in vivo*, the infection is usually already established. Nystrom-Rosander and colleagues [34] demonstrated that when azithromycin was added to HEp-2 cells 24 h after infection, the mean MIC increased to 1 mg/l, compared with 0.05 mg/l when the drug was added 1 h after infection. Gnarpe and colleagues [35] reported that even after exposure to concentrations of azithromycin up to 50 mg/l, viable *C. pneumoniae* could be recovered after several passages in tissue culture without antibiotic.

Several studies have used a mouse model of *C. pneumoniae* pneumonitis to assess the efficacy of antimicrobial therapy [36–38]. Various inbred mice have been used. After intranasal inoculation, the animals develop a subacute pneumonitis; however, most of the mice recover spontaneously without treatment. Masson and colleagues [37] attempted to compensate for this problem by immunosuppressing the mice with cyclophosphamide. Despite these variations in the model, the results obtained have been very similar. Treatment with various antibiotics, including azithromycin, despite different *in vitro* activity and pharmacokinetics, reduced but did not eliminate *C. pneumoniae* from the lungs of all infected animals [36–38]. Malinverni and colleagues [36] also reported that they could detect *C. pneumoniae* DNA in lung tissue after apparently successful treatment. A subsequent study also found that three days of treatment with a combination of azithromycin and rifampin appeared to be more effective in eliminating *C. pneumoniae* from the lungs of infected mice than azithromycin alone [38]. At 20 days after infection, lungs from 19% of the mice who were treated with the combination were culture positive, compared with 32% of those who were treated with azithromycin alone and 43% who were treated with phosphate buffered saline (PBS).

Similar data also have been reported by Kutlin and colleagues [39] using HEp-2 cells continuously infected with *C. pneumoniae*. The cells were infected for ≥ 2 years and were maintained without centrifugation, the addition of cycloheximide, fresh host cells, or chlamydia. Treatment with azithromycin and ofloxacin at concentrations up to four times the MIC (0.5 mg/l and 4 mg/l, respectively) reduced but did not completely eliminate the organism from the cells. In a subsequent study, 30 days treatment with azithromycin at a concentration of 50 mg/l or with clarithromycin at 500 mg/l (which are the concentrations achieved in the pulmonary epithelial lining fluid) reduced the infectious load from 10^6 to 10^2 inclusion-forming units (IFU)/ml but, again, did not eliminate the organism (unpublished results).

Use of macrolides for treatment of respiratory infection due to *C. pneumoniae*

There has been little published data describing the response of *C. pneumoniae* infection to antibiotic therapy. Optimum dose and duration of therapy are uncertain. Anecdotal data suggest that prolonged therapy (*i. e.*, at least 2 weeks) may be desirable since recrudescent symptoms and persistent positive cultures have been described following two-week courses of erythromycin and even after 30 days of tetracycline or doxycycline [14, 15]. Practically all treatment studies presented or published to date have used serology alone for diagnosis [2]. An example of the limitations of serology when used to assess efficacy is illustrated in the study of File and colleagues [40], which reported a clinical cure rate of 98% among patients who were treated with levofloxacin compared with 93% of those treated with ceftriaxone and/or cefuroxime axitil; the latter two compounds have little or no activity against *C. pneumoniae in vitro*. Either erythromycin or doxycycline could be added at the discretion of the investigator. In the latter group, the response rate of those with serologic evidence of *C. pneumoniae* infection did not differ between those patients who had erythromycin or doxycycline added to their treatment regimen. There was also no difference in the response rate among those patients who were felt to have serologic evidence of definite infection, *i. e.* a four-fold rise in anti-*C. pneumoniae* IgG or IgM as determined by the microimmunofluorescence (MIF) test, compared with those who had probable infection, *i. e.*, a single IgG ≥ 512 or IgM ≥ 32. A recent study by Leophonte and colleagues [41] comparing two trovafloxacin regimens to amoxicillin-clavulanate for treatment of acute exacerbations of chronic bronchitis found a similar clinical response rate for all three regimens, and they claimed that *C. pneumoniae* was successfully eradicated from 80% to 100% at the end of treatment, with all three regimens. The investigators stated that "Atypical respiratory pathogens, which were identified by serological testing (a 4-fold increase in antibody titer) were presumed eradicated if the patient's clinical response was cure or improvement." The apparent success of regimens using antibiotics that have poor or no activity against *C. pneumoniae in vitro*, such as amoxicillin and cephalosporins, raises a number of questions about the specificity of the serologic criteria used to diagnose *C. pneumoniae* infection. Several recent studies have found a poor correlation between the results of MIF serology and culture, especially in children [8, 9, 14].

The only published studies that have utilized culture and assessed microbiological efficacy have been with macrolides. Block and colleagues [8] found that treatment with erythromycin and clarithromycin suspensions eradicated *C. pneumoniae* from the nasopharynx of 86% and 79% of culture-positive children with community-acquired pneumonia, respectively. All children improved clinically despite persistence of the organism. Persistence was not related to the development of antibiotic resistance, as all the isolates remained susceptible to erythromycin and clarithromycin during and after treatment [25]. Clarithromycin is 10- to 100-fold more active than erythromycin *in vitro* and has superior pharmacokinetics and tissue penetration, yet it was not more effective than erythromycin in eradicating *C. pneumoniae* from the respiratory tract. The experience with azithromycin has been similar. In an open, non-comparative, multicenter pneumonia treatment study [30], adolescents and adults ≥ 12 years of age were given 1.5 g of azithromycin orally over five days. *C. pneumoniae* was eradicated from the nasopharynx of 7 (70%) of the 10 culture-positive patients after treatment. Harris and colleagues [9] reported eradication of *C. pneumoniae* after treatment from the nasopharynx of 19 of 23 (83%) evaluable children who were treated with a 5-day course of azithromycin; 4 of 4, and 7 of 7 who were treated with 10 days of amoxicillin-clavulanate and erythromycin, respectively ($p = 0.9$, Chi square). The MICs and MBCs of 3 of 9 isolates of *C. pneumoniae* obtained after treatment from 2 of 7 persistently infected patients in both studies who were treated with azithromycin increased four-fold after treatment, although they were still within the range considered susceptible to the antibiotic [30]. It is not clear whether this result is an isolated event or is suggestive of possible development of resistance. All patients improved clinically despite persistence of the organism. These studies illustrate several important issues dealing with the treatment of *C. pneumoniae* infections. *In vitro* activity does not always predict microbiological efficacy. Unless cultures are done and microbiological efficacy is assessed, we may never be able to survey for, or document, the emergence of resistance.

C. pneumoniae and asthma and atherosclerosis: role of macrolides

Infection with *C. pneumoniae* has also been implicated in a number of chronic diseases, most notably asthma and atherosclerosis. Detailed analyses of the evidence supporting these associations has been presented in detail elsewhere [42, 43]. Here we shall concentrate on the potential role of macrolide antibiotics in the management of asthma and atherosclerosis associated with *C. pneumoniae* infection.

Studies of the association of asthma and *C. pneumoniae* infection have been predominantly based on serology except for one study in children [11, 44–47]. Emre and colleagues [11], isolated *C. pneumoniae* from the nasopharynx of 11%

of children, 5 to 16 years old, who presented with acute exacerbations of asthma. The culture-positive children were treated with either erythromycin and/or clarithromycin for 10 to 14 days. In terms of efficacy, erythromycin successfully eradicated *C. pneumoniae* from nasopharyngeal cultures of all six children who were treated with the drug, compared with five of six children who were treated with clarithromycin. One child failed two 10-day courses of clarithromycin and became culture-negative after an additional three weeks of erythromycin. In terms of clinical outcome, 9 of 12 (75%) children with positive cultures demonstrated laboratory and clinical improvement of their asthma symptoms following eradication of the *C. pneumoniae* infection. The response to therapy was related to the severity of the asthma, as all four children with moderate asthma improved after antibiotic treatment, whereas only three of five children with chronic severe asthma, improved after treatment. Determination of improvement was based on pulmonary-function tests and quality-of-life assessments. Several children with moderate asthma were able to discontinue their asthma medications after treatment of their *C. pneumoniae* infection. Aside from this study, there are no others that have evaluated the effect of treatment that have used culture. Similar to what was found in children with community-acquired pneumonia who were culture positive, over 50% of the culture-positive children seen by Emre and colleagues [11] were seronegative by MIF, including one child who was culture positive on four occasions over a five-month period. There have been no controlled studies of treatment of asthma. Given the results of the pneumonia treatment that have evaluated microbiological efficacy, one cannot assume that a clinical "response" after therapy with a particular antibiotic implies that *C. pneumoniae* or another organism has been eradicated. An important confounding variable of macrolide therapy is that these drugs have anti-inflammatory activity that is independent of their antimicrobial activity [48, 49]. Anti-inflammatory activity attributed to macrolides includes inhibition of neutrophil oxidant burst, inhibition of neutrophil chemotaxis, reduced production of cytokines (IL-6, IL-8, IL-1β, and TNF-α), and suppression of granulocyte-macrophage stimulating factor. However, all macrolides may not have equivalent anti-inflammatory activity. Azithromycin and clarithromycin have been demonstrated to have only slight anti-inflammatory activity in the rat carrageenian paw edema model when compared with roxithromycin [48].

Studies of the use of antibiotics in atherosclerosis also have been subject to the same limitations as asthma. Most studies have used serology with the MIF assay to determine the presence of *C. pneumoniae* infection [42, 43, 50, 51]. The serologic criteria used have varied from study to study and were often selected post-hoc [42]. Overall, comparison of those individuals judged to have serologic evidence of *C. pneumoniae* infection with those felt to be seronegative yielded a combined risk ratio for coronary heart disease of 1.22 (95% confidence interval 0.96 to 1.54) [51]. Identification of the organism in atheromas by polymerase chain reaction, immunocytochemical staining, and electron microscopy has been reported, ranging from 0% to over 90% of lesions [52]. A major problem is that these methods are not yet standardized. In studies where more than one method has been used, discordant results are frequent [53]. *C. pneumoniae* occasionally has been isolated by culture from atherosclerotic plaques, but these patients often do not meet the serologic criteria for infection or may be seronegative [53–55]. We do not have an accurate way of identifying which patients are really infected. Two recent small secondary prevention studies have suggested a beneficial effect of short-term macrolide antibiotic therapy, intended to be specifically directed against *C. pneumoniae*. The first of these studies was presented by Gupta and colleagues [56]. They screened male patients who had prior mycocardial infarction (MI) for anti-*C. pneumoniae* antibody by MIF. Seropositivity was defined as an IgG ≥ 64. Seropositive patients were randomized to receive either azithromycin 500 mg/d for 3 or 6 days or placebo. After six months follow-up, the odds ratio for seropositive patients who were treated with azithromycin was the same as that of the seronegative group. The investigators also demonstrated a decrease in anti-*C. pneumoniae* IgG titers after treatment, which they suggested implied successful treatment of *C. pneumoniae* infection. Subsequently, Gurfinkel and colleagues [57] assessed the effect of 30 days treatment with roxithromycin, 150 mg orally twice a day, or placebo in patients with unstable angina or non-Q-wave MI. MIF serology for *C. pneumoniae* was performed but not presented in the preliminary publication. At 30 days there was a statistically significant reduction in a triple endpoint, severe recurrent ischemia, MI, and death, in the treated compared to the placebo group. Although no data on chlamydial serology was presented, the authors concluded that "antichlamydial antibiotics" may be useful in this setting. The final report, which was published two years later, analyzed the response at 90 and 180 days and found again that the rates of severe recurrent ischemia, MI, and death were higher in the placebo compared with the roxithromycin group [58]. There was no significant difference in response in those patients who had anti-*C. pneumoniae* IgG ≥ 64 or who were seronegative. Anti-*C. pneumoniae* IgG titers did not decrease in the seropositive patients who were treated with roxithromycin. Although ischemic events occurred more frequently in the patients with higher anti-*C. pneumoniae* IgG titers independent of therapy, there was no demonstrable association between the efficacy of roxithromycin therapy and IgG titers.

There are several problems with these studies. In addition to lacking power, *i. e.*, both studies enrolled approximately 200 patients each, an MIF IgG ≥ 64 may not be an accurate indicator of active chlamydial infection. The background rate of seropositivity may be very high in some populations. Hyman and colleagues [14] found that 84% of subjectively healthy adults in one population had anti-*C. pneumoniae* IgG ≥ 32. The dosage of azithromycin used by Gupta and colleagues [56], 500 mg once a day for three days, repeated six months later, would be unlikely to eradicate *C. pneumoniae*. The results of a pneumonia treatment study found that 1.5 g of azithromycin over five days had only a 70% eradication rate in adults with pneumonia [30]. Data from the mouse model and the continuously infected cell line also suggest that complete eradication may not be feasible even with prolonged treatment with very high doses of drug. There are no data on the microbiological efficacy of roxithromycin for treatment of any *C. pneumoniae* infection. Roxithromycin is also one of the less active macrolides *in vitro*. Thus, one cannot determine whether the dosage or duration of treatment used by Gurfinkel and colleagues [57] would have been effective.

One cannot assume that reduction of anti-*C. pneumoniae* IgG implies eradication of the organism. More recently, Anderson and colleagues [59] presented the results of another secondary prevention study evaluating longer duration of therapy with azithromycin. They screened patients with coronary artery disease, documented by previous MI, bypass surgery, or > 50% angiographic stenosis of ≥ 1 major coronary artery, for anti-*C. pneumoniae* antibody. Patients with an MI within five days were excluded. Patients with IgG ≥ 16 were eligible. They were then randomized to receive either azithromycin, 500 mg/day for three days, then 500 mg/week for three months, or placebo. At six months, there was no difference in the number of clinical cardiac events between the patients who received azithromycin and placebo (6% in the azithromycin group *versus* 4.6% in the placebo group). There was a trend towards reduced inflammmatory markers (C-reactive protein, IL-1, IL-6, and TNF-α) in the azithromycin group. Unlike the results reported by Gupta and colleagues [56], there was no change in the antibody titers. It is again unlikely that the dosage and duration of therapy was adequate to eradicate *C. pneumoniae*. It is also possible that 500 mg/week could lead to prolonged periods of sub-inhibitory concentrations of azithromycin which could select for resistant organisms. This has been demonstrated with *Streptococcus pneumoniae* [60]. In a small pilot study, Jackson and colleagues [61] randomized 88 patients with coronary artery disease to receive a one-month course of azithromycin or placebo, 500 mg/d for two days followed by 250 mg/d for 26 days (total 7.5 g). Safety and compliance were assessed at two and four weeks, and serological testing was performed at six months post-enrollment. Although azithromycin was well tolerated, the majority of patients had no change in their anti-*C. pneumomiae* IgG, IgM, or IgA antibodies after treatment. A small number of patients had titers that increased or decreased. Currently underway is a much larger study, with 3500 patients enrolled, evaluating azithromycin *versus* placebo at essentially the same dosage and duration evaluated by Anderson and colleagues [62]. Patients will receive 600 mg/d for three days followed by 600 mg/week for 11 weeks. To be eligible, patients had to have an MI within six weeks, no recent bypass surgery or angioplasty, and an anti-*C. pneumoniae* IgG ≥ 16. The investigators assume the numbers are large enough to detect a 25% reduction in the presumed 8% placebo event rate (time to a composite all-cause death, MI, a revascularization procedure, or hospitalization for angina) with 90% power.

There have been two studies that have sought to assess the effect of therapy with azithromycin in a rabbit model of atherosclerosis [63, 64]. Rabbits fed either a cholesterol-free or cholesterol-supplemented feed developed atheromatous lesions in the aorta after intranasal inoculation with *C. pneumoniae*. However, this effect may not be specific for *C. pneumoniae,* as similar lesions have been described in rabbits after natural and laboratory infection with *Pasteurella multocida* [65]. Although respiratory infection with *P. multocida* appears to stimulate development of these lesions, the organism cannot be isolated from them. Similarly, *C. pneumoniae* has not been isolated from these lesions in rabbits after intranasal inoculation. Muhlstein and colleagues [63] reported that weekly treatment with azithromycin for seven weeks after inoculation with *C. pneumoniae* prevented accelerated intimal thickening in the rabbit aortas when compared with untreated controls. However, chlamydial antigen, detected by staining with a fluorescein-conjugated, genus-specific monoclonal antibody, could be detected in the same proportion of treated and untreated animals. Fong and colleagues [64] reported that only 4.2% of rabbits treated for 10 to 11 weeks starting five days after inoculation developed early signs of atherosclerosis, compared with 34.8% of untreated control rabbits. However, if treatment was initiated two weeks after infection, 33.3% developed early changes of atherosclerosis. As in the first study, the organism was not isolated from the aorta, but antigen was detected by immunocytochemical staining with a species-specific monoclonal antibody. Treatment with azithromycin did not decrease the prevalence of antigen between untreated controls and early-treated rabbits. These results are in a way compatible with the studies in continuously infected cells and imply that it may be impossible to eradicate *C. pneumoniae* in established infection. However, there are questions about the specificity of the staining methods, especially since the organism has not been isolated from the tissue of the rabbits. In contrast, dissemination after intranasal infection with *C. pneumoniae* has been demonstrated in several mouse pneumonia models with isolation of the organism from buffy coats, peripheral blood monocytes, and spleen [66]. There are also concerns about the specificity of histochemical staining for identification of *C. pneumoniae* in tissue. The prevention or regression of intimal thickening observed in the rabbits treated with azithromycin could be a direct effect of the antibiotic rather than a result of treating *C. pneumoniae* infection.

Two studies have attempted to determine if prior antibiotic therapy decreases the risk of developing a first-time acute MI [67,68]. Meier and colleagues [67], using a population-based, case-control analysis, examined the medical records of 3315 patients in the United Kingdom, ≤ 75 years of age, with a diagnosis of a first MI. Exposure to antibiotics was considered if any antibiotic was used within three years of the index event, the MI. They found that patients were significantly less likely to have used tetracycline antibiotics or quinolones, but, surprisingly, no effect was found for previous use of macrolides (primarily erythromycin), penicillins, and cephalosporins. The discrepancy of the effect between tetracyclines and macrolides was attributed to "poor" efficacy of erythromycin for treatment of *C. pneumoniae* infection. The study had some major problems because the investigators did not control for duration of treatment or dose. Only eight patients had prior treatment with quinolones, including norfloxacin and ciprofloxacin, which are relatively inactive against *C. pneumoniae in vitro* and known to also be ineffective for treatment of *C. trachomatis* infection. A subsequent study found no association between the use of erythromycin, tetracycline, or doxycycline within five years and the risk for first MI among 1 796 cases and 4 882 controls seen in a large health maintenance organization in Seattle [68]. Unlike in the study of Meier and colleagues, the investigators did attempt to determine the duration of therapy. The general conclusion reached was that exposure to antibiotics in routine clinical care may be insufficient to reduce risk; however, no effect on risk was seen in patients who were treated for ≥ 29 days with antibiotics, including erythromycin, which is a similar or greater duration of therapy than was used by Gupta and colleagues [56] and Gurfinkel and colleagues [57]. The authors also hypothesized that the failure to see an effect with erythromycin when compared with the prior results with azithromycin and roxithromycin may have been due to superior activity and tissue penetration of these drugs. However, azithromycin has not been demonstrated to be more effective than erythromycin for eradication of *C. pneumoniae* from the nasopharynx of patients with pneumonia [30]. As stated earlier, there are no data on the microbiological efficacy of roxithromycin.

Conclusions

Macrolide antibiotics, especially erythromycin, azithromycin, clarithromycin, and the new ketolides are very active against *C. pneumoniae in vitro*. Unfortunately, data are limited on the efficacy of any of these agents for the treatment of *C. pneumoniae* infection, including pneumonia. Anecdotal experience suggests that *in vitro* activity may not always correlate with efficacy *in vivo*.

The majority of published treatment studies have relied on serologic diagnosis; thus, microbiological efficacy has not been assessed. Several studies of the use of macrolides for secondary prevention of cardiac morbidity in patients with coronary artery disease have been reported, but the results have been conflicting and inconclusive. One of the major problems with these studies has been the inability to accurately determine who is really infected with *C. pneumoniae*, making any assessment of efficacy difficult. The development of standardized non-culture and serologic methods for diagnosis of *C. pneumoniae* infection are necessary before we can truly understand the role of this organism in chronic disease and determine the most effective therapy.

References

1 Grayston JT, Kuo CC, Wang SP, Altman J (1986) A new *Chlamydia psittaci* strain, TWAR, isolated in acute respiratory tract infections. *N Engl J Med* 315: 161–168
2 Hammerschlag, MR (1994) Antimicrobial susceptibility and therapy of infections caused by *Chlamydia pneumoniae*. *Antimicrob Agents Chemother* 38: 1873–1878
3 Jackson M, White N, Giffard P, Timms P (1999) Epizootiology of chlamydia infections in two free-range koala populations. *Vet Microbiol* 65: 255–264
4 Grayston JT, Campbell LA, Kuo CC, Mordhorst CH, Saikku P, Thom DH, Wang SP (1990) A new respiratory tract pathogen: *Chlamydia pneumoniae* strain TWAR. *J Infect Dis* 161: 618–625
5 Hammerschlag MR (1999) Community-acquired pneumonia due to atypical organisms in adults: diagnosis and treatment. *Infect Dis Clin Pract* 8: 232–240
6 Marston BJ, Plouff JF, File Jr. TM, Hackman BA, Salstrom SJ, Lipman HB, Kolczak MS, Breiman RF (1997) Incidence of community-acquired pneumonia requiring hospitalization. *Arch Intern Med* 157: 1709–1718

7 Norrby SR (1997) Atypical pneumonia in the nordic countries: aetiology and clinical results of a trial comparing fleroxacin and doxycycline. *J Antimicrob Chemother* 39: 499–508

8 Block S, Hedrick J, Hammerschlag MR, Cassell GH, Craft JC (1995) *Mycoplasma pneumonie* and *Chlamydia pneumoniae* in pediatric community-acquired pneumonia: comparative efficacy and safety of clarithromycin vs. erythromycin ethylsuccinate. *Pediatric Infect Dis J* 14: 471–477

9 Harris JS, Kolokathis A, Campbell M, Cassell GH, Hammerschlag MR (1998) Safety and efficacy of azithromycin in the treatment of community-acquired pneumonia in children. *Pediatr Infect Dis* 17: 865–871

10 Wubbel L, Muniz L, Ahmed A, Trujillo M, Carubelli C, McCoig C, Abramo T, Leinonen M, McCracken GH (1999) Etiology of community-acquired pneumonia in ambulatory children. *Pediatr Infect Dis J* 18:98–104

11 Emre U, Roblin PM, Gelling M, Dumornay W, Rao M, Hammerschlag MR, Schachter J (1994) The association of *Chlamydia pneumoniae* infection and reactive airway disease in children. *Arch Pediatr Adolesc Med* 148: 727–732

12 Block S, Hammerschlag MR, Hedrick J, Tyler R, Smith A, Robin P, Gaydos C, Pham D, Quinn TC, Palmer R et al (1997) *Chlamydia pneumoniae* in acute otitis media. *Pediatr Infect Dis J* 16: 858–862

13 Grayston JT, Aldous MB, Easton A, Wang SP, Kuo CC, Campbell LA, Altman J (1993) Evidence that *Chlamydia pneumoniae* causes pneumonia and bronchitis. *J Infect Dis* 168: 1231–1235

14 Hyman CL, Roblin PM, Gaydos CA, Quinn TC, Schachter J, Hammerschlag MR (1995) Prevalence of asymptomatic nasopharyngeal carriage of *Chlamydia pneumoniae* in subjectively healthily adults: assessment of polymerase chain reaction-enzyme immunoassay and culture. *Clin Infect Dis* 20: 1174–1178

15 Hammerschlag MR, Chirgwin K, Roblin PM, Gelling M, Dumornay W, Mandel L, Smith P, Schachter J (1992) Persistent infection with *Chlamydia pneumoniae* following acute respiratory illness. *Clin Infect Dis* 14:178–182

16 Dean D, Roblin PM, Mandel L, Schacter J, Hammerschlag MR (1998) Molecular evaluation of serial isolates from patients with persistent *Chlamydia pneumoniae* infections. In: Stephens RS, Byrne GI, Christiansen G, Eds. Chlamydia infections: Proceedings of the Ninth International Symposium on Human Chlamydia Infection. San Francisco: USCF, 219–223

17 Wong YK, Gallagher PJ, Ward ME (199) *Chlamydia pneumoniae* and atherosclerosis. *Heart* 82:232–238

18 Fenelon LE, Mumtaz G, Ridgway GL (1990) The *in vitro* antibiotic susceptibility of *Chlamydia pneumoniae. J Antimicrob Chemother* 26: 763–767

19 Cooper MA, Baldwin D, Matthews RS, Andrews JM, Wise R (1991) *In vitro* susceptibility of *Chlamydia pneumoniae* (TWAR) to seven antibiotics. *J Antimicrob Chemother* 28: 407–413

20 Ridgway GL, Mumtaz G, Fenelon L (1991) The *in vitro* activity of clarithromycin and other macrolides against the strain of *Chlamydia pneumoniae* (TWAR). *J Antimicrob Chemother* 27: 43–45

21 Agacfidan A, Moncada J, Schachter J (1993) *In vitro* activity of azithromycin (CP-62,993) against *Chlamydia trachomatis* and *Chlamydia pneumoniae. Antimicrob Agents Chemother* 37: 1746–1748

22 Hammerschlag MR, Khaldoon KQ, Roblin PM (1992) *In vitro* activities of azithromycin, clarithromycin, L-ofloxacin, and other antibiotics against *Chlamydia pneumoniae. Antimicrob Agents Chemother* 36: 1573–1574

23 Welsh LE, Gaydos CA, Quinn TC (1992) *In vitro* evaluation of activities of azithromycin, erythromycin, and tetracycline against *Chlamydia trachomatis* and *Chlamydia pneumoniae. Antimicrob Agents Chemother* 36: 291–294

24 Niki Y, Kimura M, Miyashita N, Soejima R (1994) *In vitro* and *in vivo* activities of azithromycin, and new azalide antibiotic, against chlamydia. *Antimicrob Agents Chemother* 38: 2296–2299

25 Roblin PM, Montalban G, Hammerschlag MR (1994) Susceptibilities to clarithromycin and erythromycin of isolates of *Chlamydia pneumoniae* from children with pneumonia. *Antimicrob Agents Chemother* 38: 1588–1589

26 Welsh L, Gaydos C, Quinn TC (1996) *In vitro* activities of azithromycin, clarithromycin, erythromycin and tetracycline against 13 strains of *Chlamydia pneumoniae. Antimicrob Agents Chemother* 40: 212–214

27 Kuo CC, Jackson LA, Lee A, Graystron JT (1996) *In vitro* activities of azithromycin, clarithromycin, and other antibiotics against *Chlamydia pneumoniae. Antimicrob Agents Chemother* 40: 2669–2670

28 Miyashita N, Niki Y, Kishimoto T, Nakajima M, Matsushima T (1997) *In vitro* and *in vivo* activities of AM-1155, a new fluoroquinolone, against *Chlamydia* spp. *Antimicrob Agents Chemother* 41: 1331–1334

29 Roblin PM, Kutlin A, Sokolovskaya N, Hammerschlag MR (1997) *In vitro* activity of dirithromycin against *Chlamydia pneumoniae. J Antimicro Chemother* 39: 647–649

30 Roblin PM, Hammerschlag MR (1998) Microbiologic efficacy of azithromycin and susceptibilities to azithromycin of isolates of *Chlamydia pneumoniae* from adults and children with community-acquired pneumonia. *Antimicrob Agents Chemother* 42: 194–196

31 Roblin PM, Hammerschlag MR (1998) *In vitro* activity of a new ketolide antibiotic, HMR 3647, against *Chlamydia pneumoniae. Antimicrob Agents Chemother* 42: 1515–1516

32 Strigil S, Roblin PM, Reznik T, Hammerschlag MR (2001). *In vitro* activity of ABT 773, a new ketolide antibiotic, against *Chlamydia pneumoniae. Antimicrob Agents Chemother; in press.*

33 Freidank HM, Losch P, Vogele H, Weidmann-Al-Ahmad M (1999) *In vitro* susceptibilities of *Chlamydia pneumoniae* isolates from German patients and synergistic activity of antibiotic combinations. *Antimicrob Agents Chemother* 43: 1808–1810

34 Nystrom-Rosander C, Hulten K, Gustavson I, Cars O, Engstrand L, Hjelm E (1997) Susceptibility of *Chlamydia pneumoniae* to azithromycin and doxycycline: methodological aspects on the determination of minimal inhibitory and minimal bactericidal concentrations. *Scand J Infect Dis* 29: 513–516

35 Gnarpe J, Eriksson K, Gnarpe H (1996) *In vitro* activities of azithromycin and doxycycline against 15 isolates of *Chlamydia pneumoniae. Antimicrob Agents Chemother* 40: 1843–1845

36 Malinverni R, Kuo CC, Campbell LA, Lee A, Grayston JT (1995) Effects of two antibiotic regimens on course and persistence of experimental *Chlamydia pneumoniae* TWAR pneumonitis. *Antimicrob Agents Chemother* 39: 45–49

37 Masson ND, Toseland CDN, Beale AS (1995) Relevance of *Chlamydia pneumoniae* murine pneumonitis model to evaluation of antimicrobial agents. *Antimicrob Agents Chemother* 39: 1959–1964

38 Wolf K, Malinverni R (1999) Effect of azithromycin plus rifampin *versus* that of azithromycin alone on the eradication of *Chlamydia pneumoniae* from lung tissue in experimental pneumonitis. *Antimicrob Agents Chemother* 43: 1491–1493

39 Kutlin A, Roblin PM, Hammerschlag MR (1999) *In vitro* activities of azithromycin and ofloxacin against *Chlamydia pneumoniae* in a continuous-infection model. *Antimicrob Agents Chemother* 43: 2268–2272

40 File Jr. TM, Segrett J, Dunbar L, Player R, Kohler R, Williams RR, Kojak C, Rubin A (1997) A multicenter, randomized study comparing the efficacy and safety of intravenous and/or oral levofloxacin versus ceftriaxone and/or cefuroxime axetil in treatment of adults with community-acquired penumonia. *Antimicrob Agents Chemother* 41: 1965–1972

41 Leophonte P, Baldwin RJT, Pluck N (1998) Trovafloxavin versus amoxicillin/clavulanic acid in the treatment of acute exacerbations of chronic obstructive bronchitis. *Eur J Clin Microbiol Infect Dis* 17: 434–440

42 Danesh J, Collins R, Peto R (1997) Chronic infections and coronary heart disease: is there a link? *Lancet* 350: 430–436

43 Hammerschlag MR (1998) Current knowledge of *Chlamydia pneumoniae* and atherosclerosis. *Eur J Clin Microbiol Infect Dis* 17 305–308

44 Hahn DL (1999) *Chlamydia pneumoniae*, asthma and COPD: what is the evidence? *Ann Allergy Asthma Immun* 83: 271–292

45 Cook PJ, Davies P, Tunnicliffe W, Ayres JG, Honeybourne D, Wise R (1998) *Chlamydia pneumoniae* and asthma. *Thorax* 53: 254–259

46 Larsen FO, Norn S, Mordhorst CH, Skov P, Stahl P, Milman N, Clementsen P (1998) *Chlamydia pneumoniae* and possible relationship to asthma: serum immunoglobulins and histamine release in patients and controls. *APMIS* 106: 928–934

47 Hahn DL (1995) Treatment of *Chlamydia pneumoniae* infection in adult asthma: a before-after trial. *J Fam Pract* 41:345–351

48 Scaglione F, Rossoni G (1998) Comparative anti-inflammatory effects of roxithromycin azithromycin and clarithrommycin. *J Antimicrob Chemother* 41: 47–50

49 Takizawa H, Desaki M, Ohtoshi T, Kawasaki S, Kohyama T, Sato M, Nakajima J, Yanagisawa M, Ito K (1999) Erythromycin and clarithromycin attenuate cytokine-induced endothelin-1 expression in human bronchial epithelial cells. *Thorax* 54: S58–S62

50 Ridker P (1999) Are associations between infection and coronary disease causal or due to confounding? *Am J Med* 106: 376–377

51 Danesh, J (1999) Coronary heart disease, *Helicobacter pylori*, dental disease, *Chlamydia pneumoniae*, and cytomegalovirus: Meta-analyses of prospective studies. *Am Heart J* 138: S434–S437

52 Weiss SM, Hammerschlag, MR (1997) Are heart attacks infectious? A critical look at the link between *Chlamydia pneumoniae* and atherosclerosis. *Bull Institut Pasteur* 95:107–113

53 Ramirez JA (1996) Isolation of *Chlamydia pneumoniae* from the coronary artery of a patient with coronary atherosclerosis. *Ann Intern Med* 125: 979–982

54 Jackson LA, Campbell LA, Kuo CC, Rodriguez DI, Lee A, Grayston JT (1997) Isolation of *Chlamydia pneumoniae* from a carotid endarterectomy specimen. *J Infect Dis* 176: 292–295

55 Maass M, Gieffers J, Krause E, Engel PM, Bartels C, Solbach W (1998) Poor correlation between microimmunofluorescence serology and polymerase chain reaction for detection of vascular *Chlamydia pneumoniae* infection in coronary artery disease patients. *Med Microbiol Immunol* 187: 103–106

56 Gupta S, Leatham EW, Carrington D, Mendall MA, Kaski JC, Camm J (1997) Elevated *Chlamydia pneumoniae* antibodies, cardiovascular events, and azithromycin in male survivors of myocardial infarction. *Circulation* 96: 404–407.

57 Gurfinkel E, Bozovich G, Darcoa A, Beck E, Mautner B (1997) Randomised trial of roxithromycin in non-Q-wave coronary syndromes: ROXIS pilot study. *Lancet* 350: 404–407

58 Gurfinkel E, Bozovich G, Beck E, Testa E, Livellara B, Mautner B (1999) Treatment with the antibiotic roxithromycin in patients with acute non-Q-wave coronary syndromes. *Eur Heart J* 20: 121–127

59 Anderson JL, Muhlestein JB, Carlquist J, Allen A, Trehan S, Nielson C, Hall S, Brady J, Egger M, Horne B et al (1999) Randomized secondary prevention trial of azithromycin in patients with coronary artery disease and serological evidence for *Chlamydia pneumoniae* infection: the azithromycin in coronary artery disease: elimination of myocardial infection with chlamydia (ACADEMIC) study. *Circulation* 99: 1540–1547

60 Leah AJ, Shelby-James TM, Mayo M, Gratten M, Laming AC, Currie BY, Matthews JD (1997) A prospective study of the impact of community-based azithromycin treatment of trachoma on carriage and resistance of *Streptococcus pneumoniae. Clin Infect Dis* 24: 356–362

61 Jackson LA, Stewart DK, Wang SP, Cooke DB, Cantrell T, Grayston JT (1999) Safety and effect on anti-*Chlamydia pneumoniae* antibody titres of a 1 month course of daily azithromycin in adults with coronary artery disease. *J Antimicrob Chemother* 44: 411–414

62 Michael Dunne (1999) WIZARD and the design of trials for secondary prevention of atherosclerosis with antibiotics. *Am Heart J* 138: S542–S544

63 Muhlestein JB, Anderson JL, Hammon EH, Zhao L, Trehan S, Schwobe BS, Carlquist JF (1998) Infection with *Chlamydia pneumoniae* accelerates the development of artherosclerosis and treatment with azithromycin prevents it in a rabbit model. *Circulation* 97: 633–636

64 Fong IW, Chiu B, Vira E, Jang D, Fong MW, Peeling R, Mahony JB (1999) Can an antibiotic (macrolide) prevent *Chlamydia pneumoniae* induced atherosclerosis in a rabbit model? *Clin Diag* 6:891–894

65 Richardson M, De Reske M, Delaney K, Fletch A, Wilcox LH, Kinlough-Rathbone RL (1997) Respiratory infection in lipid-fed rabbits enhances sudanophilia and the expression of VCAM-1. *Am J Pathol* 151: 1009–1017

66 Moazed TC, Kuo CC, Grayston JT, Campbell LA (1998) Evidence of systemic dissemination of *Chlamydia pneumoniae* via macrophages in the mouse. *J Infect Dis* 177: 1322–1325

67 Meier CR, Derby LE, Jick SS, Vasilaksi C, Jick H (1999) Antibiotics and risk subsequent first-time acute myocardial infarction. *JAMA* 281: 427–431

68 Jackson LA, Smith NL, Heckbert SR, Grayston JT, Siscovick DS, Psaty BM (1999) Lack of association between first myocardial infarction and past use of erythromycin, tetracycline, or doxycycline. *Emerg Infect Dis* 5: 281–284

Macrolide Antibiotics
ed. by W. Schönfeld and H. A. Kirst

Activity of macrolides in sexually transmitted diseases

Geoffrey L. Ridgway

Department of Clinical Microbiology, University College London Hospitals, Grafton Way, London WC1E 6DB, UK

Introduction

The *in vitro* antimicrobial spectrum of the macrolides is well suited for the treatment of many sexually transmitted bacterial infections. This activity, coupled with the established safety profile of erythromycin and the advent of newer compounds with improved pharmacokinetic and pharmacodynamic profiles of particular relevance to bacterial sexually transmitted diseases (STDs), has resulted in a recent surge of interest in their clinical use.

Erythromycin, first introduced to clinical medicine in 1952, is effective *in vitro* against *Treponema pallidum*, *Neisseria gonorrhoeae*, *Chlamydia trachomatis*, and *Ureaplasma urealyticum*. However, the oral absorption is unreliable and its therapeutic efficacy is frequently limited by gastrointestinal side effects. Erythromycin cannot be used to treat uncomplicated gonorrhoea in a single dose, and there have been problems with the emergence of resistant strains. Therefore, although theoretically tailor-made to treat bacterial STDs, erythromycin is clinically disappointing.

Over the past 10 years, there have been a number of new macrolides introduced to the market, with improved acid stability, better gastro-intestinal tolerance; and extended plasma half-life, tissue affinity, and intracellular penetration, all factors that are of importance in the management of bacterial STDs.

Syphilis

Erythromycin has long been regarded as an alternative drug to penicillin or tetracyclines for the treatment of syphilis [1]. It is salutary to note that there have never been any formal clinical trials to confirm efficacy and it is universally regarded as inferior to both penicillin and tetracyclines. Erythromycin is ineffective in neurosyphilis and does not reliably protect the fetus. Stamm and colleagues have documented a strain of *T. pallidum* resistant to erythromycin and roxithromycin [2]. Patients treated with erythromycin require close monitoring, and the 1998 Guidelines for Treatment of STDs from the Centers for Disease Control

(CDC) no longer recommends its use for this purpose, preferring desensitising to avoid acute allergic reactions and treatment with penicillin if necessary [3].

Encouraging anti-treponemal activity in animal models has been demonstrated for both roxithromycin and clarithromycin [4, 5]. Human trials of these agents have not been reported.

The activity of azithromycin in a rabbit model of syphilis was demonstrated by Lukehart and colleagues [6]. Clinical trials are difficult to carry out. In a preliminary study using 500 mg once daily, orally for 10 days, 11 of 13 patients with primary or secondary syphilis were cured [7]. The largest treatment study to date was reported from Moscow by the late Mashkilleyson and colleagues in 1996. They treated 89 patients with seropositive syphilis with 0.5 g azithromycin orally daily for 10 days and a further 11 patients with 0.5 g on alternate days for 11 days. Results were compared with erythromycin (2 g daily for 15 days), benzylpenicillin (300 000 IU intramuscularly 8 times daily for 16 to 30 days), or benzathine penicillin (2.4 mega IU once or twice at 7-day interval). Clinical signs resolved much faster in these cases than with penicillin or erythromycin, and treponemes could not be demonstrated after a mean of 26 hours in patients treated with azithromycin [8]. Ennis and colleagues reported that azithromycin (1 g orally) was as effective as benzathine penicillin (2.4 mega IU) in post-exposure prophylaxis [9]. Further evidence of efficacy is required before azithromycin can be recommended formally for the treatment of syphilis.

Chancroid

Erythromycin base and erythromycin stearate, given as 500 mg 6 hourly for 7 days, are both effective regimens for the treatment of chancroid [10, 11]. Azithromycin shows high *in vitro* activity against *Haemophilus ducreyi*, and the pharmacokinetics of oral medication suggest that single-dose therapy may be effective. Clinical trial results have confirmed this suggestion. Thus, Tyndall and colleagues reported an 89% (73 of 82) cure rate [12] and Martin and colleagues a 100% (all of 32) cure rate with a single 1-g dose of azithromycin [13]. Martin and colleagues also noted that azithromycin was as effective as 250 mg of ceftriaxone for culture negative ulcers (*H. ducreyi* or herpes viruses not isolated or detected by other means). All patients in both studies had negative serological tests for syphilis. Tyndall, working in Kenya, noted a correlation between failure to respond, lack of circumcision, and HIV-1 seropositivity. Ballard and colleagues, working in South Africa, found a similar cure rate (92% *versus* 89%) but did not find such an association [14].

Donovanosis (Granuloma inguinale)

Donovanosis is caused by the bacterium *Calymmatobacterium granulomatis*, which cannot be cultured on conventional media. The treatment of donovanosis is unsatisfactory. Erythromycin stearate or base given as 500 mg 6 hourly for two to three weeks is accepted therapy. However, relapse is likely. Reported clinical trials are few; therefore, the results of the study by Bowden and co-workers using azithromycin is of interest [15]. The study was conducted in the Northern Territories of Australia. Eleven patients with histologically confirmed donovanosis were enrolled into an open-label study. Seven patients received 1 g of azithromycin weekly for 4 weeks, and 4 patients received 500 mg daily for 7 days. At 6 weeks assessment, 4 patients receiving intermittent therapy and one patient receiving continuous therapy were healed. The remaining 6 were improved. At 7 months follow-up, none required retreatment. An additional 17 patients with clinical donovanosis also were treated successfully during the study.

Gonorrhoea

The *in vitro* activity of erythromycin against *Neisseria gonorrhoeae* has long been appreciated [16]. However, clinical experience is less satisfactory, and erythromycin is not reliable in a single dose for the treatment of uncomplicated gonococcal infection. This fact alone disallows the use of erythromycin for routine treatment. Because of the established safety of erythromycin, it was long used to treat gonococcal infection during pregnancy [17]. Brown and colleagues treated 152 men with gonorrhoea, using a total dose of 9 g over 5 days. Persistent or recurrent gonorrhoea was recorded in 23.6% of men [18]. As is the case with syphilis, careful monitoring of progress is required, and the drug is no longer recommended for routine use [3]. Oriel and colleagues examined the efficacy of erythromycin stearate (1 g) plus rifampicin (900 mg) as a single dose treatment for gonococcal urethritis in men [19]. The organism was re-isolated from 4 of 108 men returning for first follow-up and from 0 of 68 returning for second follow-up. A similar study of women with gonorrhoea showed similar efficacy, with re-isolation of the gonococcus from the pharynx of 1 patient out of 100 treated [20].

Although less active than erythromycin *in vitro*, the greater half-life of spiramycin may allow more reliable therapy. Its use for gonorrhoea has been investigated by a number of workers [21]. Doses ranged from a single dose of 2.5 g to 4–12 g over 2 days. Single-dose cure rates were of the order of 80% to 85%.

Rosaramicin (rosamicin) also showed *in vitro* promise, with a reported MIC_{90} of 0.1 mg/l [22]. A clinical study using 1.5 g or 2 g daily for 4 days cured 39 of 40 men with acute uncomplicated gonorrhoea. Gastrointestinal side effects occurred in 5% [23]. The clinical use of this antibiotic has not been pursued.

Interest in macrolide anti-gonococcal activity persists, and Table 1 lists the activity of the more prominent macrolides [24]. Most interest has focused on azithromycin, with the appreciation that particularly high intracellular levels made this compound attractive as a single-dose oral agent for treating uncomplicated gonorrhoea. Handsfield [25] reported abandonment of a multicentre study of the treatment of gonorrhoea with a single 1 g oral dose when a cure rate of only 85% to 90% was documented. However Waugh [26] found that this dose was effective against gonorrhoea in 95% (78 of 82) of men with acute gonorrhoea, including 4

Table 1. Activity of macrolides and azalides against *Neisseria gonorrhoeae* (after [23])

Antimicrobial	MIC_{50} (mg/l)	MIC_{90} (mg/l)
Erythromycin	0.06	2.0
Azithromycin	0.12	0.25
Josamycin	0.25	1.0
Roxithromycin	0.25	1.0
Midecamycin acetate	1.0	1.0
Clarithromycin	1.0	2.0

rectal and 2 pharyngeal infections, and in 100% (9) of women patients with cervicitis and rectal and pharyngeal infection. Clinical cure was reported in 72 (90%) of the men, and improvement was reported in 5 of the remaining 8 initially symptomatic men. All women with symptoms were cured. The minimal inhibitory concentration (MIC) of azithromycin for the strains isolated from the treatment failures was 0.25 mg/l; that is at the top end of the expected range of MIC reported as clinically effective (0.003 to 0.25 mg/l). It would therefore appear that 1 g of azithromycin is effective against *N. gonorrhoeae* infection, provided that the prevalence of macrolide-resistant gonorrhoea is not high in the population being treated. Side effects were low in Waugh's study, with one patient vomiting the tablets. A further study reported by Handsfield [27] found that 2 g azithromycin cured 370 of 374 patients with culture-confirmed gonorrhoea (99%), including all patients infected with β-lactamase producing strains. However, of 431 patients receiving the 2 g dose, 152 (35%) complained of gastrointestinal effects, reported as moderate in 10.1%, and severe in 2.9%, compared with 2.9% side effects to ceftriaxone, the comparator in this study. Several further studies of the single 1 g oral dose have been reported, including Gruber and colleagues [28]. They treated 50 patients with 1 g of azithromycin and 51 patients with 500 mg of ciprofloxacin. Cure rates were 96% (48 of 50) in the azithromycin group and 92% (47 of 51) in the ciprofloxacin group.

Resistance of *N. gonorrhoeae* to macrolides is not well understood. It is apparent, however, that cross-resistance is to be expected. Erythromycin, although highly active against the gonococcus *in vitro*, cannot be used to treat gonorrhoea in a single oral dose. Apart from the treatment failures noted in Waugh's study [26], Ehret and colleagues reported an erythromycin MIC of 32 mg/l, and an azithromycin MIC of 2 mg/l against a single isolate of *N. gonorrhoeae* [29]. Examination of a further 500 strains yielded MICs of 0.015 to 2 mg/l for erythromycin, and 0.015 to 0.5 mg/l for azithromycin. There was a strong correlation between raised MICs for either drug. A treatment failure with 1 g of azithromycin yielded an increase in MIC of erythromycin from 1 mg/l pre-treatment to 32 mg/l post-treatment and from 0.125 mg/l to 3 mg/l for azithromycin [30]. The authors speculated that the prolonged half-life of azithromycin may increase the selection pressure on *N. gonorrhoeae* for resistance. There is no doubt that azithromycin is very effective as a 1 g dose, provided that macrolide resistance is not a significant epidemiological problem. The need for continued surveillance of susceptibility patterns cannot be overemphasised.

Chlamydia trachomatis and non-specific (non-gonococcal) genital infection (NSGI)

Erythromycin has long been known to be clinically effective in the management of NSGI [31]. It was not until *Chlamydia trachomatis* was appreciated as the major cause of NSGI that any scientific basis could be applied to the clinical findings. That said, the results of therapy for NSGI, whether caused by *C. trachomatis* or truly non-specific, remain less than satisfactory. There is no doubt that eradication of *C. trachomatis* correlates with clinical resolution, but the relationship is not simple. Whether the cause is *C. trachomatis* or unknown, the clinical response is seldom better than 85% to 90%, even with eradication of the known pathogen. Chlamydial genital infection and NSGI seem to respond equally well to the same antibiotic regimens and, for this reason, must be considered together.

The isolation of *C. trachomatis* in cell culture led to the development of techniques for investigating the activity of antibiotics against it [32], and the high activity of erythromycin was confirmed. Treatment studies soon followed. Oriel and colleagues compared erythromycin stearate 500 mg 12 hourly with oxytetracycline 250 mg 6 hourly, both given for 2 weeks in the treatment of non-gonococcal urethritis (NGU) [33]. The organism was eradicated from 39 of 40 men with chlamydia-positive NGU. Clinical improvement assessed at two weeks was found in 86% of chlamydia-positive men and in 89% of chlamydia-negative men. In a similar study involving chlamydial infection of the cervix, the organism was not re-isolated from any of 70 women examined 2 weeks after completion of therapy [34]. Erythromycin continues to be recommended as alternative treatment for NSGI, but problems with the pharmacokinetics and the resulting number of preparations (base, lactobionate, stearate, ethylsuccinate, estolate) have resulted in confusion over optimal dosage and duration [3]. Coupled with the widespread problem of gastrointestinal side effects with erythromycin, the possibility to use alternative macrolides became attractive.

Table 2 lists the *in vitro* antimicrobial activity of various macrolides against *C. trachomatis* [35]. Many other macrolides have been evaluated both *in vitro* and in animal models, but they have not been further pursued in human clinical trials for NSGI or chlamydial genital infection. As stated above, it is also necessary to bear in mind the activity of anti-chlamydial agents against other potential pathogens. Foremost amongst such organisms are the mycoplasmas and ureaplasmas, and the activity of the macrolides against these organisms is shown in Table 3 [36]. With the possible exception of midecamycin acetate, the macrolides have no clinically useful activity against *Mycoplasma hominis*. Whilst this organism is not implicated in NGU, its role in Pelvic Inflammatory Disease (PID) may have an

Table 2. Activity of various macrolides and azalides against *Chlamydia trachomatis* (after [36])

Antimicrobial	MIC (mg/l)
Clarithromycin	0.007
Josamycin	0.03
Roxithromycin	0.03
Midecamycin acetate	0.06
Erythromycin	0.06
Azithromycin	0.125
Spiramycin	0.5

Table 3. Activity of various macrolides and azalides against *Mycoplasma hominis* and *Ureaplasma urealyticum* (after [37])

Antimicrobial	*M. hominis* MIC (mg/l)	*U. urealyticum* MIC (mg/l)
Midecamycin acetate	0.008–0.12	0.03–0.25
Clarithromycin	8.0–64.0	0.025–1.0
Josamycin	Not available	0.02–0.5
Roxithromycin	8.0– > 64	0.06–1.0
Azithromycin	2.0–16.0	0.12–1.0
Erythromycin	> 32.0	0.12–2.0

important bearing on the use of macrolides for therapy of this condition. The role of *Ureaplasma urealyticum* in NGU and NSGI is far from clear, and the correlation between treatment failure and persistence of this organism after macrolide therapy is poor.

Amongst the first of the newer macrolides to be evaluated clinically was rosaramicin. In a dose of 250 mg orally 6 hourly for 7 days, rosaramicin eradicated *C. trachomatis* from the urethras of 95% of men. Clinical cure at 87% compared favourably with the tetracycline comparator response of 77% [37].

Spiramycin is the least active of this group of macrolides against *C. trachomatis*. However, Dylewski and colleagues evaluated its clinical use *versus* doxycycline for chlamydial genital infection [38]. A microbiological cure of 100% was obtained in 133 men and women, using 1 g orally twice daily for 14 days.

Enthusiasm to use the more recent macrolides for chlamydial genital infection and NSGI has been dampened by the intracellular pharmacokinetics of the azalide macrolide azithromycin and by the discovery that a single oral dose of this drug is as effective as a conventional course of doxycycline against genital chlamydial infection and NSGI. A few studies with these other macrolides have however been reported. Roxithromycin in doses of 150 mg twice daily, or 300 mg or 450 mg daily for 7 to 10 days, is as effective as doxycycline or erythromycin [39, 40]. A study of the activity of roxithromycin against chlamydia-negative NGU, using

300 mg once daily compared with erythromycin 500 mg twice daily for one week, found clinical cure rates of 88% and 98% on day 8, falling to 84% and 86%, respectively, by day 21 [41]. Reported interest in josamycin has largely surrounded its use for chlamydial infection in pregnancy. Söltz-Szöts and colleagues treated pregnant women with either 500 mg 2 times daily for 12 days (Group A) or with 500 mg 3 times daily for 8 days (Group B). Respective microbiological failure rates were 17% and 9%. They attributed most failures to errors in dosage or reinfection and recommended the routine use of the Group B regimen [42].

Clarithromycin is the most active macrolide against *C. trachomatis*. Few published trials exist on the use of this drug for chlamydial genital infection and NSGI. Stein and Mummaw treated 20 adult patients with NSGI with oral clarithromycin 250 mg 2 times daily for 7 days. All cases of proven chlamydial infection (14 of 20) were microbiologically cured. At 3 weeks follow-up, 2 patients had clinical relapse but tested chlamydia-negative [43].

Uncomplicated gonococcal infection is almost universally treated with a single dose of an effective antibiotic. The 48- to 72-h life cycle of *C. trachomatis* suggested that such a treatment regimen would be difficult to achieve for chlamydial genital infection. Indeed, the findings of Oriel and colleagues that single-dose erythromycin plus rifampicin for gonorrhoea had little effect on concomitant chlamydial infection was of interest in this respect (5 of 9 and 26 of 36 men and women, respectively, were still chlamydia-positive on follow-up) [19, 20]. The unique pharmacological profile of azithromycin, coupled with its *in vitro* activity against both *C. trachomatis* and the ureaplasmas, suggested the possibility of treating genital infections caused by these bacteria with a single dose of the antibiotic. Worldwide clinical studies have confirmed that this is indeed the case, thus revolutionising the treatment of these conditions.

One of the earliest studies with azithromycin was carried out by Steingrimsson and colleagues [44]. They treated patients with chlamydial genital infection with either a single dose of 1 g, 500 mg x 2, or 500 mg on day 1 followed by 250 mg on days 2 and 3. The total dose was thus the same. They demonstrated cure in 91 of 96 patients, including 43 of 44 treated with the single dose. They also noted that the single dose eradicated *Ureaplasma urealyticum* from 11 of 14 patients. Whatley and colleagues treated men with NGU (chlamydial and non-chlamydial) with either a single 1 g dose of azithromycin, or 500 mg on day one followed by 250 mg on days 2 and 3. They followed patients for 21 days and found that all patients with chlamydial urethritis were microbiologically cured. The authors commented that although both groups received the same total dose, clinical cure was subjectively better with the three-day dose [45]. Both these studies are notable for the low incidence of side effects, with only 1% of patients in the Steingrimsson study complaining of diarrhoea.

Nilsen and colleagues used placebo to blind their study on the therapy of chlamydial urethritis such that all patients took the same number of capsules [46]. A single 1 g oral dose of azithromycin was compared with standard doxycycline therapy (100 mg x 2 daily for 7 days). Patients were followed up at 6 to 12 days and 13 to 21 days post-commencement of therapy. *C. trachomatis* was eradicated from all patients in both groups at first follow-up and 100% (35/35) and 97% (34/35), respectively, at second follow-up. Clinical cure rates, again reflecting the difference between persistence of symptoms and eradication of the organism when identified, were not significantly different between the two groups at either first or second follow-up (64% *versus* 69% and 89% *versus* 94%, respectively). Side effects were reported by 30% in the azithromycin group and were mainly mild gastrointestinal.

The treatment of chlamydial cervical infection in women was investigated by Ossewarde and colleagues [47]. Fourteen women were treated with standard doxycycline therapy for one week, and 17 women were treated with a single 1 g oral dose of azithromycin. *C. trachomatis* was not re-isolated from any patient examined 1 or 4 weeks post-therapy.

The first multicentre study was reported by Martin and colleagues in 1992 [48]. A single oral dose of 1 g azithromycin was again compared with standard oral doxycycline for treatment of laboratory-confirmed chlamydial urethritis or cervicitis. Cumulative results for eradication of *C. trachomatis* (*i. e.,* attendance at one or more follow-up clinics) were 41/43 (95%) men and 95/98 (97%) women with azithromycin compared with 37/38 (97%) men and 185/187 (99%) women in the doxycycline group. Clinical cure rates varied between centres within the range 91% to 98% for either sex or treatment.

As indicated previously, the symptoms of NSGI are indistinguishable between chlamydial or non-chlamydial forms. However, it is important that empirical treatment is equally effective. Two studies looked at both chlamydia-positive and chlamydia-negative NSGI. Laurahanta and colleagues [49] treated 120 patients, divided into 4 groups of 30, with two chlamydia-positive groups and 2 chlamydia-negative. One group in each category received 1 g azithromycin, and the other group received standard doxycycline therapy. Patients were followed for up to 35 days post-treatment, and those who might have been reinfected were excluded from the final analysis. *C. trachomatis* was eradicated overall from 87% of the azithromycin and from 93% of the doxycycline groups. Clinical cure rates (resolved or improved) were similar at 91% and 96%, respectively, at late follow-up. Of particular note was the trend for a better clinical cure rate with azithromycin in the *C. trachomatis*-negative group, 79% (15 of 19), compared with 47% (8 of 17) receiving doxycycline, at the 35-day follow-up. In the second study [50], 72 men with non-gonococcal urethritis were treated with azithromycin and 71 with doxycycline. Of the 128 evaluable men, 51 (39.8%) were positive for *C. trachomatis*. Follow-up at 14 to 21 days after treatment found that the organism was eradicated from 100% of those treated with doxycycline (12 of 12) and from 81% (13 of 16) in the azithromycin group. However, there was evidence that 2 of 3 failures in the latter group had become reinfected. This problem bedevils trials in STDs and is probably underestimated. Again, there was no statistical difference for clinical resolution of either *C. trachomatis*-positive or -negative NGU between the two treatments. The conclusion that azithromycin is an effective and convenient alternative to doxycycline for the treatment of chlamydial or non-chlamydial NGU is reflected in the Recommendations for Prevention and

Management of *Chlamydia trachomatis* Infections, 1993 [51]), the 1998 Sexually Transmitted Diseases Treatment Guidelines [3], and the UK National Guidelines for the Management of Sexually Transmitted Infections Closely Related Conditions [52].

One attraction of the single-dose approach is compliance, particularly where high-risk groups less likely to be compliant to conventional therapy are concerned, for example adolescents. Hammerschlag and colleagues treated 73 adolescents (65 female) with either 1 g azithromycin or conventional doxycycline. All patients had either urethral or cervical chlamydial infection. At 4 weeks follow-up, 4 of 46 (8.7%) who received azithromycin were positive, all female, and 3 were probable reinfections. There was no difference in clinical efficacy for the two treatments. Side effects were mild gastrointestinal only in both groups [53].

The aetiological diagnosis of NSGI is, to say the least, imprecise, with *C. trachomatis* being isolated in up to 50% of cases. The specific role of *U. urealyticum* in either chlamydial or non-chlamydia urethritis is still unclear. Stamm and colleagues addressed this problem with a multicentre study involving over 400 patients [54]. Study design was a 2 to 1 randomisation of single-dose azithromycin with standard dose doxycycline. Cultures were performed for both *C. trachomatis* and *U. urealyticum*. Overall eradication rates were similar for chlamydiae and ureaplasmas (83% *versus* 90% and 45% *versus* 47%, respectively). Cumulative clinical cure rates also were not significantly different between the treatment groups, with 81% in the azithromycin group and 77% in the doxycycline group. Further, clinical cure rates were not dissimilar irrespective of the presence or absence of either *C. trachomatis* or *U. urealyticum*. There was no correlation between persistence of ureaplasmas and persistence of symptoms. Side effects (23% *versus* 29%) were generally mild. The convenience and efficacy of azithromycin in community care of STDs was demonstrated in another study where 347 patients with uncomplicated chlamydial genital infection received single-dose azithromycin [55]. Bacteriological cure was demonstrated in 338 (99%), with clinical cure at 86% after 2 weeks follow-up. These results were similar to the doxycycline comparator. Side effects were particularly high in this study, at 41% and 37%, respectively, but were largely mild gastrointestinal.

The established safety of erythromycin has led to a number of appraisals of azithromycin for chlamydial infection in pregnancy. Although not yet licensed for this purpose there is a reasonable body of evidence supporting its use and confirming its efficacy [56–58].

C. trachomatis is the most common pathogen associated with Pelvic Inflammatory Disease [59]. A course of azithromycin (500 mg intravenously on day one, followed by 250 mg orally days 2 to 7, *i. e.*, a total dose 2 grams) with or without additional metronidazole is effective therapy for this disease, eradicating both *N. gonorrhoeae* and *C. trachomatis* when present (Bevan and Ridgway, personal communication). The results of further studies are awaited with interest.

Conclusion

Bacterial STDs continue to be a major source of morbidity worldwide, and the macrolides have an antimicrobial spectrum that is ideally suited for the chemotherapy of many sexually transmitted bacterial infections. The *in vitro a*ctivity of these agents against *Gardnerella vaginalis* and *Mobiluncus* spp., agents predominating in bacterial vaginosis, is high, but preliminary studies with azithromycin have proved clinically disappointing in this condition (Ridgway personal communication).

Azithromycin dominates the field of macrolide use in STDs. It has revolutionised the management of chlamydial genital infection, but the cost of a one gram oral dose is considerably more expensive than doxycycline at 100 mg twice daily for 7 days. Several studies have examined the economics of chlamydial genital infection, demonstrating that when other factors such as clinic attendances, follow-up, side effects, and cost of sequelae are taken into account, azithromycin single-dose therapy is more cost-effective than doxycycline [60–62]. However, the problem of apportioning costs across a healthcare system to realise the value of azithromycin use was highlighted in the extensive review by Lea and Lamb [63].

The use of macrolides for treating STDs has come a long way from the empirical use of erythromycin 40 years ago. Most recent studies have concentrated on the use of azithromycin, almost to the exclusion of other agents. The use of a single agent in a single dose to treat concurrent gonococcal and chlamydial infection, plus activity against incubating syphilis, is exciting [64] However, there is still room for improvement, both with regard to efficacy and side effects. It will be sad if clinicians are denied the opportunity to test newer macrolides and derivatives in clinical trials for the treatment of STDs.

References

1 Report 1993. Sexually Transmitted Diseases Treatment Guidelines (1993) *Morbidity and Mortality Weekly Report* 42: (RR-14) 47–52

2 Stamm LV, Stapleton JT, Bassford PJ Jr (1988) *In vitro* assay to demonstrate high-level erythromycin resistance of a clinical isolate of *Treponema pallidum. Antimicrob Agents Chemother* 32: 164–169

3 Report 1998. Sexually Transmitted Diseases Treatment Guidelines (1998) *Morbidity and Mortality Weekly Report* 47: (RR-1)

4 Lukehart SA, Baker-Zander SA (1987) Roxithromycin (RU 965): effective therapy for experimental syphilis infection in rabbits. *Antimicrob Agents Chemother* 31: 187–190

5 Alder J, Jarvis K, Mitten, Shipkowitz NL, Gupta P, Clement J (1993) Clarithromycin therapy of *Treponema pallidum* infections in hamsters. *Antimicrob Agents Chemother* 37: 864–867

6 Lukehart SA, Fohn MJ, Baker-Zander SA (1990) Efficacy of azithromycin for therapy of active syphilis in the rabbit model. *J Antimicrob Chemother* 25 (suppl A): 91–99.

7 Verdon MS, Handsfield HH, Johnson RB (1994) Pilot study of azithromycin for treatment of primary and secondary syphilis. *Clin Infect Dis* 19: 484–488

8 Mashkilleyson AL, Gomberg MA, Mashkilleyson N, Kutin SA (1996) Treatment of syphilis with azithromycin. *Int J STD Aids* 7 (Suppl 1): 13–15

9 Hook EW, Stephens J, Ennis DM (1999) Azithromycin compared with penicillin G benzathine for the treatment of incubating syphilis. *Ann Intern Med* 131: 434–437
10 Duncan MO, Bilgeri YR, Fehler HG, Ballard RC (1983) Treatment of chancroid with erythromycin. A clinical and microbiological appraisal. *Brit J Vener Dis* 59: 265–268
11 Plummer NA, D'Costa LJ, Nsanze H, Maclean IW, Karasira P, Piot P, East MV, Ronald AR (1983) Antimicrobial therapy of chancroid. *J Infect Dis* 148: 726–731
12 Tyndall MW, Agoki E, Plummer FA, Malisa W, Ndinya-Achola JO, Ronald AR (1994) Single dose treatment of chancroid: a randomised comparison with erythromycin. *Sex Transm Dis* 21:231–234
13 Martin DH, Sargent S, Wendel GD, McCormack WM, Spier NA, Johnson RB (1995) Comparison of azithromycin and ceftriaxone for the treatment of chancroid. *Clin Infect Dis* 21: 409–414
14 Ballard RC, Ye H, Matta A, Dangor Y, Radebe F (1996) Treatment of chancroid with azithromycin. *Int J STD Aids* 7 (suppl 1): 9–12
15 Bowden FJ, Mein J, Plunkett C, Bastian I (1996) Pilot study of azithromycin in the treatment of genital donovanosis. *Genitourin Med* 72: 17–19
16 Phillips I, Ridley M, Rimmer D, Lynn R, Warren C (1970) *In vitro* activity of twelve antibacterial agents against *Neisseria gonorrhoeae*. *Lancet* I (7641) 263–265
17 Report (1974) Gonorrhea-CDC recommended treatment Schedules, 1974. *J Amer Vener Dis* 1: 67–69
18 Brown ST, Pedersen AHB, Holmes KK (1977) Comparison of erythromycin base and estolate in gonococcal urethritis. *J Amer Med Assoc* 238: 1371–1373
19 Oriel JD, Ridgway GL, Goldmeier D, Felmingham D (1982) Treatment of gonococcal urethritis in men with a rifampicin-erythromycin combination. *J Amer Vener Dis* 9: 208–211
20 Boakes AJ, Loo PS, Tovey S, Oriel JD (1984) Treatment of uncomplicated gonorrhoea in women with a combination of rifampicin and erythromycin. *Brit J Vener Dis* 60: 309–311
21 Leading Article (1970). *Brit J Med* 258: 129
22 Dillon JR, Duck PD, Eidus L (1978) A comparison of the *in vitro* activity of rosamicin, erythromycin, penicillin and tetracycline against *N. gonorrhoeae, including* β-lactamase producing isolates. *J Antimicrob Chemother* 4: 477–480
23 Dasco C, Greenberg S, Martin RR (1980) Rosaramicin treatment of gonococcal urethritis in men. *Sex Transm Dis* 7: 133–134
24 Ridgway GL (1995) Chlamydia and other sexually transmitted diseases. In: HC Neu, LS Young, S Zinner (eds): *The new macrolides, azalides and streptogramins.* Marcel Dekker, New York, 147–154
25 Handsfield HH (1993) Sexually transmitted chlamydial infections, gonorrhoea and syphilis. In: HC Neu, LS Young, S Zinner (eds): *The new macrolides, azalides and streptogramins.* Marcel Dekker, New York, 167–172
26 Waugh MA (1993) Open study of the safety and efficacy of a single oral dose of azithromycin for the treatment of uncomplicated gonorrhoea in men and women. *J Antimicrob Chemother* 31 (suppl E): 193–198
27 Handsfield HH, Dalu Z A, Martin DH, Douglas JM, McCarty JM, Schlossberg D, and the Azithromycin Study Group (1994) Multicentre trial of single dose azithromycin *versus* ceftriaxone in the treatment of uncomplicated gonorrhoea. *Sex Transm Dis* 21: 107–111
28 Gruber F, Brajac I, Jonjic A, Grubišic-Greblo H, Lenkovic M, Stasic A (1997) Comparative trial of azithromycin and ciprofloxacin in the treatment of gonorrhoea. *J Chemother* 9: 263–266
29 Erhret JM, Nims LJ, Judson FN (1996) A clinical isolate of *Neisseria gonorrhoeae* with *in vitro* resistance to erythromycin, and decreased susceptibility to azithromycin. *Sex Transm Dis* 23: 270–272
30 Young H, Moyes A, McMillan A (1997) Azithromycin and erythromycin resistant *Neisseria gonorrhoeae* following treatment with azithromycin. *Int J STD Aids* 8: 299–302
31 Willcox RR (1968) Erythromycin in treatment of non-gonococcal urethritis. *Brit J Vener Dis* 44: 157–159
32 Ridgway G, Owen JM, Oriel JD (1976) A method for testing the antibiotic susceptibility of *Chlamydia trachomatis* in a cell culture system. *J Antimicrob Chemother* 2: 71–79
33 Oriel JD, Ridgway, GL, Tchamouroff S (1977) Comparison of erythromycin stearate and oxytetracycline in the treatment of non-gonococcal urethritis. *Scot Med J* 22: 375–379

34 Oriel JD, Ridgway GL (1980) Comparison of erythromycin and oxytetracycline in the treatment of cervical infection by *Chlamydia trachomatis. J Infect* 2: 259–262.
35 Ridgway GL (1992) Advances in the antimicrobial therapy of chlamydial genital infections. *J Infect* 25 (suppl 1): 51–59
36 Ridgway GL (1993) *In vitro* activity against *Mycoplasma* spp. and intracellular organisms. In: HC Neu, LS Young, S Zinner (eds): *The new macrolides, azalides and streptogramins.* Marcel Dekker, New York, 25–30
37 Darne JF, Ridgway GL, Oriel JD (1982) Rosaramicin and tetracycline in the treatment of non-gonococcal urethritis. *Brit J Vener Dis* 58: 117–120
38 Dylewski J, Clecner B, Dubois J, St. Pierrre C, Murray G, Bouchard C, Phillips R (1993) Comparison of spiramycin and doxycycline for treatment of *Chlamydia trachomatis* genital infection. *Antimicrob Agents Chemother* 37: 1373–1374
39 Lassus A, Seppala A (1987) Roxithromycin in nongonococcal urethritis. *J Antimicrob Chemother* 20 (suppl B): 157–165
40 Worm AM, Hoff G, Kroon S, Petersen CS, Christensen JJ (1989) Roxithromycin compared with erythromycin against genitourinary chlamydial infections. *Genitourin Med* 65: 35–38
41 Worm AM (1990) Roxithromycin and erythromycin in chlamydia negative non-gonococcal urethritis. *Acta Derm Venerol* 70: 269–71
42 Söltz-Szöts J, Schneider S, Niebauer B, Knobler RM, Lindmaier A (1989) Significance of the dose of josamycin in the treatment of chlamydia infected pregnant patients. *Z Hautkr* 64: 129–131
43 Stein GE, Mummaw N, Havlichek DH (1995) A preliminary study of clarithromycin *versus* doxycycline in the treatment of nongonococcal urethritis and mucopurulent cervicitis. *Pharmacotherapy* 15: 727–731
44 Steingrimsson O, Olfsson JH, Thorarinsson H, Ryan RW, Johnson RB, Tilton RC (1990) Azithromycin in the treatment of sexually transmitted disease. *J Antimicrob Chemother* 25 (Suppl. A): 109–114
45 Whatley JD, Thin RNT, Mumtaz G, Ridgway GL (1991) Azithromycin vs doxycycline in the treatment of non-gonococcal urethritis. *Int J STD Aids* 2: 248–251
46 Nilsen A, Halsos A, Johansen A, Hansen E, Torud E, Moseng D, Anestad G, Storvold G (1992) A double blind study of single dose azithromycin and doxycycline in the treatment of chlamydial urethritis in males. *Genitourin Med* 68: 325–327
47 Ossewaarde JM, Plantema FHF, Rieffe M, Nawrocki RP, de Vries A, van Loon AM (1992) Efficacy of single-dose azithromycin *versus* doxycycline in the treatment of cervical infections caused by *Chlamydia trachomatis. Eur J Clin Microbiol Infect Dis* 11: 693–697
48 Martin DH, Mroczdowski TF, Dalu ZA McCarty J, Jones RB, Hopkins SJ, Johnson RB and the Azithromycin for Chlamydial Infections Study Group (1992) A controlled trial of a single dose of azithromycin for the treatment of chlamydial urethritis and cervicitis. *N Engl J Med* 327: 921–925
49 Lauharanta J, Saarinen K, Mustonen M-T, Happonen H-P (1993) Single oral azithromycin *versus* seven day doxycycline in the treatment of nongonococcal urethritis in males. *J Antimicrob Chemother* 31 (suppl E): 177–183
50 Lister PJ, Balechandran T, Ridgway GL, Robinson AJ (1993) Comparison of azithromycin and doxycycline in the treatment of non-gonococcal urethritis in men. *J Antimicrob Chemother* 31 (suppl E): 185–192
51 Report 1998. Recommendations for the prevention and management of *Chlamydia trachomatis* infections (1993) *Morbidity and Mortality Weekly Report* 42: (RR-12)
52 Report 1999. UK National Guidelines on Sexually Transmitted Infections and Closely Related Conditions. *Sex Transm Infect* 75, (suppl 1): S4–11
53 Hammerschlag MR, Golden MH, Oh MK Gelling M, Sturdeven M, Brown PR, Aras Z, Neuhoff SM Dumornay W, Roblin P (1993) Single dose of azithromycin for the treatment of genital chlamydial infection in adolescents. *J Paediatrics* 122: 961–965
54 Stamm WE, Hicks CB, Martin DH, Leone P, Hook EW, Cooper RH, Cohen MS, Batteiger BE, Workowski K, McCormack WM et al (1995) Azithromycin for empirical treatment of the non-gonococcal urethritis syndrome in men. *J Amer Med Assoc* 274: 545–549
55 Thorpe EM, Stamm WE, Hook EW, Gall SA, Jones RB, Henry K, Whitworth G, Johnson RB (1996) *Genitourin Med* 72: 93–97

56 Bush M, Rosa C (1994) Azithromycin and erythromycin in the treatment of cervical chlamydial infection during pregnancy (1994) *Obstet Gynecol* 84: 61–63

57 Miller JM (1995) Efficacy and tolerance of single dose azithromycin for the treatment of chlamydial cervicitis during pregnancy. *Infect Dis Obstet Gynecol* 3: 189–192

58 Rosenn MF, Macones G, Silverman NS (1995) Randomized trial of erythromycin and azithromycin for the treatment of chlamydial infection in pregnancy. *Infect Dis Obstet Gynecol* 3: 241–244

59 Bevan C, Johal BJ, Mumtaz G, Ridgway G, Siddle NC (1995) Clinical, laparoscopic and microbiological findings in acute salpingitis: report on a UK cohort. *Brit J Obstet Gynaecol* 102: 407–414

60 Carlin EM, Barton SE (1996) Azithromycin as the first line treatment of non-gonococcal urethritis (NGU): a study of follow-up rates, contact attendances and patients' treatment preference. *Int J STD Aids* 7: 185–189

61 Genç M, Mårdh P-A. A cost-effectiveness analysis of screening and treatment for *Chlamydia trachomatis* infection in asymptomatic women. *Ann Intern Med* 124: 1–7

62 Magid D, Douglas JM, Schwartz JS (1996) Doxycycline compared with azithromycin for treating women with genital *Chlamydia trachomatis* infections: an incremental cost effectiveness study. *Ann Intern Med* 124: 389–399

63 Lea A, Lamb HM (1997) Azithromycin. A pharmacokinetic review of its use as a single-dose regimen in the treatment of uncomplicated urogenital *Chlamydia trachomatis* infections in women. *Pharmacoeconomics* 12: 596–611

64 Robinson AJ, Ridgway GL (2000) Concurrent gonococcal and chlamydial infection: how best to treat. *Drugs* 59: 801–813

Macrolide Antibiotics
ed. by W. Schönfeld and H. A. Kirst

Helicobacter pylori and macrolides

Francis Mégraud

Laboratoire de Bactériologie, Hôpital Pellegrin, Place Amélie Raba-Léon, 33076 Bordeaux cedex, France

Introduction

A considerable amount of data gathered since 1982 has shown that *Helicobacter pylori* infection is responsible for most stomach diseases [1]. The *primum movens* of *H. pylori* is the most common type of gastritis found. This condition constitutes the background for diseases such as gastric and duodenal ulcers [2], as well as gastric lymphoma and carcinoma [3], which may occur when additional factors from either the host or the environment are present.

This new understanding has transformed these chronic diseases into infectious diseases, and therefore the treatment of choice has become antibiotics. While most antibiotics are effective against this bacterium *in vitro* [4], the majority have reduced activity *in vivo* as a result of the special nature of the stomach niche. Very few compounds can be employed, but among them, the group of choice is the macrolides. In this chapter, we will review macrolides as related to *H. pylori*.

Activity and pharmacology of macrolides

The eradication of *H. pylori* is dependent on the MICs and on the pharmacological properties of the antibiotics where the bacterium is located, *i. e.,* in the gastric mucosa. The fact that less favorable conditions for the activity of antibiotics, *e. g.,* low pH, exist in this particular niche must be taken into account.

Macrolides with the best MIC against *H. pylori* at neutral pH are clarithromycin (MIC_{50}=0.03 mg/l), azithromycin (MIC_{50}=0.12 mg/l), roxithromycin (MIC_{50}=0.25 mg/l), and erythromycin (MIC_{50}=0.5 mg/l) (Tab. 1) [5]. Other macrolides of the 16-membered ring group such as josamycin, miokamycin, and rokitamycin have been tested by Hardy and colleagues but did not show superior activity [6]. The MIC for clarithromycin is lower due to faster intrabacterial penetration [7] compared with that of erythromycin, which has similar binding properties.

While topical action of the drugs has been hypothesized, it is now accepted that antibiotics act essentially systemically. Experimental studies performed *in vitro* on epithelial cells with tight junctions and using labeled clarithromycin have shown that this antibiotic can cross the epithelium from the basal to the apical side [8]. In contrast

Table 1. MIC_{50} of various macrolides against susceptible *Helicobacter pylori* at different pH [5].

	pH 7.5	pH 6.5	pH 5.5
14-membered macrolides			
Erythromycin	0.5	2.0	16.0
Dirithromycin	1.0	4.0	16.0
Clarithromycin	0.03	0.06	0.25
Roxithromycin	0.25	1.0	4.0
15-membered macrolide (azalide)			
Azithromycin	0.12	1.0	8.0
16-membered macrolides			
Spiramycin	2.0	8.0	32.0
Midecamycin	1.0	2.0	4.0

to amoxicillin, clarithromycin accumulates intracellularly and is progressively released on the apical side. This mechanism probably allows this antibiotic to be constantly present in the gastric mucus despite a twice-daily regimen, while amoxicillin, which diffuses paracellularly, may be present for only a few hours after drug consumption. In addition, the intracellular penetration of clarithromycin may allow the killing of the few bacteria present inside the cells [9]. A model designed by Hulten and colleagues showed a 3 $\log_{10}$ reduction of *H. pylori* using azithromycin and 4 $\log_{10}$ reduction using clarithromycin, while no intracellular effect was seen when amoxicillin was used [10]. Despite its large molecular size, clarithromycin is highly lipophilic, which may explain its good diffusion.

The pH gradient in the gastric mucus ranges from 7.4 to 1.5. Studies have shown that clarithromycin is stable at pH 5 to 8 in aqueous solution. In gastric juice, the half-life of clarithromycin is 1.0 h ± 0.04 h at pH 2 *versus* > 68 h at pH 7 [11]. Furthermore, macrolide activity decreases significantly when the pH decreases from 7.5 to 5.5. As is shown in Table 1, the MIC_{50} on susceptible strains increases 4 to 32 times and even more for azithromycin. At pH 5.5 only clarithromycin has a MIC in the range of that achieved *in vivo* [5]. Similar results have been obtained in other studies [6, 12]. These data indicate the additional need to increase the pH of the stomach by using antisecretory agents. Goddard and colleagues studied the effect of omeprazole, a proton pump inhibitor, on the distribution of clarithromycin in gastric juice in 24 healthy men. Clarithromycin concentrated significantly in gastric juice compared with plasma in both the placebo and omeprazole groups, but no significant difference was found between the two groups [13] (Fig. 1). In contrast, Gustavson and colleagues, who studied gastric tissue rather than gastric juice, reported higher concentrations in the omeprazole group. The results were especially dramatic in the gastric mucus where the clarithromycin concentration (mean ± standard deviation) increased from 4.2 ± 7.7 µg/g in the placebo group to 39.3 ± 32.8 µg/g in the omeprazole group [14]. All of these studies indeed concerned *H. pylori* negative subjects. It is

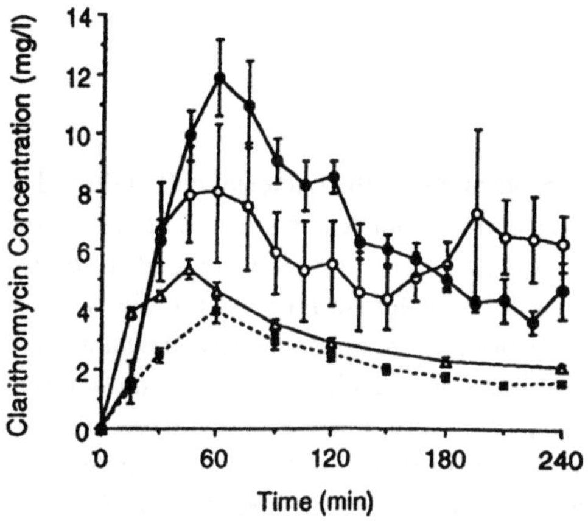

Figure 1. Clarithromycin concentration (mean ± SEM) in gastric juice, plasma and saliva according to time in subjects treated with clarithromycin [13].

- ● gastric juice in placebo group
- ○ gastric juice in omeprazole group
- △ plasma
- ■ saliva

likely that *H. pylori*-positive patients may behave differently because of the inflammation present, which may improve drug delivery across the blood-stomach barrier.

The distribution of azithromycin in gastric tissues also has been studied, but only in patients who were submitted to gastric cancer resection. High levels of the drug were found in gastric tissue 24 h after a 500 mg oral dose, and these levels persisted over a five-day period. Concentrations in the gastric mucus were 5- to 10-fold lower but were still significant [15]. The results of Blandizzi and colleagues in *H. pylori*-positive patients also showed a good gastric mucosal distribution [16].

Roxithromycin is another macrolide for which pharmocokinetics in the stomach and interaction with proton pump inhibitors have been studied in a crossover study in *H. pylori*-negative volunteers. Proton pump inhibitors increased the roxithromycin concentration significantly in gastric juice (3.0 to 5.0 mg/l *versus* 0.3 to 0.4 mg/l) and to a lesser extent in gastric tissue [17]. Furthermore, proton pump inhibitors also have an anti-*H. pylori* activity [18]. Macrolides are bactericidal to *H. pylori* [19, 20], and proton pump inhibitors may exhibit a synergistic activity, or at least an additive effect, when combined with macrolides [21–23]. A possible synergy was investigated also by testing clarithromycin and its metabolite 14-hydroxyclarithromycin with other antibiotics (amoxicillin, metronidazole) or bismuth subsalicylate. No synergy was demonstrated, but an additive effect was observed [24, 25].

Ranitidine bismuth citrate (RBC) is another drug designed specifically to treat *H. pylori* infection. It combines the antisecretory activity of ranitidine with the antimicrobial activity of bismuth salts in the same drug. A synergistic effect was reported by Osato and Graham when they tested RBC with clarithromycin on clarithromycin-resistant strains [26, 27]. This synergy was also found *in vivo* by using an RBC-clarithromycin dual therapy [28]. Clarithromycin also induces a dose dependent post-antibiotic effect (*i. e.,* delayed regrowth after brief exposure to antibiotics) [29].

Macrolide resistance in *H. pylori*

Mechanism of resistance

In order to be active, a macrolide must penetrate into the bacterial cell and bind to its target, the ribosomes. However, there is no evidence for the role of ribosomal proteins in this binding. It has been shown that the target is indeed a special domain of the 23S rRNA, *i. e.,* the peptidyl transferase loop in domain V. This binding leads to an interruption in protein elongation; consequently, the bacterium can no longer synthesize protein. Goldman and colleagues have shown that clarithromycin, its parent compound, erythromycin, and its 14-hydroxy metabolite have the tightest binding interaction observed to date for a macrolide-ribosome complex [7]. This mechanism of action is not specific to *H. pylori* and is described further in another chapter.

The principal mechanism of resistance discerned many years ago, especially in *Staphylococcus aureus,* is a post-transcriptional modification of the 23S rRNA. In *Escherichia coli*, it is due to a methylation of an adenine residue in position 2058 under the command of methylase genes usually transferred on plasmids (*erm* genes) [30]. This mechanism has been named MLS (for macrolides, lincosamides and streptogramin B, which are the antibiotics concerned). The methylation leads to an important change in the conformation of the ribosome, with the result that the macrolide can no longer bind. Neither *erm* genes nor any erythromycin-modifying enzymes have been found in *H. pylori* [31, 32].

Another mechanism achieving the same goal has been described more recently, first in *E. coli* [33] and later in other species such as *Mycobacterium avium, Mycobacterium intracellulare,* and *Mycoplasma pneumoniae*. Versalovic and colleagues were the first to demonstrate that this mechanism was indeed involved in *H. pylori* resistance [34]. They showed that point mutations (adenine → guanine) in two positions, namely 2142 and 2143 (formerly designated as the 2058 and 2059 cognates in *E. coli*, then 2143 and 2144 in *H. pylori* nomenclature before being renamed correctly based on the ribosomal sequence of *H. pylori* [35]), were associated with macrolide resistance. Later, Occhialini and colleagues showed that these mutations also were associated with a lack of binding of macrolides to isolated ribosomes: the amount of bound antibiotic increases proportionally with the amount of purified ribosomes from the susceptible strain but not from the resistant strain [36] (Fig. 2). Therefore, a causal association is most likely involved and the mutations are target-structural mutations.

Originally, two transition mutations were described, A2142G and A2143G, essentially found in clinical specimens. Another mutation has been described, the transversion A2142C, but it seldomly occurs. Debets-Ossenkop and colleagues were able to obtain other kinds of mutations (A2143C, A2142T, A2143T) *in vitro* by site-directed mutagenesis of a clarithromycin susceptible strain. However, these mutant strains were unstable and had a reduced growth rate. In addition, the mutant A2143T had a MIC of only 0.5 mg/l. It has been hypothesized that the change in nucleotide sequence induces a change in free energy and conformation

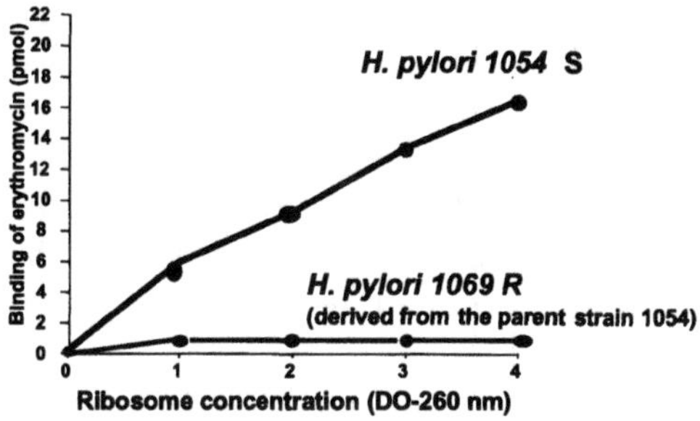

Figure 2. Binding of labeled erythromycin on increasing concentrations of *Helicobacter pylori* ribosomes [36].

within the ribosome greater than for A2142G and A2143G, which has an impact on bacterial fitness. It is not clear why the mutant A2142C, which is apparently of the same type as the two previous ones, is found so seldomly [37]. Similar results, especially with regard to the growth rate of laboratory induced mutants, also were described in another study [38]. The mutations that are not found are most likely lethal. The simultaneous mutations A2115G and G2141 A, which were described once by Hulten and colleagues, have never been found again [32].

The impact of the arising mutation on the MIC of the strain also has been studied. In most but not all studies, A2142G mutations were significantly more likely to be present in isolates with MICs > 64 mg/l than in those with MICs < 64 mg/l (65% *versus* 30%, $p = 0.01$) [39, 40]. MICs of clarithromycin are usually lower than MICs of erythromycin and, even in rare cases, strains with the A2143G mutation may have a MIC against *H. pylori* under the cut-off for clarithromycin resistance while they are clearly resistant to erythromycin [38, 41]. However, we do not think that it is advisable to use clarithromycin for treatment in such cases.

The question of the number of 23S rRNA operons present on the chromosome of *H. pylori* has been answered following the complete sequencing of *H. pylori* [42, 43]. Two operons are present and, therefore, when the mutation is present, it concerns both. Heterozygosity has been detected only four times [32, 34, 44].

It is now understood that mutations occur spontaneously and are selected after exposure to the drug. Indeed, the presence of a low number of bacterial cells with a given point mutation has been shown within a population of otherwise susceptible bacteria, even though the patient was not supposed to have previously consumed macrolides [40, 45–47]. Both main mutations can also be observed in the bacterial population of a given strain.

The frequency of mutations inducing spontaneous resistance to erythromycin was found to be in the range of 3.2×10^{-7} to 6×10^{-8} *in vitro* [6, 48]. However, this figure may be different *in vivo*. Indeed, the bacterial mutation rate increases under stress conditions (antibiotic or pathogenic stress) [49]. Furthermore, a homolog of the *mutS* gene, which encodes for mutation repair in *E. coli,* may have a different role in *H. pylori*, leading to the hypothesis that *H. pylori* is a spontaneously hypermutable bacterium [50]. No association was found with known pathogenic properties of the strains (*cagA*, *vacA* genotype) [40].

The question of the stability of mutants A2142G and A2143G also has been raised, since resistance is usually known to have a biological cost [51]. In two studies, where the strains were subcultured 10 to 50 times *in vitro* or obtained from a given patient after several months interval, and the identity of the pre- and post-isolates confirmed by Random Amplified Polymorphic DNA (RAPD), resistance was still present, indicating the stability of the mutations [32, 52]. In contrast, the authors of another study claimed that a reversion toward the susceptible phenotype was possible [53].

Resistance by efflux did not seem to play a role in *H. pylori* when the three putative restriction–nodulation–division efflux system operons present in the genome were submitted to mutagenesis. No effect on the *in vitro* susceptibility of *H. pylori* to 19 antibiotics including macrolides was noted [54].

2-Prevalence of resistance

One must be reminded that, when resistance is selected by one macrolide, it concerns all of the compounds in the group. Resistance by point mutation, as is the case here, is not transmitted horizontally but only to the descendants of the bacterium. Nevertheless, natural transformation is possible in *H. pylori* and could lead to horizontal transfer. Clarithromycin-resistant determinants introduced into a clarithromycin susceptible *H. pylori* strain by natural transformation confer MICs equal to the donor cell [35]. But *H. pylori* lives alone in its niche, so the risk of transformation with DNA from other bacterial species is unlikely. Transformation with DNA released from *H. pylori* cells could nevertheless increase the population of resistant strains.

The consequence is that an epidemic diffusion of macrolide resistance has not been observed, but a progressive increase does exist. This progression most likely parallels the use of macrolides in each country, but there are no studies showing a parallel between increased resistance and increased consumption of macrolides in the community. Only one such study has been published for *Streptococcus pyogenes* and macrolides in Finland [55]. In addition to the mechanism of resistance, another factor that limits the spread of resistance is the low transmission rate of *H. pylori*, at least in developed countries.

Because of these characteristics, the resistance rate is now between 0% and 20% in most countries. However, it is difficult to obtain a precise picture of this resistance rate. Most of the studies have important drawbacks, especially with regard to the epidemiological approach [56]. The studies were performed in special settings where gastroenterologists were interested in *H. pylori* infection; therefore, patients were more likely to be referral patients with possibly higher rates of resistance. Furthermore, the number of strains studied was limited, leading to large 95% CI limits.

A study was undertaken in France involving more than 500 gastroenterologists, constituting a representative sample of gastroenterologists in the country. They were asked to send biopsies from the first *H. pylori*-positive patient endoscoped on a randomly selected day. The *H. pylori* strains from this large sample were tested over a 15-month period in 1996 to 1997. Resistance to clarithromycin, determined by agar dilution, was 14.1% (95% CI ± 11.5 to 17.6) [57]. Since 1999, we are continuing the study in order to estimate the evolution of resistance. Based on available data, macrolide resistance seems to be higher in countries in Southern Europe than in Northern Europe. In the MACH2 study, for example, in which patients were essentially included from Scandinavia, Germany, and the UK, the resistance rate was only 3% [58]. In large studies performed in the Netherlands, the rate was in the range of 1% to 2% with no increase over the years [59, 60]. Countries such as Germany and the UK are in an intermediary position. These data were confirmed recently in a European survey involving 22 centers from 17 countries. A standardized E-test protocol was used to test 1305 strains. The overall rate of resistance to clarithromycin was 9.8% (95% CI 8.3 to 11.5), with a marked difference between Northern Europe (4.5%) and Southern Europe (18.1%), and with Eastern and Central Europe being in between (8.5% and 9.2%, respectively). Clarithromycin resistance was higher in children (< 10 years old) than in other age groups ($p < 0.05$), probably due to a more frequent use of macrolides during childhood [61]. In the French study, antibiotic consumption was also a significant risk factor [57]. In the United States, the pooled results from four large multicenter trials, including 836 isolates, showed an overall resistance rate of 8%, with no significant variation between the six defined regions [62].

In two monocentric studies, the evolution of *H. pylori* macrolide resistance was monitored over several years and an increase was found in both, from 2.2% to 11.1% (Belgium) [63] and from 1.3% to 7.7% (England) [64].

The results shown previously represent so-called primary resistance, *i. e.,* the patients were not supposed to have previously received anti-*H. pylori* treatment, or at least not recently. The situation is different when considering secondary resistance, *i.e.*, following failure of a current treatment, which may reach 60% or more [65]. For this reason, treatments including clarithromycin as the only antibiotic must be avoided because the success rate is low and when the rate of acquired resistance is expressed in relation to the total number of patients included, it may reach 25% *versus* 2% when a triple therapy is administered [65].

However, the selection of resistant mutants may be lower with other macrolides such as azithromycin [66]. *In vitro*, selection occurs for sub-inhibitory concentrations of the drug. Assuming that the same phenomenon occurs *in vivo*, it is possible that the concentration of antibiotics in the mucosa may be lower than the sub-inhibitory concentration, which will be a reason for increasing the dose usually prescribed for this antibiotic.

Susceptibility testing

H. pylori susceptibility to antimicrobial agents can be evaluated by the usual phenotypic methods and also by recently developed molecular methods. Because of the gap between MICs from susceptible and resistant strains, all phenotypic methods can be used accurately and, because of the existence of a very limited number of point mutations, genotypic methods are also easy to apply.

Phenotypic methods

The reference method is the agar dilution method. Two very similar protocols have been published recently. The first one, developed by an American group, has been approved by the National Committee for Clinical Laboratory Standards (NCCLS) in the USA [67]. The second one was developed by a European group and has not yet been officially published [68]. The difference concerns essentially the type of blood to be used (Tab. 2).

Table 2. Recommended protocol to test macrolides against *Helicobacter pylori* by the agar dilution method.

	NCCLS protocol [67]	European protocol [68]
Medium	Mueller Hinton + 5% aged sheep blood	Mueller Hinton + 10% horse blood
Inoculum	saline suspension (McFarland 2)	saline suspension (10^8 UFC/ml)
Incubation	37°C, 3 days microaerobic atmosphere	37°C, 3 days microaerobic atmosphere

Breakpoints have been validated based on the correlation between the MICs determined *in vitro* and the outcome of clinical trials. Strains with MICs $\geq$ 1 mg/l are considered resistant, MICs $\leq$ 0.25 mg/l susceptible, and the others in the intermediary state.

The Etest also has been used frequently [69]. It has the advantage of offering precise information on the MIC using a simpler technique, which is adapted for routine testing. The correlation with MICs performed by agar dilution is usually perfect [58, 70].

Macrolide susceptibility testing also can be performed by disk diffusion. In a French study, a disk of erythromycin was found to have the best correlation with reference methods, with a threshold diameter of 17 mm [71]. Methods such as broth dilution [70] or a breakpoint method on agar also can be used.

Genotypic methods

Numerous techniques have been developed to detect the point mutations in positions 2142 and 2143. They are all polymerase chain reaction (PCR)-based methods. First, a fragment of the 23S rRNA gene flanking the 2142 and 2143 nucleotides must be amplified. Different methods can then be applied to study the amplicons. The reference method is sequencing of the amplicon, but it cannot be performed routinely in most settings.

An easy method is based on the occurrence of restriction sites within the amplified fragment when one of the two most frequent mutations is present. These restriction sites can be recognized by the enzymes *Bsa*I (A2142G mutation) and *Bsb*I (A2143G mutation), and lead to the presence of two bands instead of one on the gel. If an incomplete cleavage is observed, the presence of a mixed population is likely [31, 34, 36, 47, 72]. This method (PCR-restriction fragment length polymorphism) has the disadvantage of not being able to detect the A2142C mutation.

3'- mismatch primers can also be used for all point mutations including the A2142C mutation [73]. However, the mutations are identified by the absence of a band, which is a less preferable endpoint than a positive endpoint.

Other methods, such as the PCR oligonucleotide ligation assay [44] or the PCR/DNA enzyme immunoassay, include an additional step after the PCR. To perform the second method, oligonucleotide probes complementary to the DNA fragment containing the different mutations and the wild type have to be constructed. The amplified products are added to probe-coated microtiter wells. The DNA-enzyme immunoassay consists of a colorimetric hybridization in liquid phase [74]. This test has been applied to detect *H. pylori* and its eventual clarithromycin resistance directly on biopsy specimens and has given a perfect correlation with the other methods tested [45].

A similar approach has been developed in a solid phase instead of liquid phase. This reverse hybridization line probe assay (INNO-LiPA) is already available to detect point mutations in other areas. Oligonucleotide probes corresponding to the different possible point mutations are immobilized on a nitrocellulose strip and are hybridized with the amplified products. Results were highly concordant and, as with the previous method, this assay appears to be significantly more sensitive than other methods in detecting several genotypes in the same sample [75].

The preferential homoduplex formation assay (PHFA) has been applied to the direct detection of *H. pylori* and clarithromycin resistant mutants in gastric juice samples by Maeda and colleagues [46]. This assay may be more sensitive than the previous ones since it detected more mixed populations and, in half of them, the resistant population was present at a concentration so low that the phenotypic method did not detect them. The authors argue that testing gastric juice gives a better picture of what happens in the whole stomach than does testing only biopsy specimens.

However, the most appealing method to detect *H. pylori* mutations stems from the development of the LightCycler® (Roche), an apparatus designed to perform quantitative PCR [76]. The method includes the use of fluorescent probes. It is very simple and quick. The only disadvantage is the need for the expensive apparatus. In addition, it has provided excellent results [77] and is now being applied directly to biopsy specimens.

Another approach has been proposed that consists of an rRNA-based whole cell *in situ* hybridization using a set of fluorescent-labeled oligonucleotide probes (FISH method). Labeling of intact single bacteria is monitored by fluorescence microscopy. This approach allows the detection of *H. pylori* using a 16S rRNA probe and resistant mutant using a 23S rRNA probe simultaneously. This technique holds great promise because it avoids not only culture but also PCR, but it has yet to be evaluated in the field [78]. These genotypic methods of identification of *H. pylori* and antibiotic resistance are likely to be further developed in the future. Rapid detection of bacteria and resistance profiles will no doubt modify the habits of the prescribers and should contribute to a reduction of the dissemination of antimicrobial resistance [79].

Macrolides in *H. pylori regimens*

By analogy to the treatment of *Campylobacter jejuni /Campylobacter coli* infections, in 1986 a study was performed in Bordeaux that aimed to eradicate *H. pylori* with the 16-membered ring macrolide josamycin given as the only drug. This attempt was unsuccessful [80]. Azithromycin was also unsuccessfully used as a monotherapy [81], and erythromycin cleared the infection in only 1 out of 15 patients in another trial [82].

It is the merit of Graham and colleagues to have performed the first clinical trial with clarithromycin given alone to treat *H. pylori* infection where they were able to obtain an eradication rate of 42% with 250 mg given four times daily [83].

At this moment, the concept of acid inhibition had already been introduced, and, therefore, further clinical trials including clarithromycin (500 mg t.i.d.) and a proton pump inhibitor for 2 weeks have been undertaken. The results were satisfactory, with an eradication rate of 60% to 80%, which was within the range of that obtained with amoxicillin, but they were more consistent from one study to another [84].

During this period, triple therapies became popular, especially those including amoxicillin and metronidazole. They shortened the treatment period and increased the success rate.

Two clarithromycin-based triple therapies were originally proposed, one by Bazzoli and colleagues which consisted of a low dose of clarithromycin, metronidazole, and a low dose of proton pump inhibitor administered for 7 days [85]; the other was proposed by Lamouliatte and colleagues, with a higher dose of clarithromycin, amoxicillin, and a double dose of proton pump inhibitor administered for 10 days [86]. Following several monocentric studies with good results, a multi-center study, namely the MACH1 study, was carried out using a 7-day treatment with a double dose of proton pump inhibitor. The eradication rates were above 90% [87]. To better understand the roles of antisecretory drugs and antibiotic resistance, the MACH2 study was then performed. The study indicates that when amoxicillin, rather than metronidazole, was involved as the second antibiotic, the antisecretory drug played a major role, probably because the two drugs require a high pH to be active. However, there were not enough cases with

Table 3. Recommended clarithromycin based regimens for *Helicobacter pylori* eradication [89].

Proton pump inhibitor	double dose (or Ranitidine bismuth citrate)
Clarithromycin	500 mg b.i.d.
Amoxicillin	1 g b.i.d.
	for 7 days (Europe) or 10 days (USA)
Proton pump inhibitor	**double dose (or Ranitidine bismuth citrate)**
Clarithromycin	250 mg or 500 mg b.i.d.
Metronidazole	500 mg b.i.d.
	for 7 days (Europe) or 10 days (USA)

resistant strains to draw a definitive conclusion on the impact of clarithromycin resistance in this trial [88].

The two regimens, recommended by several consensus conferences [89–91] and approved by the authorities of most European countries and elsewhere, are presented in Table 3.

In a meta-analysis comparing two doses of clarithromycin (500 mg b.i.d. *versus* 250 mg b.i.d.) the higher dose showed the best results when combined with amoxicillin ($p < 0.0001$), while the difference was not significant for the combination with metronidazole [92].

Another meta-analysis comparing different lengths of treatment concluded that there was significant improvement of the eradication rate (7% to 9%) when treatment was given for 14 days compared to 7 days. There were too few cases to make conclusions on the 10-day regimen [93]. The eradication rates are excellent in clinical trials but seem to be lower in the community. In France, where the combination of amoxicillin-clarithromycin is used in 90% of cases, a survey of 1270 patients showed an eradication rate of 70% [94]. In the UK, the eradication rate was 61% in an intention-to-treat analysis and 70% in evaluable patients in a community study of asymptomatic subjects, using clarithromycin and tinidazole [95].

The main drawback of clarithromycin-based regimens seems to be the resistance to clarithromycin; given the low resistance rate observed to date, only a tendency was observed in the clinical trials performed with regard to the impact of resistance to clarithromycin [65, 96]. Two meta-analyses have been published recently on this topic. In the study of Dore and colleagues resistance reduced efficacy by an average of 55% (95% CI 33 to 78), but this analysis was not limited to triple therapies and only 501 patients were considered [97]. A similar drop in efficacy was found in the meta-analysis of Houben and colleagues who differentiated between the different lengths of treatment regimens. In the four arms that received ranitidine bismuth citrate (RBC) instead of a proton pump inhibitor, there was no drop in efficacy, but the data were too limited to draw a definitive conclusion [98]. An analysis of the individual data of all clinical trials undertaken in France over the last 10 years has been performed recently. More than 2 700 patients were analyzed; unfortunately, information on clarithromycin resistance was available for only 436 cases. Treatment was not successful for any of the patients harboring a clarithromycin-resistant strain and suffering from non-ulcer dyspepsia, and only 20% of those with a peptic ulcer disease were treated successfully, highlighting that macrolide resistance is the primary factor for failure of *H. pylori* therapy [99].

Azithromycin is another macrolide that has been studied in triple therapies, but to a much lesser extent than clarithromycin. A 1998 review [100] identified 17 arms including a proton pump inhibitor, azithromycin and a second antibiotic: amoxicillin or metronidazole/tinidazole. There was too much variability with regard to the drug dosages and treatment duration to perform a meta-analysis. The most successful combination of antibiotics was azithromycin (500 mg once daily) and tinidazole (2 g once daily), both given as a single dose after breakfast for 6 days. The treatment led to 95% *H. pylori* eradication and only 15% of the patients reporting side effects. However, it must be emphasized that this was not a controlled trial and that the number of patients was small. Other data, such as the absence of acquired resistance in the case of failure, also argue that low doses of azithromycin should not be prescribed. Several large trials conducted in Europe with apparently promising results included high doses of azithromycin. Dirithromycin tested, in a dual therapy with omeprazole was not successful in a single patient and was not tested further [101]. Other macrolides (spiramycin, roxithromycin) have also been tested, but the results were less convincing. Clarithromycin gives probably the best combination of low MIC, even at a low pH, and gastric concentration.

Macrolides, especially clarithromycin, often induce adverse events such as a bad taste in the mouth at high doses, but this does not lead to interruption of the treatment.

It is also interesting to consider the ecological impact of these treatments. Only one study has been carried out on this topic. The authors compared the effect of the standard treatment of proton pump inhibitor, clarithromycin, and metronidazole with the same treatment including amoxicillin instead of clarithromycin. Marked ecological disturbances were seen in the intestinal microflora in both groups. The numbers of anaerobic bacteria decreased while enterococci increased in those receiving clarithromycin. In the latter group, 74% of the *Streptococcus* sp from saliva, 90% of *Enterococcus* sp, and 74% of *Bacteroides* sp from feces became resistant at the end of the treatment, and 4 weeks later, the percentages of resistance were still 26%, 29%, and 59%, respectively [102].

In conclusion, the introduction of macrolides, and especially clarithromycin, in the regimens aiming to eradicate *H. pylori* has been an important breakthrough. Clinical trials have reported high rates of eradication. However, it seems that they are difficult to reproduce in clinical practice, and selection of clarithromycin-resistant *H. pylori* strains is the major cause of eradication failure. However, this resistance can be easily detected by standard techniques and by molecular methods. Currently, detection of resistance is not performed routinely before administrating a treatment. Methods that could give quick results without the necessity of culturing the organism will be available soon and should allow the physician to adapt treatment to improve the success rate. Compliance should also be stressed and macrolide resistance monitored in each region in order to limit its spread. Another solution could come from the development of related compounds such as the ketolides, which have been shown to be active against macrolide-resistant strains.

References

1 Warren JR, Marshall BJ (1983) Unidentified curved bacilli on gastric epithelium in active gastritis. *Lancet* i: 1273

2 Mégraud F, Lamouliatte H (1992) *Helicobacter pylori* and duodenal ulcer: evidence suggesting causation. *Dig Dis Sci* 37: 769–772

3 International Agency for Research on Cancer (1994) Monographs on the evaluation of carcinogenic risk to humans: schistosomes, liver flukes and *Helicobacter pylori*. International Agency for Research on Cancer, Lyon: 177–241

4 Lambert T, Mégraud F, Gerbaud G, Courvalin P (1986) Susceptibility of *Campylobacter pyloridis* to 20 antimicrobial agents. *Antimicrob Agents Chemother* 30: 510–511

5 Darmaillac V, Bouchard S, Lamouliatte H, Mégraud F (1995) Macrolides and *Helicobacter pylori* determination of MICs and effect of pH. *Gut* 37 (supl.1): A91

6 Hardy DJ, Hanson CW, Hensey DM , Beyer JM, Fernandes PB (1988) Susceptibility of *Campylobacter pylori* to macrolides and fluoroquinolones. *J Antimicrob Chemother* 22: 631–636

7 Goldman RC, Zakula D, Flamm R, Beyer J, Capobianco J (1994) Tight binding of clarithromycin, its 14-(R)-hydroxy metabolite, and erythromycin to *Helicobacter pylori* ribosomes. *Antimicrob Agents Chemother* 38: 1496–1500

8 Matysiak-Budnik T, Puzin C, Heyman M, Mégraud F (2001) *In vitro* transfer of clarithromycin and amoxycillin across the epithelial barrier using labeled antibiotics. *J Antimicrob Chemother* (submitted)

9 Evans DG, Evans D Jr, Graham DY (1992) Adherence and internalization of *Helicobacter pylori* by Hep-2 cells. *Gastroenterology* 102: 1557–1567

10 Hulten K, Rigo R, Gustafsson I, Engstrand L (1996) New pharmacokinetic *in vitro* model for studies of antibiotics activity against intracellular microorganisms. *Antimicrob Agents Chemother* 40: 2727–2731

11 Erah PO, Goddard AF, Barrett DA, Shaw PN, Spiller RC (1997) The stability of amoxicillin, clarithromycin and metronidazole in gastric juice: relevance to the treatment of *Helicobacter pylori* infection. *J Antimicrob Chemother* 39: 5–12

12 Malanoski GJ, Eliopoulos GM, Ferraro MJ, Moellering RC Jr (1993) Effect of pH variation on the susceptibility of *Helicobacter pylori* to three macrolide antimicrobial agents and temafloxacin. *Eur J Clin Microbiol Infect Dis* 12: 131–133

13 Goddard AF, Jessa MJ, Barrett DA, Shaw PN, Idström JP, Cederberg C, Spiller RC (1996) Effect of omeprazole on the distribution of of metronidazole, amoxycillin and clarithromycin in human gastric juice. *Gastroenterology* 111: 358–367.

14 Gustavson LE, Kaiser JF, Edmonds AL, Locks CS, DeBartolo ML, Schneck DW (1995) Effect of omeprazole on concentrations of clarithromycin in plasma and gastric tissue at steady state. *Antimicrob Agents Chemother* 39: 2078–2083

15 Harrison JD, Jones JA, Morris DL (1991) Azithromycin levels in plasma and gastric tissue, juice and mucus. *Eur J Clin Microbiol Infect Dis* 10: 862–864

16 Blandizzi C, Malizia T, Gherardi G, Costa F, Marchi S, Marveggio C, Natale G, Senesi S, Bellini M, Maltini G et al (1998) Gastric mucosal distribution and clinical efficacy of azithromycin in patients with *Helicobacter pylori* related gastritis. *J Antimicrob Chemother* 42: 75–82

17 Kees F, Holstege A, Ittner KP, Zimmermann M, Lock G, Scölmerich J, Grobecker H (2000) Pharmacokinetic interaction between proton pump inhibitors and roxithromycin in volunteers. *Aliment Pharmacol Ther* 14: 407–412

18 Mégraud F, Boyanova L, Lamouliatte H (1991) Activity of lansoprazole against *Helicobacter pylori*. *Lancet* 337: 1486
19 Goodwin CS, Blake P, Blincow E (1986) The minimum inhibitory and bactericidal concentrations of antibiotics and anti-ulcer agents against *Campylobacter pyloridis*. *J Antimicrob Chemother* 17: 309–314
20 Nagate T, Numata K, Hanada K, Kondo I (1990) The susceptibility of *Campylobacter pylori* to anti-ulcer agents and antibiotics. *J Clin Gastroenterol* 12 (suppl 1): S135–S138
21 Midolo PD, Turnbridge JD, Lambert JR (1997) Bactericidal activity and synergy studies of proton pump inhibitors and antibiotics against *Helicobacter pylori in vitro*. *J Antimicrob Chemother* 39: 331–337
22 Mégraud F, Darmaillac V, Brügmann D (1995) *Helicobacter pylori* et azithromycine. *Path Biol* 43: 555–560
23 Malizia T, Tejada M, Marchetti F, Favini P, Pizzarelli G, Campa M, Senesi S (1998) Synergic interactions of macrolides and proton-pump inhibitors against *Helicobacter pylori*: a comparative in-vitro study. *Antimicrob Agents Chemother* 41 (suppl B): 29–35
24 Cederbrant G, Kahlmeter G, Schalén C, Kamme C (1994) Additive effect of clarithromycin combined with 14-hydroxyclarithromycin, erythromycin, amoxicillin, metronidazole or omeprazole against *Helicobacter pylori*. *J Antimicrob Chemother* 34: 1025–1029
25 Meyer JM, Ryu SY, Pendland SL, Danziger LH (1997) *In vitro* synergy testing of clarithromycin and 14-hydroxyclarithromycin with amoxicillin or bismuth subsalicylate against *Helicobacter pylori*. *Antimicrob Agents Chemother* 41: 1607–1608
26 Osato MS, Graham DY (1997) Ranitidine bismuth citrate enhances clarithromycin activity against clinical isolates of *H. pylori*. *Gastroenterology* 112: A1057
27 Midolo PD, Lambert JR, Ken TG (1997) Ranitidine bismuth citrate can overcome *in vitro* antibiotic resistance in *Helicobacter pylori*. *Gut* 41 (suppl.1): A12
28 Mégraud F, Roberts P, Williamsson R (2000) Ranitidine bismuth citrate can help overcome *Helicobacter pylori* resistance to clarithromycin *in vivo*. *Helicobacter* 5: 196–201
29 Sörberg M, Hanberger H, Nilsson M, Nilsson LE (1997) Pharmacodynamic effects of antibiotics and acid pump inhibitors on *Helicobacter pylori*. *Antimicrob Agents Chemother* 41: 2218–2223
30 Weisblum B (1995) Erythromycin resistance by ribosome modification. *Antimicrob Agents Chemother* 39: 577–585
31 Debets-Ossenkopp YJ, Sparrius M, Kusters JG, Kolkman JJ, Vandenbroucke-Grauls CMJE (1996) Mechanism of clarithromycin resistance in clinical isolates of *Helicobacter pylori*. *FEMS Microbiol Lett* 142: 37–42
32 Hulten K, Gibreel A, Sköld O, Engstrand L (1997) Macrolide resistance in *Helicobacter pylori*: Mechanism and stability in strains from clarithromycin-treated patients. *Antimicrob Agents Chemother* 41: 2550–2553
33 Sigmund CD, Morgan EA (1992) Erythromycin resistance due to a mutation in a ribosomal RNA of *Escherichia coli*. *Proc Natl Acad Sci USA* 79: 5602–5606
34 Versalovic J, Shortridge D, Kliber K, Griffy V, Beyer J, Flamm RK, Tanaka SK, Graham DY, Go MF (1996) Mutations in 23S rRNA are associated with clarithromycin resistance in *Helicobacter pylori*. *Antimicrob Agents Chemother* 40: 477–480
35 Taylor DE, Ge Z, Purych D, lo T, Hiratsuka K (1997) Cloning and sequence analysis of two copies of a 23S rRNA gene from *Helicobacter pylori* and association of clarithromycin resistance with 23S rRNA mutations. *Antimicrob Agents Chemother* 41: 2621–2628
36 Occhialini A, Urdaci M, Doucet-Populaire F, Bébéar CM, Lamouliatte H, Mégraud F (1997) Macrolide resistance in *Helicobacter pylori*: rapid detection of point mutations and assays of macrolide binding to ribosomes. *Antimicrob Agents Chemother* 41: 2724–2728
37 Debets-Ossenkopp YJ, Brinkman AB, Kuipers EJ, Vandenbroucke-Grauls CMJE, Kusters JG (1998) Explaining the bias in the 23S rRNA gene mutations asociated with clarithromycin resistance in clinical isolates of *Helicobacter pylori*. *Antimicrob Agents Chemother* 42: 2749–2751
38 Wang GE, Rahman SM, Humayun MZ, Taylor DE (1999) Multiplex sequence analysis demonstrates the competitive growth advantage of the A-to-G mutants of clarithromycin-resistant *Helicobacter pylori*. *Antimicrob Agents Chemother* 43: 683–685

39 Versalovic J, Osato MS, Spakovsky K, Dore MP, Reddy R, Stone GG, Shortridge D, Flamm RK, Tanaka SK, Graham DY (1997) Point mutations in the 23S rRNA gene of *Helicobacter pylori* associated with different levels of clarithromycin resistance. *J Antimicrob Chemother* 40: 283–286

40 van Doorn LJ, Glupczynski Y, Kusters JG, Mégraud F, Midolo P, Piffaretti JC, Queiroz D, Nouhan N, Stet E, Quint W (2001) Accurate prediction of macrolide resistance in *Helicobacter pylori* by a PCR line probe assay for detection of mutations in the 23S RNA gene. Multicenter validation study. *Antimicrob Agents Chemother* 45: 1500–1504

41 Garcia-Arata MI, Baquero F, de Rafael L, de Argila CM, Gisbert JP, Mermjo F, Boixeda D Canton R (1999) Mutations in 23S rRNA in *Helicobacter pylori* conferring resistance to erythromycin do not always confer resistance to clarithromycin. *Antimicrob Agents Chemother* 43: 374–376

42 Alm RA, Ling LSL, Moir DT, King BL, Brown ED, Doig PC, Smith DR, Noonan B, Guild BC, deJonge BL et al (1999) Genomic-sequence comparison of two unrelated isolates of the human gastric pathogen *Helicobacter pylori*. *Nature* 397: 176–180

43 Tomb JF, White O, Kerlavage AR, Clayton RA, Sutton GG, Fleischmann RD, Ketchum KA, Klenk HP, Gill S, Dougherty BA et al (1997) The complete genome sequence of the gastric pathogen *Helicobacter pylori*. *Nature* 388: 539–547

44 Stone GG, Shortridge D, Versalovic J, Flamm RK, Beyer J, Ghoneim AT, Graham DY, Tanaka SK (1997) A PCR-oligonucleotide ligation assay to determine the prevalence of 23S rRNA gene mutations in clarithromycin-resistant *Helicobacter pylori*. *Antimicrob Agents Chemother* 41: 712–714

45 Marais A, Monteiro L, Occhialini A, Pina M, Lamouliatte H, Mégraud F (1999) Direct detection of *Helicobacter pylori* resistance to macrolides by a polymerase chain reaction/DNA enzyme immunoassay in gastric biopsy specimens. *Gut* 44: 463–467

46 Maeda S, Yoshida H, Matsunaga H, Ogura K, Kawamata O, Shiratori Y, Omata M (2000) Detection of clarithromycin-resistant *H. pylori* strains by a preferential homoduplex formation assay. *J Clin Microbiol* 38: 210–214

47 Matsuoka M, Yoshida Y, Hayakawa K, Fukuchi S, Sugona K (1999) Simultaneous colonisation of *Helicobacter pylori* with and without mutations in the 23S rRNA gene in patients with no history of clarithromycin exposure. *Gut* 45: 503–507

48 Haas CE, Nix DE, Schentag JJ (1990) *In vitro* selection of resistant *Helicobacter pylori*. *Antimicrob Agents Chemother* 34: 1637–1641

49 Martinez JL, Baquero F (2000) Mutation frequencies and antibiotic resistance. *Antimicrob Agents Chemother* 44: 1771–1777

50 Burucoa C, Blasac G, Solnick JV, Fauchère JL (2000) *Helicobacter pylori*: une bactérie spontanément hypermutatrice? *Lett Infect* 15 (suppl 3): 30

51 Lenski RE (1997) The cost of antibiotic resistance from the perspective of a bacterium. *Ciba Found Symp* 207: 131–140

52 Mégraud F, Camou-Juncas C, Occhialini A, Birac C (1996) *Helicobacter pylori* resistance levels to clarithromycin remain stable. *Gastroenterology* 110 (4):A192

53 Xia H, Buckley M, Keane CT, O'Morain CA (1996) Clarithromycin resistance in *Helicobacter pylori*: prevalence in untreated dyspeptic patients and stability *in vitro*. *J Antimicrob Chemother* 37: 473–481

54 Bina JE, Alm RA, Uria-Nickelsen M, Thomas SR, Trust TJ, Hancock REW (2000) *Helicobacter pylori* uptake and efflux: Basis for intrinsic susceptibility to antibiotics *in vitro*. *Antimicrob Agents Chemother* 44: 248–254

55 Seppälä H, Klaukka T, Vuopio-Varkila J, Muotiala A, Helenius DH, Lager K, Huovinen P (1997) The effect of changes in the consumption of macrolide antibiotics on erythromycin resistance in group A streptococci in Finland. *N Engl J Med* 337: 441–446

56 Mégraud F (1998) Epidemiology and mechanism of antibiotic resistance in *Helicobacter pylori*. *Gastroenterology* 115: 1278–1282

57 Broutet N, Guillon F, Sauty E, Lethuaire D, Mégraud F (1998) Survey of the *in vitro* susceptibility of *Helicobacter pylori* to antibiotics in France. Preliminary results. *Gut* 43 (suppl.2): A11

58 Mégraud F, Lehn N, Lind T, Bayerdörffer E, O'Morain C, Spiller R, Unge P, van Zanten SV, Wrangstadh M, Burman CF (1999) Antimicrobial susceptibility testing of *Helicobacter pylori* in a large multicenter trial. The MACH 2 study. *Antimicrob Agents Chemother* 43: 2747–2752

59 van Zwet AA, de Boer WA, Schneeberger PM, Weel J, Jansz AR, Thijs JC (1996) Prevalence of primary *Helicobacter pylori* resistance to metronidazole and clarithromycin in the Netherlands. *Eur J Clin Microbiol Infect Dis* 15: 861–864

60 Debets-Ossenkopp YJ, Herscheid AJ, Pot RGJ, Kuipers EJ, Kusters JG, Vandenbroucke-Grauls CMJE (1999) Prevalence of resistance to metronidazole, clarithromycin, amoxicillin, tetracycline and trovafloxacin in *Helicobacter pylori* in The Netherlands. *J Antimicrob Chemother* 43: 511–515

61 Glupczynski Y, Mégraud F, Lopez-Brea M, Andersen LP (2001) Zool-Results of a multicenter European Survey of *in vitro* antibacterial resistance in *Heliobacter pylori* (1997–1998) *Eur J Clin Microbiol Inf Dis (in press)*

62 Weissfeld A, Haber M, Rose P, Kidd S, Siepman N (1997) Geographical distribution in the United States of primary resistance to clarithromycin and metronidazole in patients infected with *Helicobacter pylori. Gastroenterology* 112: A328

63 de Koster E, Cozzoli A, Vandenbroucke C, Jonas C, Denis P, Oters J, Deltenre M (1997) *Helicobacer pylori* resistance to macrolides increases, to imidazole remains stable. *Gastroenterology* 112: A99

64 Morton D, Bardhan KD (1998) A six-year assessment of tinidazole, metronidazole, clarithromycin, tetracycline and amoxicillin resistance in *Helicobacter pylori* clinical isolates: a rising tide of antibiotic resistance? *Gastroenterology* 114: A235

65 Wurzer H, Rodrigo L, Stamler D, Archambault A, Rokkas T, Skandalis N, Fedorak R, Bazzoli F, Hentschel E, Mora P et al (1997) Short-course therapy with amoxicillin-clarithromycin triple therapy for 10 days (ACT-10) eradicates *Helicobacter pylori* and heals duodenal ulcer. ACT-10 Study Group. *Aliment Pharmacol Ther* 11: 943–952

66 Laurent J, Mégraud F, Fléjou JF, Caekert A, Barthélémy P (2001) A randomized comparison of four omeprazole-based triple therapy regimens for the eradication of *Helicobacter pylori* in patients with non-ulcer dyspepsia. *Aliment Pharmacol Ther,* in press

67 NCCLS (1999) Performance standards for antimicrobial susceptibility testing. VIth Informational supplement. M100S9 19, 1

68 Glupczynski Y (1998) Toward standardisation of antimicrobial susceptibility testing of *H. pylori*: preliminary results by a European multicentre study group. *Gut* 43 (suppl 2): A47

69 Glupczynski Y, Labbé M, Hansen W, Crokaert F, Yourassowsky E (1991) Evaluation of the Etest for quantitative antimicrobial susceptibility testing of *Helicobacter pylori. J Clin Microbiol* 29: 2072–2075

70 Piccolomini R, Di Bonaventura G, Catamo G, Carbone F, Neri M (1997) Comparative evaluation of the Etest, agar dilution, and broth microdilution for testing susceptibilities of *Helicobacter pylori* strains to 20 antimicrobial agents. *J Clin Microbiol* 35: 1842–1846

71 Fauchère JL, Burucoa C, Grignon B (2000) Tests in vitro de la sensibilité *de Helicobacter pylori* aux antibiotiques. *Lett Infect* 15 (suppl): 5–6

72 Szczebara F, Dhaemens L, Vincent P, Husson MO (1997) Evaluation of rapid molecular methods for detection of clarithromycin resistance in *Helicobacter pylori. Eur J Clin Microbiol Infect Dis* 16: 162–164

73 Alarcón T, Domingo D, Prieto N, Lopez-Brea M (2000) PCR using 3'-mismatched primers to detect A2142C mutation in 23S rRNA conferring resistance to clarithromycin in *Helicobacter pylori* clinical isolates. *J Clin Microbiol* 38: 923–925

74 Pina M, Occhialini A, Monteiro L, Doermann HP, Mégraud F (1998) Detection of point mutations associated with resistance of *Helicobacter pylori* to clarithromycin by hybridization in liquid phase. *J Clin Microbiol* 36: 3285–3290

75 van Doorn LJ, Debets-Ossenkopp YJ, Marais A, Sanna R, Mégraud F, Kusters JG, Quinnt WGV (1999) Rapid detection, by PCR and reverse hybridization, of mutations in the *Helicobacter pylori* 23S rRNA gene, associated with macrolide resistance. *Antimicrob Agents Chemother* 43: 1779–1782

76 Wittwer CT, Ririe KM, Andrew RV, David DA, Gundry RA, Balis UJ (1997) The Lightcycler™: a microvolume multisample fluorimeter with rapid temperature control. *BioTechniques* 22: 176–181
77 Gibson JR, Saunders NA, Burke B, Owen RJ (1999) Novel method for rapid determination of clarithromycin sensitivity in *Helicobacter pylori*. *J Clin Microbiol* 37: 3746–3748
78 Trebesius K, Panthel K, Strobel S, Vogt K, Faller G, Kirchner T, Kist M, Heeseman J, Haas R (2000) Rapid and specific detection of *Helicobacter pylori* macrolide resistance in gastric tissue by fluorescent *in situ* hybridisation. *Gut* 46: 608–614
79 Bergeron MG, Ouelette M (1998) Preventing antibiotic resistance through rapid genotypic identification of bacteria and of their antibiotic resistance genes in the clinical microbiology laboratory. *J Clin Microbiol* 36: 2169–2172
80 Lamouliatte H, Mégraud F, de Mascarel A, Quinton A (1987) Placebo-controlled trial of josamycin in *Campylobacter pylori* associated gastritis. In: Kaijser B, Falsen E (eds) Campylobacter IV. University of Göteborg, Göteborg, 388–389
81 Glupczynski Y, Burette A (1990) Failure of azithromycin to eradicate *Campylobacter pylori* from the stomach because of acquired resistance during treatment. *Am J Gastroenterol* 85: 98–99
82 McNulty CA, Gearty JC, Crump B, Davis M, Donovan IA, Melikian V, Lister DM , Wise R (1986) *Campylobacter pyloridis* and associated gastritis: investigator blind, placebo controlled trial of bismuth salicylate and erythromycin ethylsuccinate. *Br Med J* 293: 645–649
83 Graham DY, Opekun AR, Klein PD. (1993) Clarithromycin for the eradication of *Helicobacter pylori*. *J Clin Gastroenterol* 16: 292–294
84 Axon ATR, Moayyedi P (1996) Eradication of *Helicobacter pylori*: omeprazole in combination with antibiotics. *Scand J Gastroenterol* 31 (suppl 215): 82–89
85 Bazzoli F, Zagari RM, Fossi S, Pozzato P, Roda A, Roda E (1993) Efficacy and tolerability of a short term, low dose triple therapy for eradication of *Helicobacter pylori*. *Gastroenterology* 104: A40
86 Lamouliatte H, Cayla R, Mégraud F, Zerbib F, Stablo M, Bouchard S, Quinton A (1993) Amoxicillin-clarithromycin-omeprazole: the best therapy for *Helicobacter pylori* infection? *Acta Gastroenterol Belg* 56: 140
87 Lind T, van Zanten SV, Unge P, Spiller R, Bayerdörffer E, O'Morain C, Bardhan KD, Bradette M, Chiba N, Wrangstadh M et al. (1996) Eradication of *Helicobacter pylori* using one-week triple therapies combining omeprazole with two antimicrobials: the MACH1 study. *Helicobacter* 3: 138–144
88 Lind T, Mégraud F, Unge P, Bayerdörffer E, O'Morain C, Spiller R, van Zanten SV, Bardhan KD, Hellblom M, Wrangstadh M et al (1999) The MACH2 study: Role of omeprazole in eradication of *Helicobacter pylori* with 1-week triple therapies. *Gastroenterology* 116: 248–253
89 The European *Helicobacter pylori* Study Group.Current European concepts on the management of *Helicobacter pylori* infection. (1997) The Maastricht Consensus Report. *Gut* 41:8–13
90 The Report of the Digestive Health Initiative International Update Conference on *Helicobacter pylori* (1997) *Gastroenterology* 113 (suppl): S4–S8
91 Lam SK, Talley NJ (1998) Report of the 1997 Asia Pacific Consensus Conference on the management of *Helicobacter pylori* infection. *J Gastroenterol Hepatol* 13: 1–12
92 Huang JQ, Hunt RH (1999) The importance of clarithromycin dose in the management of *Helicobacter pylori* infection: a meta-analysis of triple therapies with a proton pump inhibitor, clarithromycin and amoxicillin or metronidazole. *Aliment Pharmacol Ther* 13: 719–729
93 Calvet X, Garcia N, Lopez T, Gisbert JP, Gené E, Roque M (2000) A meta-analysis of short *versus* long therapy with a proton pump inhibitor, clarithromycin and either metronidazole or amoxicillin for treating *Helicobacter pylori* infections. *Aliment Pharmacol Ther* 14: 603–609
94 Delchier JC, Roudot-Thoraval F, Guisau IM et le Groupe d'Etudes Français de Hélicobacters (GEFH) (2000) Evaluation de l'efficacité du traitement éradicateur de l'infection à *Helicobacter pylori* en France: résultats préliminaires de l'enquête du GEFH. *Lett Infect* 15 (suppl): 9–10
95 Moayyedi P, Feltbower R, Crocombe W, Mason S, Athas P, Brown J, Dowell AC, Richards IDG, Axon ATR on behalf of the Leeds Help Study Group (2000) The effectiveness of omeprazole, clarithromycin and tinidazole in eradicating *Helicobacter pylori* in a community screen and treat programme. *Aliment Pharmacol Ther* 14: 719–728

96 Lamouliatte H and the Aquitaine Gastro Association, Samoyeau R, de Mascarel A, Mégraud F (1999) Double *versus* single dose of pantoprazole in combination with clarithromycin and amoxicillin for 7 days in eradication of *Helicobacter pylori* in patients with non-ulcer dyspepsia. *Aliment Pharmacol Ther* 13: 1523–1530

97 Dore MP, Leandro G, Realdi G, Sepulveda AR, Graham DY (2000) Effect of pretreatment antibiotic resistance to metronidazole and clarithromycin on outcome of *Helicobacter pylori* therapy – A meta-analytical approach. *Dig Dis Sci* 45: 68–76

98 Houben MHMG, van de Beek D, Hensen EF, De Craen JM, Rauws EAJ, Tytgat GNJ (1999) A systematic review of *Helicobacter pylori* eradication therapy-the impact of antimicrobial resistance on eradication rates. *Aliment Pharmacol Ther* 13: 1047–1056

99 Broutet N, Tchamgoué S, Pereira E, Mégraud F (2000) Risk factors for failure of *Helicobacter pylori* therapy. *In:* Hunt RH, Tytgat GNJ. *Helicobacter pylori*: Basic mechanisms to clinical cure (2000) Kluwer, Dordrecht, 601–607

100 Dohmen W, Seelis REA (1998) The role of azithromycin in the treatment of *Helicobacter pylori* infection. A retrospective report. *Infection* 28: 256–261

101 Laine L, Stein C, Garcia F, Trujillo M, Estrada R (1996) Prospective evaluation of the macrolide antibiotic dirithromycin for the treatment of *Helicobacter pylori. Aliment Pharmacol Ther* 10: 269–273

102 Adamsson I, Nord CE, Lundquist P, Sjöstedt S, Edlund C (1999) Comparative effects of omeprazole, amoxycillin plus metronidazole versus omeprazole, clarithromycin plus metronidazole on the oral, gastric and intestinal microflora in *Helicobacter pylori*-infected patients. *J Antimicrob Chemother* 44: 629–640

Macrolide Antibiotics
ed. by W. Schönfeld and H. A. Kirst

Effects of macrolide antibiotics on ribosome function

Norris E. Allen

Animal Science Discovery and Development Research, Elanco Animal Health, 2001 West Main Street, Greenfield, IN 46140, USA

Introduction

The ribosome is the biochemical target of numerous antimicrobial agents. As a result of the conformational complexity inherent in the ribonucleoprotein composition of this organelle, a disproportionately large number of structurally diverse agents target the ribosome. The ribosome catalyzes polymerization of amino acids in the sequence dictated by the nucleotide sequence in mRNA. The process of protein biosynthesis requires a spatial and temporal recognition between mRNAs, tRNAs (aminoacyl-, peptidyl-, deacyl-tRNAs), and ribosomes. At the heart of the process lies a unidirectional movement of tRNAs through the peptidyltransferase center of the ribosome where the peptide bond is formed. Both weak and strong interactions contribute to the binding of tRNAs to the peptidyltransferase region [1]. Many ribosome inhibitors (e. g., chloramphenicol, puromycin, erythromycin, sparsomycin, gougerotin, and clindamycin among others) interfere with the relatively weak interactions between the 3'-CCA-aminoacyl terminus of tRNA and the peptidyltransferase center. Agents that disrupt the much stronger codon-dependent interactions include streptomycin and other aminoglycoside antibiotics.

The macrolide group of antibiotics inhibits ribosome function. For purposes of this chapter, the group comprises the naturally occurring polyketides consisting of 12-, 14-, and 16-membered-lactone structures wherein the lactone rings are typically substituted with one or more sugars including amino sugars. The group includes azithromycin, which is a semi-synthetic, 15-membered-ring derivative of the 14-membered macrolactone ring. The mechanism of action of macrolides shares similarity with two distinct classes of antibiotics, namely lincosamide and streptogramin B agents. The three classes are referred to collectively as the MLS group. Although structurally distinct [2], all three classes appear to bind to the ribosomal peptidyltransferase center on the large 50S ribosomal subunit and interfere with peptide elongation.

The mechanism of action of macrolide antibiotics may be considered in two parts: 1) recognition of the ribosomal binding site and 2) effects on polypeptide elongation. Ribosome-binding studies and footprinting experiments coupled with analyses of macrolide-resistant mutations have provided an explanation for how and where macrolides bind to the peptidyltransferase site. However, many of the details of how macrolides, by virtue of binding to this site, interfere with polypeptide elongation remain to be elucidated. Results of both early (prior to 1980) and more recent studies in which the effects of macrolide antibiotics on ribosome function were examined will be reviewed in this chapter.

Early studies (before 1980)

Spectrum of activity

Erythromycin inhibits growth of gram-positive bacteria, including but not limited to *Staphylococcus*, *Streptococcus*, and *Enterococcus* (3). *Mycoplasma* are also susceptible. Erythromycin and other macrolides can inhibit growth of certain gram-negative bacteria, *e. g.*, *Bordetella, Neisseria, Haemophilus, Campylobacter, Legionella,* and *Bacteroides. Escherichia coli* and *Salmonella* are poorly susceptibile to the macrolides [3]. The lack of activity against *E. coli* and other outer membrane-containing gram-negative bacteria has been attributed to lack of intracellular accumulation due to presence of an outer membrane [4, 5]. In recent years there has been an increasing awareness that many gram-negative bacteria harbor efflux pumps. These pumps effectively prevent the intracellular accumulation of a variety of antibacterial agents, which has led to the opinion that lack of susceptibility in these bacteria may be due to both outer membrane exclusion and efflux [6].

Effects on ribosomes: general

MLS antibiotics inhibit ribosome function and block protein synthesis. This has been demonstrated by measuring incorporation of radiolabeled amino acids into protein by intact bacteria [7–9], as well as in cell-free polypeptide synthesizing systems that measure synthetic polynucleotide-directed amino-acid polymerization by isolated ribosomes [10, 11]. Macrolides are generally bacteriostatic, although bacteriocidal activity has been observed at very high drug concentrations [2]. Stasis is typical of the majority of antibacterial agents that target protein synthesis.

Erythromycin binds to the large 50S subunit of bacterial ribosomes [12, 13] with a 1:1 stoichiometry [14]. Results of other studies (see [15] for review) directly demonstrated binding of other macrolides to the 50S subunit of bacterial ribosomes. Dissociation constants for binding are in the range of 10^{-8} M to 10^{-7} M [2, 14]. Binding occurs to ribosomes isolated from both gram-positive and gram-negative bacteria, indicating that the relatively poor activity of erythromycin against some gram-negative bacteria is not explained by a lack of ribosome affinity. Erythromycin binds very poorly to polyribosomes [16]. Macrolides do not bind to cytoplasmic ribosomes from eukaryotic organisms but do bind to the procaryotic-like ribosomes of mitochondria and chloroplasts [15]. In general, the 12-, 14-, and 16-membered-ring macrolides (MRMs), as well as members of the lincosamide and streptogramin B classes, are thought to bind to closely, possibly overlapping, sites on the 50S ribosomal subunit. The data supporting this notion derive from binding studies in which competition between MLS and other agents including chloramphenicol were measured and from examination of mutants demonstrating cross resistance to MLS antibiotics [2, 15].

Ribosomes from mutants resistant to erythromycin have reduced binding affinity for erythromycin [17, 18], an early observation that helped identify the ribosome as the primary target of macrolide inhibition. Results of studies with resistant mutants of *E. coli* revealed that a 50S ribosomal protein (designated L4) was altered in the mutants [18–20]. These mutants were cross-resistant to other 14- and 16-MRMs. Moreover, peptide bond formation by the mutants having an altered L4 protein was reduced [18, 21]. These findings implicated a specific ribosomal protein as being associated with the erythromycin binding site and were consistent with the idea that macrolides bind to closely related sites, possibly involving ribosomal proteins. Despite evidence that ribosomal proteins play a role in ribosome binding, examination of ribosomes from inducibly macrolide-resistant *S. aureus* revealed the presence of N^6, N^6-dimethyladenine in 23S rRNA [22, 23]. The dimethylation mechanism represents a postranscriptional modification of rRNA and derives from clinical isolates having acquired genes belonging to a class called *erm* (erythromycin ribosome methylation) [23]. No alteration of ribosomal proteins was detected in these isolates, and N^6, N^6-dimethyladenine was not present in uninduced cells. Demonstration of a causal relationship between the presence of dimethyladenine in 23S rRNA and the macrolide (MLS)-resistance phenotype [24], combined with earlier data [13], suggested the possibility that rRNA served an equally if not more significant role in the binding of macrolide antibiotics to ribosomes.

Effects on ribosomes: specific

According to the classic two-site model for polypeptide elongation [25], aminoacyl-tRNA (complexed with EF-Tu [elongation factor Tu] and GTP) binds into the acceptor site (A site) on the 70S ribosome. This process is followed by GTP hydrolysis and dissociation of EF-Tu · GDP. Peptide bond formation results from transfer of the nascent peptide moiety of peptidyl-tRNA bound in the adjacent donor site (P site), to the 3'-amino acid of the aminoacyl-tRNA (acceptor substrate) in the A site. Peptidyl transfer is followed by translocation, which accomplishes movement of the peptidyl-tRNA (with the nascent peptide extended now by one amino acid) from the A site to the P site with subsequent removal of the deacylated tRNA from the A site. Translocation facilitates addition of the next amino acid to the elongating peptide from another aminoacyl-tRNA and requires EF-G and hydrolysis of GTP.

Most studies prior to 1980 were consistent with the notion that macrolide antibiotics bind to the peptidyltransferase center and interfere with the elongation process [15]. There was no evidence that erythromycin blocked initiation, or for an effect on aminoacylation of tRNA, and erythromycin did not inhibit ribosome-dependent GTP hydrolysis in the presence of elongation factors and aminoacyl-tRNA. Yet the fact that erythromycin did not inhibit actively elongating ribosomes (polysomes) indicated that its effect was not directly on peptidyltransferase activity [2, 15]. Several studies [11, 26, 27] revealed that erythromycin and other 14- and 16-MRMs did not affect all cell-free polypeptide-synthesizing systems to the same extent. The extent of inhibition was dependent on the synthetic polynucleotide employed and, thus, the composition of the polypeptide synthesized in these assays. For example, polyphenylalanine polymerization directed by polyU was inhibited by 16-MRMs [26]; however, there was little or no inhibition by erythromycin [11, 15, 26, 27]. Erythromycin inhibited polyA-directed polymerization of polylysine and the polyC-directed polymerization of proline [15]. It was stated [15, 26] that the differential activity seen with various macrolides could be determined, at least in part, by the sugar constituents. Additionally, macrolides differed in their ability to block synthesis of short *versus* longer polypeptides in cell-free systems directed by synthetic polynucleotides of different lengths [28]. In general, erythromycin and other 14-MRMs prevent synthesis of longer polypeptides and have little effect and may even stimulate synthesis of tri and tetra-peptides; 16-MRMs tend to block synthesis of all polypeptides [28, 29].

Results of other studies showed that erythromycin and other macrolides could inhibit binding of chloramphenicol (an inhibitor of the peptidyl transferase reaction [2]) to bacterial ribosomes [26, 30, 31]. These observations were consistent with the concept that macrolide antibiotics act on the 50S subunit, and implied that, similar to chloramphenicol, macrolides exerted their inhibitory effects at the peptidyltransferase center [2, 32]. However, data from more detailed studies showed that erythromyin did not affect binding of chloramphenicol to polyribosomes [16] and that erythromycin and chloramphenicol were bound to separate sites on 70S ribosomes [33].

The ribosome-dependent reaction between puromycin (acting as a surrogate for aminoacyl-tRNA) and either peptidyl-tRNA (including Fmet-tRNA and *N*-acetyl-aminoacyl-tRNAs) or *N*-acetyl-aminoacyl-oligonucleotides has been used extensively to evaluate antibiotics to determine effects on the peptidyltransferase reaction, *i. e.*, peptide bond formation [2, 15, 34]. The latter of these puromycin reactions is known as the fragment reaction. Using *N*-acetylated aminoacyl-oligonucleotides as donor and puromycin as acceptor substrates in fragment reactions, 16-MRMs inhibited transfer, but 14-MRMs, including erythromycin, were without effect [34]. Both 14- and 16-MRMs affected the puromycin reaction when a variety of peptidyl-tRNAs were employed as donor substrates [28, 35, 36]; however, the extent of the effect depended on the nature of the donor substrates. In general, erythromycin inhibited the puromycin reaction only when polypeptidyl-tRNA substrates exceeded a minimum number of amino acid residues implicating a selective interaction between the antibiotic and nascent peptide chains. In experiments examining macrolide effects on binding of aminoacyl-oligonucleotide fragments into the A and P sites, only 16-MRMs inhibited binding [37–40]. Erythromycin either stimulated or had no effect on binding. Although the results of these studies and others revealed that macrolide antibiotics had some effect on peptidyltransferase and were likely acting at the peptidyltransferase center, the data did not support a direct effect on actual peptide bond formation, at least for all macrolide antibiotics.

Several early attempts to understand the action of macrolides on the peptidyltransferase reaction provided results consistent with an inhibitory effect on the translocation step of elongation. Pretreatment of *Bacillus megaterium* protoplasts with erythromycin stabilized polysomes and left them unreactive towards puromycin, *i. e.,* puromycin was unable to serve as an acceptor, indicating that, as a result of pretreatment with erythromycin, peptidyl-tRNA could be blocking the A site [41]. If the protoplasts were pretreated with chlortetracycline to block entry of aminoacyl-tRNA into the A site, the puromycin reaction proceeded normally. These results and those from other *in vitro*, cell-free studies [28, 42–44] could be explained as an erythromycin-induced inhibitory effect on the translocation step following peptide bond formation, perhaps by preventing proper positioning of peptidyl-tRNA in the donor site [42, 44, 45]. In some cases, peptidyl-tRNA was released from the ribosomes [44]. An erythromycin-induced accumulation of di-, tri- and tetra-peptides, along with the inhibition of synthesis of longer peptides [28, 45] was consistent with translocation as the target.

16-MRMs caused rapid polyribosome breakdown in protoplasts [46, 47]. In contrast, erythromycin stabilized polyribosomes in protoplasts and failed to inhibit elongation [48]. Similar observations were derived from experiments in intact cells [46]. Other data demonstrated that erythromycin inhibited the puromycin-induced release of nascent peptides from polyribosomes unless polyribosomes were pretreated with chlortetracycline [41], inhibited the EF G-dependent release of deacyl-tRNA following or subsequent to peptide bond formation [42], and induced release of peptidyl-tRNA from ribosomes [44]. These observations were generally compatible with inhibition of the translocation step, possibly by sequestering deacylated-tRNA in the ribosomal P site [2]. Alternatively, the results did not rule out inhibition of elongation immediately subsequent to polypeptide initiation [48]. Results from the early studies, taken together, indicated that macrolide antibiotics bind to the peptidyltransferase center and interfere with polypeptide elongation, but the data did not provide for a simple explanation of how inhibition occurred.

Effects on the peptidyl transferase center

Based on results published in the early 1980s (see [49] for review), the two-site model for polypeptide elongation was reexamined and modified to account for the identification of a third tRNA-binding site (E site) on the elongating ribosome. The three-site model for polypeptide elongation [49, 50], along with recent advances in our understanding of the three-dimensional structure of the ribosome and its components from x-ray crystallography [51] and cryo-electron microscopy [52], provides for deeper insight into the structural basis of polypeptide elongation

[53, 54]. The elongation process has been described as the movement of tRNA molecules through, and the nascent polypeptide away from, the peptidyltransferase center [1]. Antibiotics that inhibit elongation, including the macrolides, seemingly interfere with one or the other of these processes. RNA footprinting (chemical protection of nucleotides detected by primer-directed reverse transcription [55]), affinity labeling, and molecular genetic analyses of antibiotic-resistance mutations all have been employed in recent years to better understand where and how these agents bind and inhibit at the target site.

Ribosome binding site

Role of rRNA.

The atomic resolution structure of the 50S ribosomal subunit at 2.4 Å resolution was published recently [51], along with an examination of the structural basis of peptide bond formation derived from the structure of the 50S subunit complexed with substrate analogs [54]. This work confirms that highly conserved nucleotide residues within domain V of 23S rRNA form the active site region of peptidyltransferase. The ribosome is thus a ribozyme. No proteins are located close to the site where peptide bond formation occurs and none appears to directly contribute to the catalytic activity. Rather, ribosomal proteins of the large subunit more likely stabilize RNA (5S and 23S) in a catalytically active and/or functional conformation [54].

It has long been proposed and debated that macrolides (and other antibiotic inhibitors of ribosome function) bind directly to rRNA rather than to ribosomal protein [13, 56, 57]. The absence of proteins at the catalytic center [51] argues against direct binding of macrolides to ribosomal protein. Nevertheless, because mutations in ribosomal proteins can affect macrolide binding and polypeptide elongation, ribosomal proteins appear to play a role, although perhaps indirectly, in determining the mechanism of action of macrolide antibiotics.

Data from numerous studies have established that the central loop portion of domain V of 23S rRNA is critical for macrolide binding [56, 57]. Residue A2058 plays a key role in binding, as N^6-dimethylation of A2058 in *Saccharopolyspora erythraea* (the erythromycin-producing organism [58]) and N^6-monomethylation in *Streptomyces celestis* (the celesticetin [a lincosamide antibiotic]-producing organism [59]) confer resistance to MLS antibiotics. The same residue is N^6-dimethylated in MLS-resistant strains of *S. aureus* [22, 23]. In *E. coli*, base substitutions at residue A2058 and other nucleotide positions in the central loop were shown to confer resistance to macrolides and lincosamides [60]. A point mutation (G→A) in residue 2057 confers resistance in *E. coli* to both erythromycin and chloramphenicol, an indication of the close proximity of binding sites for these compounds [60, 61]. In addition to bacterial systems, an A→G transition at A2058 confers ribosomal resistance to erythromycin in ribosomes of yeast mitochondria [62]. The same change confers resistance to lincomycin in chloroplast ribosomes of *Nicotiana plumbaginifolia* [63].

Results from RNA footprinting studies [55] demonstrated direct binding by macrolide and other MLS antibiotics to specific nucleotides in domain V of 23S rRNA. Residues A2058, A2059, G2061, A2062, A2439, A2451, and G2505 exhibited altered chemical reactivities in experiments with MLS antibiotics in *E. coli* [64]. Based on the secondary structure map for 23S rRNA, these nucleotides all lie in the central loop or proximal to it. It is noteworthy that the universally conserved adenosine at nucleotide position 2451 was recently specified as the active site residue for peptide bond formation [65]. The MLS antibiotics share common binding sites in the region of residues 2057–2062. Since this general region forms the entrance to a peptide channel or exit tunnel, MLS agents are thought to perturb binding and hinder movement of the nascent peptide [1]. This process also could lead to destabilization of the peptidyl-tRNA bound to the ribosome.

Although the available data clearly point to the central loop of domain V as a critical site of erythromycin action, regions in domain V outside the central loop as well as regions in domain II are known to influence binding of erythromycin. A 12-base pair deletion in domain II affords low-level resistance to erythromycin in *E. coli* [66, 67]. Base substitutions at the highly conserved residue G2032, which is part of a stem-loop structure adjacent to the central loop of domain V, confer hypersusceptibility to erythromycin [60]. The hypersusceptibilty to erythromycin can be relieved by a point mutation at residue A2057 in the central loop of domain V or by the 12 base-pair deletion in domain II, either one conferring a resistance phenotype. Labeling of nucleotides in domain II with a photoaffinity-labeled derivative of aminoacyl-tRNA has been noted as indication that the peptidyl-transferase center is influenced by nucleotides in domain II [68].

Additionally, 5S rRNA is thought to serve as a structural if not functional link between domains II and V [69]. In ribosome reconstitution experiments, an assortment of MLS antibiotics could substitute for 5S rRNA by partially restoring peptidyltransferase activity to the ribosome [70]. This is indicative of a functional connection between domains V and II and a complex interaction between MLS antibiotics and the ribosome.

The 16-MRMs also interact with the central loop of domain V. In nucleotide protection experiments, tylosin and carbomycin protected residues A2058 and A2059 in the central loop of domain V [71]. Carbomycin shares certain nucleotide residues with erythromycin, but carbomycin protects some residues not covered by erythromycin consistent with the notion that carbomycin covers a larger region of the ribosomal surface [55]. Photoaffinity studies using carbomycin and other 16-MRMs identified specific ribosomal proteins with which these agents interact [72, 73]. The investigators concluded that the macrolides they examined likely bind to the peptidyltransferase site near the peptide exit channel [74].

Nonradioactive 14- and 16-MRMs competed with radiolabeled dihydrorosar-amicin, a 16-MRM, for binding to ribosomes [75, 76]. Lincosamides and streptogramin B compounds competed as well; non-MLS protein synthesis inhibitors did not. Dihydrorosaramicin contains a single ring-substituted sugar and has no disaccharide as found in several other 16-MRMs. Interestingly and similar to erythromycin, dihydrorosaramicin failed to inhibit polyU-directed synthesis of polyphenylalanine, whereas several other 16-MRMs with disaccharides succeeded [75]. The results from these and other studies [15, 74, 77, 78] are supported by data in a recent report [79], which clearly demonstrates that 16-MRMs containing a disaccharide at position 5 of the lactone inhibit peptidyltransferase. Erythromycin and 16-MRMs with a monosaccharide at position 5 did not inhibit peptidytransferase. Moreover, chemical probing plus footprinting experiments show that those macrolides with a disaccharide at position 5 bind to regions of 23S rRNA known to be critical for peptide bond formation [79]. The results strongly support the idea that 16-MRMs having disaccharide ring substitutions are of sufficient size to perturb the positioning of peptidyl-tRNA and block peptide bond formation.

Role of ribosomal proteins

Inhibition of elongation by erythromycin involves a combination of rRNA and ribosomal protein interactions. Erythromycin interacts with several ribosomal proteins, particularly proteins L4 and L22 of the 50S subunit [80, 81]. A mutation in either of these two proteins confers resistance to erythromycin [18–20, 82, 83]. Moreover, chemical footprinting experiments indicate that mutations in either L4 or L22 affect chemical reactivities of nucleotides within domains II and III of 23S rRNA [81]. No effects on or in the vicinity of residue A2058 in the central loop of domain V were observed, and none of the nucleotide positions identified in this study as important for erythromycin binding had been identified previously with macrolide resistance. The findings point to an important role for both proteins and RNA in determining ribosomal susceptibility to erythromycin.

Interactions between 16-MRMs and ribosomal proteins were probed in crosslinking experiments using dihydrospiramycin [84]. Results revealed six ribosomal proteins crosslinked by this derivative. Each of the proteins was alleged to be located close to the peptidyltransferase region. One of the proteins, L27, forms crosslinks to numerous nucleotides in domain VII of 23S rRNA which is in close proximity to domain V [85]. Two of the six proteins crosslinked are known to be associated with the 30S ribosomal subunit. A radiolabeled derivative of carbomycin was used to affinity label its ribosomal binding site [72]. Most of the radioactivity was associated with protein L27. More recent crosslinking experiments examined effects of spiramycin on positioning of tRNA substrates within the P site [86]. Spiramycin decreased the extent of crosslinking of the substrates to nucleotides in the central loop of domain V. Although the P-site tRNA substrates also crosslinked to ribosomal proteins (in particular, L27), spiramycin did not disrupt this interaction. In contrast to the behavior of 16-MRMs, data obtained from affinity studies with side chain derivatives of erythromycin showed preferential interaction with L22 [80]. The results from these studies, taken together, show that 16-MRMs bind to a ribosomal region that differs to some extent from where 14-MRMs bind. Nevertheless, binding by all macrolides is influenced by both rRNA and ribosomal proteins.

Peptide exit tunnel

Nascent peptides undergoing elongation on the ribosome traverse a peptide exit tunnel or channel that is part of the 50S subunit [87]. This part of the peptidyltransferase region serves to lead the nascent peptide away from the peptidyltransferase center. A2058–A2062 and U2609 form the entrance to the peptide tunnel [71, 88]. The interaction between MLS antibiotics and these nucleotides is critical for inhibition of peptide elongation. Although part of the peptidyltransferase central loop, these nucleotides are distinct from the catalytic site [71]. Arévalo and colleagues [80] proposed in 1988 that since erythromycin was known to block the growing peptide chain, the drug binding site and protein L22 may be located close to the tunnel entrance.

The recent atomic resolution structure of the large ribosomal subunit [51] reveals an exit tunnel consisting largely of RNA but with several proteins (including L4 and L22) making significant contributions to the tunnel's structure [54]. Particularly noteworthy is the identification of a narrow constriction and bend located in the part of the exit tunnel close to the peptidyltransferase center. The constriction is formed by proteins L4 and L22, which approach the tunnel from opposite sides. The atomic resolution structure also reveals the nucleotides of 23S rRNA that form the surface of the tunnel. Domains I through V of 23S rRNA plus proteins L4 and L22 make significant contributions to the tunnel. In fact, protein L22, particularly its β-hairpin loop, is the major protein contributor to the tunnel surface [54]. It is also interesting that protein L22 is the only 50S protein that interacts directly with all six domains of 23S rRNA [51]. Nucleotides in 23S rRNA showing altered chemical reactivity as a result of erythromycin-resistance mutations in proteins L4 and L22 were reported previously [81]. Interestingly, all but one of these nucleotides are located in regions of 23S rRNA that, based on an examination of the atomic resolution structure (see Fig. 11F in reference [54]), are in regions of 23S rRNA that approach the tunnel.

Results obtained with strains harboring resistance mutations in proteins L4 and L22 [81, 82] and from rRNA footprinting studies and photoaffinity labeling experiments [72, 80], as well as the structural information described above, are consistent with the notion that these two proteins and the nucleotides in the central loop that form the entrance to the peptide exit tunnel play a role in the interaction of erythromycin with the ribosome. The lack of inhibition of elongation on polysomes by erythromycin is consistent with this notion, since the entrance to the exit tunnel would be blocked by the nascent peptide. In addition, the inability of erythromycin to inhibit synthesis of polyphenylalanine is consistent with an effect on the nascent peptide tunnel, since this homopolypeptide is believed to be synthesized on the ribosome as a hydrophobic aggregate and fails to enter the exit tunnel [89, 90]. However, data from the same studies indicated that polylysine whose synthesis is inhibited by erythromycin was not restrained in a tunnel either [90]. Properties of the polypeptides undergoing elongation likely determine how the peptides exit the peptidyl transferase center, which also could affect susceptibility to erythromycin and other macrolides. By blocking the movement of nascent peptide into or through the peptide exit channel, macrolides could destabilize peptidyl-tRNAs bound at the P site and/or inhibit translocation.

Ketolides
Replacing the L-cladinose at the 3 position of clarithromycin (the 6-*O*-methyl derivative of erythromycin) with a keto group yields a ketolide structure. Several ketolides with novel activities, many containing alkyl-aryl extensions of a carbamate group at the 11–12 position of the lactone ring, have been described [91]. A combination of chemical footprinting and resistance-mutation studies has established that the novel properties of ketolides derive from the fact that these agents demonstrate particularly strong interactions with hairpin 35 of domain II of 23S rRNA [92–94]. Specifically, substitution of the 3-cladinose of clarithromycin with a keto group reduces ribosome binding by a factor of 100. Cladinose interacts with nucleotide position A752 in hairpin 35, and loss of the sugar compromises this binding [94]. However, an alkyl-aryl extension of a carbamate group added at the 11–12 position of the lactone ring provides for a more effective interaction at A752 which, as a result of interactions between hairpin 35 and the central loop, provides for stronger binding to the central loop of domain V [94]. A single mutation in hairpin 35 of *E. coli* at position A754 confers low-level resistance to ketolides, another indication that hairpin 35 is part of the macrolide/ketolide binding site [93]. Binding to domain V remains critical, as evidenced by much reduced ribosome binding of macrolides in mutants carrying a mutation at position A2058 in the central loop. This binding is likewise critical for the activity of ketolides; however, extensions at the 11–12 position appear to facilitate interactions *via* domain II interactions, accounting for the activity of ketolides against certain MLS-resistant bacteria with methylations at A2058 [93, 95].

Effects on polypeptide elongation

An explanation of precisely how erythromycin and MLS antibiotics interfere with the polypeptide elongation process has proved elusive. As mentioned earlier in this chapter, the behavior of erythromycin as compared with 16-MRMs and other MLS agents in many of the cell-free peptidyl transferase assays gave ambiguous results that often depended on how the assays were conducted (see reference [96] for a summary of some of these studies). After more than 40 years of research, it can be said that erythromycin:

1) inhibits *in vitro* synthesis of polylysine and polyproline but not of polyphenylalanine
2) inhibits elongation of short polypeptides [97]
3) does not inhibit actively elongating ribosomes
4) does not generally block the puromycin reaction with peptidyl-tRNA in the P site, but must bind in proximity to the P site
5) causes fall-off of ribosomes from mRNA with subsequent degradation of 50S subunits, and
6) induces premature release of peptidyl-tRNA.

Kirillov and colleagues [1] have argued that MLS antibiotics likely bind to the peptide binding region at a hybrid P site (possibly the E site) because these compounds fail to bind to polysomes wherein P and E sites may be occupied. The fact that these agents fail to compete with puromycin is consistent with this idea. Despite the fact that erythromycin does not block the puromycin reaction, it must exert its effects at or near the P site, since photoactive erythromycin derivatives bind close to the peptidyl-tRNA site [56] and block the puromycin reaction [77]. Since erythromycin exerts minimal inhibitory effects during polypeptide elongation [96] and seems to exert its effect immediately post-initiation [48], it is assumed to act pre-elongation by sterically interfering with nascent peptides two to five amino acids in length [96, 97]. Results from binding studies [89] in which fluorescence methods were employed showed that erythromycin could bind to ribosomes harboring deacyl-tRNA, a peptidyl-tRNA analog and puromycin; however, binding of erythromycin was blocked by nascent peptides with more than a few amino acids. The inability of erythromycin to bind because of nascent peptide occurred regardless of whether peptidyl-tRNA was in the A or P sites. In fact, erythromycin was closest to the *N*-acetylphenylalanine of the peptidyl-tRNA. This was interpreted as indicating that erythromycin binds to a site occupied by the amino terminus of short nascent peptides [89, 90].

A mechanism consistent with much of the data on elongation, and in agreement with the mutation and footprinting studies, is that macrolides and other MLS agents inhibit movement of the nascent peptide away from the catalytic center of peptidyltransferase [64, 88]. This could destabilize peptidyl-tRNA bound into the P site and lead to release of peptidyl-tRNA, as has been observed [98].

Results of kinetic studies with spiramycin showed inhibition of the puromycin reaction with *N*-acetylphenylalanyl-tRNA bound to the P site [99]. Data from a recent follow-up study [100] showed that tylosin has the same effect in this system. Erythromycin, which competes with tylosin but generally does not block the puromycin reaction, did not block the puromycin reaction in this system. The results imply that spiramycin and tylosin, but not erythromycin, can inhibit peptide bond formation and compete with puromycin as an acceptor. Consistent with the view that 16-MRMs may have a direct effect on peptide bond formation due to size are findings showing that derivatives of erythromycin harboring lengthy side chains attached to the amine of the lactone showed increased inhibition in cell-free assays of peptide bond formation [77].

Azithromycin has a semi-synthetic 15-membered-ring structure; otherwise, azithromycin has the same sugar substitutions as erythromycin [101]. Like erythromycin, azithromycin is inactive in polyU-directed polyphenylalanine synthesis but inhibits both polyA- and polyC-directed polypeptide polymerization [74]. Thus, size of the lactone ring may exert less influence on mechanism of action at the peptidyltransferase center than do the sugar moieties. Alterations of the structure of sugar moieties on tylosin (a 16 MRM) increased antibacterial activity but did not affect ribosome binding, indicating that sugars may be influencing the effect on elongation [102].

Peptidyl-tRNA release

Menninger [103, 104] described a mutant of *E. coli* that fails to grow and dies at 40°C because of a temperature-sensitive mutation in peptidyl-tRNA hydrolase. This enzyme presumably acts as a tRNA and amino acid scavenger by hydrolyzing prematurely released peptidyl-tRNA. Exposure of the mutant to erythromycin prior to the shift to 40°C enhanced both the accumulation of peptidyl-tRNAs and lethality. In contrast, exposure to chloramphenicol reduced the rate of accumulation and prevented killing. The effect of chloramphenicol is consistent with inhibition of peptide bond formation and blocking of elongation. Destabilization and release of peptidyl-tRNA from ribosomes was demonstrated earlier [44].

The effects seen with erythromycin suggested that binding of erythromycin to the ribosome destabilized the peptidyl-tRNA/ribosome interaction and led to a loss of peptidyl-tRNA from the ribosome. This is consistent with the fact that short but not long peptide chains are synthesized in the presence of erythromycin [105] and the report that erythromycin exerts its effect shortly after initiation [48]. 16-MRMs [106] and lincosamide antibiotics [107] also were found to stimulate dissociation of peptidyl-tRNA in temperature-shift experiments with the mutant. In other studies [98, 108], erythromycin and lincomycin were shown to counteract error-inducing effects of streptomycin on protein synthesis. For example, the streptomycin-induced suppression of a nonsense mutation in the C-terminal region of β-galactosidase was reversed by erythromycin. The effects of erythromycin and lincomycin on accuracy of protein synthesis were most readily explained as resulting from stimulation of ribosome editing [109]. The data suggest that the primary mechanism of inhibition by macrolide and lincosamide antibiotics is due to stimulation of peptidyl-tRNA dissociation from the ribosome rather than blocking either peptide bond formation or translocation of peptidyl-tRNA [110]. Viomycin, an inhibitor of the translocation step, did not enhance peptidyl-tRNA dissociation or the cidal activity nor did it counteract the error-inducing effects of streptomycin in temperature-shift experiments with the mutant [111]. Destabilization of peptidyl-tRNA/ribosome interactions is consistent with some of the earlier studies that appeared to present conflicting results [98]. The attractiveness of this explanation not withstanding, the reason that elongating ribosomes are insensitive to erythromycin remains to be discovered [112].

Translational attenuation

Erythromycin and other, but not all, MLS antibiotics act as inducers of N^6-methylation of 23 S rRNA resulting in MLS resistance [113]. Induction occurs by translational attenuation. In *S. aureus*, the structural gene for the methylase (*ermC*) is preceeded by a 19-amino acid peptide encoded by a 141-nucleotide leader sequence. The leader sequence can assume several alternative conformations, only one of which appears to be favorable to translation. In the absence of erythromycin or another inducer, *ermC* exists in a translationally unfavorable conformation. Induction occurs when low concentrations of an inducer bind to a ribosome translating the leader sequence, stalling translation, and destabilizing the mRNA-ribosome complex so that the *ermC* transcript is in a translationally active form. Thus, erythromycin induces resistance to itself by virtue of inhibiting translation.

The first nine amino acids of the leader sequence are critical for induction of *ermC* [114], and only four or five residues (amino acid positions 6–9) are critical for ribosome stalling and subsequent translation of the methylase [115]. A mechanism requiring inhibition of a peptide less than nine amino acids in length is consistent with earlier studies that established a minimum peptide chain length for inhibition by erythromycin [15, 97]. *ErmC* is not induced by all macrolide antibiotics [116]. Only those macrolides and other MLS agents that cause translation of the leader sequence to pause at a critical point serve as inducers; pausing appears to be determined by the amino acid content at the critical region of the leader sequence [113]. Changes in amino acid content in the leader sequence result in changes in induction specificity of different antibiotics.

The critical nature of the leader sequence may not be unrelated to the mechanism of action proposed for certain pentapeptides that confer ribosomal resistance to macrolide and ketolide antibiotics [117, 118]. In this case, spectrum of resistance depends on both the amino acid composition of the peptide and the structure of the macrolide, implying an interaction between peptide and antibiotic on the ribosome. Chloramphenicol, which also induces resistance to itself by attenuation, interacts with an inhibitory leader peptide as part of the induction process [119]. The first eight amino acids, which footprint to the same site on 23S rRNA as erythromycin, are required for inhibition of translation. The mechanism may involve cooperativity between chloramphenicol and the inhibitory peptide to facilitate ribosome stalling [119]. The subtle relationship between the inducing antibiotic and the critical amino acids in the leader sequence responsible for attenuation remains to be elucidated.

Effects on subunit assembly

Erythromycin and azithromycin have been shown to inhibit assembly of the large 50S ribosomal subunit in gram-negative [120] and gram-positive [121] bacteria. No effect was seen on formation of the 30S subunit, and erythromycin had no effect on preformed 50S subunits. Subunit assembly in mutants of *E. coli* resistant to erythromycin as a result of alterations in ribosomal proteins L4 and L22 [82] was less susceptible to the inhibitory effects of erythromycin. However, in a separate study [122] using an erythromycin-resistant ($ermA^+$) *S. aureus*, high concentrations of antibiotic necessary to inhibit growth had a greater inhibitory effect on translation than on subunit assembly. The findings support the possibility that ribosome assembly is a second primary target of erythromycin.

In *E. coli*, differential inhibition of subunit assembly could not be demonstrated with other MLS agents tested [120]. In *S. aureus*, assembly was inhibited by other 14-MRMs [121], 16-MRMs, lincosamides, and streptogramin B antibiotics [123]. In contrast, streptogramin A did not differentially affect assembly of 50S subunits; the same response was seen with chloramphenicol. Nor did a combination of streptogramin A and B types affect subunit assembly. Comparison of concentrations of erythromycin and other macrolides needed to inhibit growth, polypeptide synthesis, and subunit assembly in *S. aureus* indicated that the effects on polypeptide synthesis plus subunit assembly are additive and can account for the inhibitory effects on growth supporting the notion of two distinct targets [124, 125].

Several ketolide antibiotics inhibited 50S subunit assembly as well as translation [126]. Most inhibited translation to a greater extent. Since ketolide antibiotics do not act as inducers of MLS resistance (*i. e.*, ribosome methylation [127]), it was proposed that macrolides and related antibiotics might have as many as three binding sites on the ribosome: one site controlling inhibition of translation, one controlling subunit assembly, and one for inducer activity [126]. Ketolides would thus recognize only two sites since they do not act as inducers. Interestingly, although 3-deoxyclarithromycin failed to show inhibition of either translation or subunit assembly, the 11, 12-carbonate derivative of 3-deoxyclarithromycin inhibited subunit assembly but was a poor inhibitor of translation [128]. This raises the possibility that the 11, 12 position of the lactone ring is an important determinant of subunit formation. If there were a distinct ribosomal binding site controlling effects on subunit assembly, one might expect to be able to isolate mutants compromised in their inhibition of assembly but retaining their ability to inhibit translation and induce resistance.

Concluding remarks

Our understanding of where erythromycin and other macrolide antibiotics bind on the ribosome is fairly well established and supported by footprinting (chemical reactivity), affinity labeling (crosslinking), and resistance mutation data [86, 129]. Macrolides interact with specific nucleotides of 23S rRNA in the central loop of the peptidyltransferase center. Examination of resistance mutants reveals that there are also important interactions with specific ribosomal proteins found in the same region of the ribosome. Our comprehension of how macrolides inhibit the translation process is less precise. There is evidence for inhibition of elongation immediately post initiation, perhaps by blocking translocation and destabilizing peptidyl-tRNA. Much of the available data is consistent with macrolides interfering with movement of short nascent peptides, possibly by interfering with positioning of peptidyl tRNA. Although macrolides bind at the peptidyltransferase center, only the larger 16-MRMs appear to have an effect on the actual peptidyltransferase reaction itself.

Many of the effects macrolide antibiotics have on the ribosome are observed also with lincosamide and streptogramin B antibiotics. The three groups are structurally distinct, yet they share a commonality of function by binding to the same general region of the 50S subunit and exerting similar effects on polypeptide elongation. A full appreciation of how these disparate structures behave on the 50S subunit must await a more complete understanding of the details of polypeptide elongation. The recent atomic resolution structure of the 50S ribosomal subunit provides a glimpse of how the 6 domains of 23S rRNA and most of the 31 proteins fit together to bring about peptide bond formation [51]. The availability of this kind of information will undoubtedly lead to further studies into the mechanisms of protein synthesis and how macrolide and MLS antibiotics exert their effects at the atomic level.

References

1 Kirillov S, Porse BT, Vester B, Wooley P, Garrett RA (1997) Movement of the 3'-end of tRNA through the peptidyl transferase center and its inhibition by antibiotics. *FEBS Lett* 406: 223–233

2 Gale E, Cundliffe E, Reynolds PE, Richmond MH, Waring MJ (1981) *The molecular basis of antibiotic action.* 2nd ed. John Wiley & Sons, London

3 Steigbigel NH (1985) Erythromycin, lincomycin and clindamycin. In: G Mandel, RG Douglas, Jr, J Bennett (eds): *Principles and practice of infectious diseases*, 2nd ed. John Wiley and Sons, New York, 224–231

4 Mao JC-H, Putterman M (1968) Accumulation in gram-positive and gram-negative bacteria as a mechanism of resistance to erythromycin. *J Bacteriol* 95: 1111–1117

5 Nikaido H, Vaara M (1985) Molecular basis of bacterial outer membrane permeability. *Microbiol Rev* 49: 1–32

6 Nikaido H (1998) Antibiotic resistance caused by gram-negative multidrug efflux pumps. *Clin Inf Dis* 27(Suppl 1):S32–41

7 Brock TD, Brock ML (1959) Similarity in mode of action of chloramphenicol and erythromycin. *Biochim Biophys Acta* 33: 274–275

8 Taubman SB, So AG, Young FE, Davie EW, Corcoran JW (1963) Effect of erythromycin on protein-biosynthesis in *Bacillus subtilis. Antimicrob Agents Chemother* 1963: 395–401

9 Vazquez D (1967) Macrolide antibiotics – spiramycin, carbomycin, angolamycin, methymycin and lankamycin. In: D Gottlieb, PD Shaw (eds): *Antibiotics* vol 1, Springer-Verlag, New York,366–377

10 Wolfe AD, Hahn FE (1964) Erythromycin: mode of action. *Science* 143: 1445

11 Vazquez D (1966) Antibiotics affecting chloramphenicol uptake by bacteria. Their effect on amino acid incorporation in a cell-free system. *Biochim Biophys Acta* 114: 289–295

12 Taubman SB, Jones N, Young F, Corcoran J (1966) Sensitivity and resistance to erythromycin in *Bacillus subtilis* 168: the ribosomal binding of erythromycin and chloramphenicol. *Biochim Biophys Acta* 123: 438–440

13 Mao JC-H, Putterman M (1969) The intramolecular complex of erythromycin and ribosome. *J Mol Biol* 44: 347–361

14 Pestka S (1974) Binding of [^{14}C]erythromycin to *Escherichia coli* ribosomes. *Antimicrob Agents Chemother* 6: 474–478

15 Vazquez D (1975) The macrolide antibiotics. In: J Corcoran, F Hahn (eds): *Antibiotics* vol III, Springer-Verlag, Berlin, 459–479

16 Pestka S (1974) Antibiotics as probes of ribosome structure: binding of chloramphenicol and erythromycin to polyribosomes; effect of other antibiotics. *Antimicrob Agents Chemother* 5: 255–267

17 Oleinick NL, Corcoran JW (1969) Two types of binding of erythromycin to ribosomes from antibiotic-sensitive and -resistant *Bacillus subtilis* 168. *J Biol Chem* 244: 727–735

18 Otaka EH, Teraoka M, Tamaki M, Tanaka K, Osawa S (1970) Ribosomes from erythromycin-resistant mutants of *Escherichia coli* Q13. *J Mol Biol* 48: 499–510

19 Tanaka K, Teraoka H, Tamaki M, Otaka E, Osawa S (1968) Erythromycin-resistant mutant of *Escherichia coli* with altered ribosomal protein component. *Science* 162: 576–578

20 Takata R, Osawa S, Tanaka K, Teraoka H, Tamaki H (1970) Genetic studies of the ribosomal proteins in *Escherichia coli* V. Mapping of erythromycin resistance mutations which lead to alteration of a 50S ribosomal protein component. *Mol. Gen Genet* 109: 123–130
21 Tanaka K, Teraoka H, Tamaki M, Takata R, Osawa S (1971) Phenotypes represented by a mutational change in a 50S ribosomal protein component, 50–8 in *Escherichia coli. Mol Gen Genet* 114: 9–13
22 Lai C-J, Weisblum B (1971) Altered methylation of ribosomal RNA in an erythromycin-resistant strain of *Staphylococcus aureus. Proc Natl Acad Sci USA* 68: 856–860
23 Weisblum B (1995) Erythromycin resistance by ribosome modification. *Antimicrob Agents Chemother* 39: 577–585
24 Lai C-J, Weisblum B, Fahnestock SR, Nomura M (1973) Alteration of 23S ribosomal RNA and erythromycin-induced resistance to lincomycin and spiramycin in *Staphylococcus aureus. J Mol Biol* 74: 67–72
25 Spahn CMT, Nierhaus KH (1998) Models of the elongation cycle: An evaluation. *Biol Chem* 379: 753–772.
26 Vazquez D (1967) Binding to ribosomes and inhibitory effect on protein synthesis of the spiramycin antibiotics. *Life Sci* 6: 845–853
27 Mao JC-H, Wiegand RG (1968) Mode of action of macrolides. *Biochim Biophys Acta* 157: 404–413
28 Mao JC-H, Robishaw EE (1971) Effects of macrolides on peptide-bond formation and translocation. *Biochemistry* 10: 2054–2061
29 Teraoka H, Tanaka K, Tamaki M, (1969) The comparative study on the effects of chloramphenicol, erythromycin and lincomycin on polylysine synthesis in an *Esherichia coli* cell-free system. *Biochim Biophys Acta* 174: 776–778.
30 Vazquez D (1966) Binding of chloramphenicol to ribosomes. The effect of a number of antibiotics. *Biochim Biophys Acta* 114: 277–288
31 Wolfe AD, Hahn FE (1965) Mode of action of chloramphenicol IX. Effects of chloramphenicol upon a ribosomal amino acid polymerizing system and its binding to bacterial ribosomes. *Biochim Biophys Acta* 95: 146–155
32 Fernandez-Munoz RRE, Monro R, Torres-Pinedo, Nazquez D (1971) Substrate- and antibiotic-binding sites at the peptidyl-tranferase centre of *Escherichia coli* ribosomes. *Biochemistry* 23: 185–193
33 Langlois R, Cantor CR, Vince R, Pestka S (1977) Interaction between the erythromycin and chloramphenicol binding sites on the *Escherichia coli* ribosome. *Biochemistry* 16: 2349–2356.
34 Monro RE, Vazquez D (1967) Ribosome-catalyzed peptidyl transfer: effects of some inhibitors of protein synthesis. *J Mol Biol* 28: 161–165
35 Cerna J, Rychlik I, Pulkrabek P (1969) The effect of antibiotics on the coded binding of peptidyl-tRNA to the ribosome and on the transfer of the peptidyl residue to puromycin. *Eur J Biochem* 9: 27–35
36 Cerna J, Jonak J, Rychlik I (1971) Efects of macrolide antibiotics on the ribosomal peptidyl transferase in cell-free systems derived from *Escherichia coli* B and erythromycin resistant mutant of *Escherichia coli* B. *Biochim Biophys Acta* 240: 109–121
37 Cerna J, Rychlik I (1972) The effect of antibiotics on the substrate binding to the acceptor and donor site of ribosomal peptidyltransferase of an erythromycin-resistant mutant of *Escherichia coli. Biochim Biophys Acta* 287: 292–300
38 Pestka S (1969) Studies on the formation of transfer ribonucleic acid-ribosome complexes. XI. Antibiotic effects on phenylalanyl-oligonucleotide binding to ribosomes. *Proc Natl Acad Sci U.S.A.* 64: 709–714
39 Celma ML, Monro RE, Vazquez D (1970) Substrate and antibiotic binding sites at the peptidyl transferase centre of *E. coli* ribosomes. *FEBS Lett* 6: 273–277
40 Celma ML, Monro RE, Vazquez D (1971) Substrate and antibiotic binding sites at the peptidyl transferase centre of *E. coli* ribosomes: Binding of UACCA-leu to 50S subunits. *FEBS Lett* 13: 247–251
41 Cundliffe E, McQuillen K (1972) Bacterial protein synthesis: The effects of antibiotics. *J Mol Biol* 30: 137–146

42 Tanaka S, Otaka T, Kaji A (1973) Further studies on the mechanism of erythromycin action. *Biocim Biophys Acta* 331: 128–140

43 Igarashi K, Ishitsuka H, Kaji A (1969) Comparative studies on the mechanism of action of lincomycin, streptomycin, and erythromycin. *Biochem Biophys Res Commun* 37: 499–504

44 Otaka T, Kaji A (1975) release of (oligo)peptidyl-tRNA from ribosomes by erythromycin A. *Proc Natl Acad Sci U.S.A.* 72: 2649–2652

45 Sharrock WJ, Gold BM, Rabinowitz JC (1979) Protein synthesis in *Bacillus subtilis* II. Selective translation of natural mRNAs and its possible relation to the species-specific inhibition of protein synthesis by lincomycin and erythromycin. *J Mol Biol* 135: 627–638

46 Ennis HL (1972) Polysome metabolism in *Escherichia coli*: Effect of antibiotics on polysome stabilty. *Antimicrob Agents Chemother* 1: 197–203

47 Cundliffe E (1969) Antibiotics and polyribosomes. II. Some effects of lincomycin, spiramycin and streptogramin A in vivo. *Biochemistry* 8: 2063–2066

48 Tai PC, Wallace BJ, Davis BD (1974) Selective action of erythromycin on initiating ribosomes. *Biochemistry* 13: 4653–4659

49 Rheinberger HJ (1991) The function of the translating ribosome: allosteric three-site model of elongation. *Biochemie* 73: 1067–1088

50 Burkhardt N, Jüneman R, Spahn CMT, Nierhaus KH (1998) Ribosomal tRNA binding sites: three-site models of translation. *Crit Revs Biochem Mol Biol* 33: 95–149

51 Ban N, Nissen P, Hansen J, Moore P, Steitz TA (2000) The complete atomic structure of the large ribosomal subunit at 2.4 Å resolution. *Science* 289: 905–920

52 Agrawal RK, Frank J (1999) Structural studies of the translational apparatus. *Curr Opin Struct Biol* 9: 215–221

53 Al-Karadaghi S, Kristensen O, Liljas A (2000) A decade of progress in understanding the structural basis of protein synthesis. *Prog Biophys Mol Biol* 73: 167–193

54 Nissen P, Hansen J, Ban N, Moore PB, Steitz TA (2000) The structural basis of ribosome activity in peptide bond synthesis. *Science* 289: 920–930

55 Moazed D, Noller HF (1987) Chloramphenicol, erythromycin, carbomycin and vernamycin B protect overlapping sites in the peptidyltransferase region of 23S ribosomal RNA. *Biochemie* 69: 879–884

56 Cundliffe E (1990) Recognition sites for antibiotics within rRNA. In: WE Hill, A Dahlberg, RA Garrett, PB Moore, D Schlessinger, JR Warner (eds): *The ribosome: structure, function and evolution.* American Society for Microbiology, Washington, DC, 479–490

57 Cundliffe E (1987) On the nature of antibiotic binding sites in ribosomes. *Biochemie* 69: 863–869

58 Skinner R, Cundliffe E, Schmidt FG (1983) Site of action of a rRNA methylase responsible for resistance to erythromycin and other antibiotics. *J Biol Chem* 258: 12702–12706

59 Calcutt M, Cundliffe E (1990) Cloning of lincosamide resistance determinant for *Steptomyces caelestis*, the producer of celesticetin, and characterization of the resistance mechanism. *J Bacteriol* 172: 4710–4714

60 Douthwaite S (1992) Functional interactions involving the peptidyl transferase center. *J Bacteriol* 174: 1333–1338

61 Ettayebi M, Prasad SM, Morgan EA (1985) Chloramphenicol-erythromycin resistance mutations in a 23S rRNA gene of *Escherichia coli*. *J Bacteriol* 162: 551–557

62 Sor F, Fukuhara H (1984) Erythromycin and spiramycin resistance mutations of yeast mitochondria: nature of the *rib2* locus in the large ribosomal RNA gene. *Nucl Acids Res* 12: 8313–8318

63 Cseplö A, Etzold T, Schell J, Schreier PS (1988) Point mutations in the 23S rRNA genes of four lincomycin resistant *Nicotiana plumbaginifolia* mutants could provide new selectable markers for chloroplast transformation. *Mol Gen Genet* 214: 295–299

64 Garrett RA, Rodriquez-Fonseca C (1996) The peptidyl transferase center. In: RA Zimmerman, A Dahlberg (eds): *Ribosomal RNA: structure, evolution, processing and function in protein synthesis.* CRC Press, Boca Raton, 327–355

65 Muth GW, Orleleva-Donnelly L, Strobel SA (2000) A single adenosine with a neutral pK_a in the ribosomal peptidyl transferase center. *Science* 289: 947–950

66 Douthwaite S, Prince JB, Noller HF (1985) Evidence for functional interactions between domains II and V of 23S rRNA from an erythromycin-resistant mutant. *Proc Natl Acad Sci U.S.A.* 82: 8330–8334

67 Douthwaite S, Powers T, Lee JY, Noller HF (1989) Defining the structural requirements for a helix in 23S ribosomal RNA that confers erythromycin resistance. *J Mol Biol* 209: 655–665
68 Barta A, Steiner G, Brosius J, Noller HF, Kuechler E (1984) Identification of a site on 23S ribosomal RNA located at the peptidyl transferase center. *Proc Natl Acad Sci USA* 81: 3607–3611
69 Bogdanov AA, Dontsova OA (1995) Structure and function of 5S rRNA in the ribosome. *Biochem Cell Biol* 73: 869–876
70 Khaitovich P, Mankin AS (1999) Effect of antibiotics on large ribosomal subunit assembly reveals possible function of 5S rRNA. *J Mol. Biol* 291: 1025–1034
71 Rodriquez-Fonseca C, Amils R, Garrett RA (1995) Fine structure of the peptidyl transferase center on 23S-like rRNAs deduced from chemical probing of antibiotic-ribosome complexes. *J Mol Biol* 247: 224–235
72 Tejeder F, Ballesta JP (1985) Ribosome structure: binding site of macrolides studied by photoaffinity labeling. *Biochemistry* 24: 467–472
73 Tejeder F, Ballesta JPG (1986) Reaction of some macrolide antibiotics with the ribosome. Labeling of the binding site compounds. *Biochemistry* 25: 7725–7731
74 Ballesta JPG, Lazaro E (1990) Peptidyltransferase inhibitors: structure-activity relationship analysis by chemical modification. In: WE Hill, A Dahlberg, RA Garrett, PB Moore, D Schlessinger, JR Warner (eds): *The ribosome: structure, function and evolution.* American Society for Microbiology, Washington, DC, 502–510
75 Siegrist S, Lagourdat J, Moreau N, LeGoffic F (1981) Mechanism of action of a 16-membered macrolide: binding of rosarimicin to the *Escherichia coli* ribosome and its subunits. *Eur J Biochem* 115: 23–327
76 Siegrist S, Velitchkovitch S, LeGoffic F, Moreau N (1982) Mechanism of action of a 16-membered macrolide. characteristics of dihydrorosarimicin binding to *Escherichia coli* ribosomes and the effects of some competitors. *J Antibiot* 35: 866–874
77 Arévalo MA, Tejeder F, Polo F, Ballesta JPG (1989) Synthesis and biological activity of photoactive derivatives of erythromycin. *J Med Chem* 32: 2200–2204
78 Fish SA, Cundliffe E (1996) Structure-activity studies of tylosin-related macrolides. *J Antibiot* 49: 1044–1048
79 Poulsen SM, Kofoed C, Vester B (2000) Inhibition of the ribosomal peptidyl transferase reaction by the mycarose moiety of the antibiotics carbomycin, spiramycin and tylosin, *J Mol Biol* 304: 471–481
80 Arévalo MA, Tejeder F, Polo F, Ballesta JPG (1988) Protein components of the erythromycin binding site in bacterial ribosomes. *J Biol Chem* 263: 58–63
81 Gregory ST, Dahlberg AE (1999) Erythromycin resistance mutations in ribosomal proteins L22 and L4 perturb the higher order structure of 23S ribosomal RNA. *J Mol Biol* 289: 827–834
82 Chittum HS, Champney WS (1994) Ribosomal protein gene sequence changes in erythromycin-resistant mutants of *Escherichia coli. J Bacteriol* 176: 6192–6198
83 Wittmann HG, Stoffler G, Apirion S, Rosen L, Tanaka K, Tamaki M, Takata R, Dekio S, Otaka E, Osawa S (1973) Biochemical and genetic studies on two different types of erythromycin resistant mutants of *Escherichia coli* with altered ribosomal proteins. *Molec Gen Genet* 127: 175–189
84 Bischof O, Urlaub H, Kruft V, Witmann-Liebold (1995) Peptide environment of the peptidyl-tranferase center from *Escherichia coli* 70S ribosomes as determined by thermoaffinity labeling with dihydrospiramycin. *J Biol Chem* 270: 23060–23064
85 Brimacombe R, Greuer B, Mitchell P, Osswald M, Rinke-Appel J, Schuler D, Stade K (1990) Three-dimensional structure and function of *Escherichia coli* 16S and 23S rRNA as studied by cross-linking techniques. In: WE Hill, A Dahlberg, RA Garrett, PB Moore, D Schlessinger, JR Warner (eds): *The ribosome: structure, function and evolution*. American Society for Microbiology, Washington, DC, 93–106
86 Kirillov SV, Porse BT, Garrett RA (1999) Peptidyl transferase antibiotics perturb the relative positioning of the 3'-terminal adenosine of P/P'-site-bound tRNA and 23S rRNA in the ribosome. *RNA* 5: 1003–1013
87 Yonath A, Leonard KR, Wittmann HG (1987) A tunnel in the large ribosomal subunit revealed by three-dimensional image reconstruction. *Science* 236: 813–816
88 Porse BT, Rodriquez-Fonseca C, Levier I, Garrett R (1995) Antibiotic inhibition of the movement of tRNA substrates through a peptidyl transferase cavity. *Biochem Cell Biol* 73: 877–885

89 Odom OW, Picking WD, Tsalkova T, Hardesty B (1991) The synthesis of polyphenylalanine on ribosomes to which erythromycin is bound. *Eur J Biochem* 198: 713–722
90 Picking WD, Odom OW, Tsalkova T, Serdyuk I, Hardesty B (1991) The conformation of nascent polylysine and polyphenylalanine peptides on ribosomes. *J Biol Chem* 266: 1534–1542
91 Agouridas C, Benedetti Y, Bonnefoy A, Collette P, Denis A, Mauvais P, Labbe G, Chantot JF (1997) Ketolides: a new class of macrolide antibacterials, structure characteristics and biological properties of RU 004. *Clin Infect Dis Ther* 21: 279–285
92 Hansen LH, Mauvais P, Douthwaite S (1999) The macrolide-ketolide antibiotic binding site is formed by structures in domain II and V of 23S ribosomal RNA. *Mol Microbiol* 31: 623–631
93 Xiong L, Shah S, Mauvais P, Mankin AS (1999) A ketolide resistance mutation in domain II of 23S rRNA reveals the proximity of hairpin 35 to the peptidyl transferase center. *Mol Microbiol* 31: 633–639
94 Douthwaite S, Hansen, Mauvais P (2000) Macrolide-ketolide inhibition of MLS-inhibition of MLS-resistant ribosomes is improved by alternative drug interaction with domain II of 23S rRNA. *Mol Microbiol* 36: 183–193
95 Agouridas C, Bonnefoy A, Chantot JF (1997) Antibacterial activity of RU 64004 (HMR 3004), a novel ketolide derivative against respiratory pathogens. *Anitmicrob Agents Chemother* 41: 2149–2158
96 Vester B, Garrett RA (1987) A plasmid-coded and site-directed mutation in *Escherichia coli* 23S RNA that confers resistance to erythromycin. *Biochemie* 69: 891–900
97 Contreras A, Vazquez D (1977) Cooperative and antagonistic interactions of peptidyl-tRNA and antibiotics with bacterial ribosomes. *Eur J Biochem* 74: 539–547
98 Menninger JR (1985) Functional consequences of binding macrolides to ribosomes. *J Antimicrob Chemother* 16 (Suppl A):23–34
99 Dinos G, Synetos D, Coutsogeorgopoulos C (1993) Interaction between the antibiotic spiramycin and a ribosomal complex active in peptide bond formation. *Biochemistry* 32: 10638–10647
100 Dinos GP, Kalpaxis DL (2000) Kinetic studies on the interaction between a ribosomal complex active in peptide bond formation and the macrolide antibiotics tylosin and erythromycin. *Biochemistry* 39: 11621–11628
101 Retsema J, Girard A, Schelkly W, Manousos M, Anderson M, Bright G, Borovoy R, Brennan L, Mason R (1987) Spectrum and mode of action of azithromycin (CP-62,993), a new 15-membered-ring macrolide with improved potency against gram-negative organisms. *Antimicrob Agents Chemother* 31: 1939–1947
102 Omura S, Inokoshi J, Matsubara H, Tanaka H (1983) Ribosome binding activities and antimicrobial activities of tylosin and its related compounds. *J Antibiot* 36: 1709–1712
103 Menninger JR (1976) Peptidyl transfer RNA dissociates during protein synthesis from ribosomes of *Escherichia coli*. *J Biol Chem* 251: 3392–3398
104 Menninger JR (1979) Accumulation of peptidyl-tRNA is lethal to *Escherichia coli*. *J Bact* 137: 694–696
105 Tanaka K, Teraoka H (1966) Binding of erythromycin to *Escherichia coli* ribosomes. *Biochim Biophys Acta* 114: 204–206
106 Menninger JR, Otto DP (1982) Erythromycin, carbomycin, and spiramycin inhibit protein synthesis by stimulating the dissociation of peptidyl-tRNA from ribosomes. *Antimicrob Agents Chemother* 21: 811–818
107 Menninger JR, Coleman RA (1993) Lincosamide antibiotics stimulate dissociation of peptidyl-tRNA from ribosomes. *Antimicrob Agents Chemother* 37: 2027–2029
108 Menninger JR, Coleman RA, Tsai L-N (1994) Erythromycins, lincosamides, peptidyl-tRNA dossociation, and ribosome editing. *Mol Gen Genet* 243: 225–233
109 Menninger JR (1977) Ribosome editing and the error catastrophe hypothesis of cellular aging. *Mech Aging Dev* 6: 131–142
110 Menninger JR (1995) Mechanism of inhibition of protein synthesis by macrolide and lincosamide antibiotics. *J Basic Clin Physiol Pharmacol* 6: 229–250
111 Menninger JR (1995) Viomycin does not stimulate peptidyl-tRNA dissociation. *J Antimicrob Chemother* 35: 593–601
112 Andersson S, Kurland CG (1987) Elongating ribosomes in vivo are refractory to erythromycin. *Biochemie* 69: 901–904

113 Weisblum B (1995) Insights into erythromycin action from studies of its activity as inducer of resistance. *Antimicrob Agents Chemother* 39: 797–805
114 Mayford M, Weisblum B (1989) *ermC* leader peptide. Amino acid sequence critical for induction by translational attenuation *J Mol Biol* 206: 69–79
115 Mayford M, Weisblum B (1990) The *ermC* leader peptide: amino acid alterations leading to differential efficiency of induction by macrolide-lincosamide-stretogramin B antibiotics. *J Bacteriol* 172: 3772–3779
116 Allen NE (1977) Macrolide resistance in *Staphylococcus aureus*: inducers of resistance. *Antimicrob Agents Chemother* 11: 661–668
117 Tenson T, DeBlasio A, Mankin A (1996) A functional peptide encoded in the *Escherichia coli* 23S rRNA. *Proc Natl Acad Sci USA* 93: 5641–5646
118 Tripathi S, Kloss PS, Mankin AS (1998) Ketolide resistance conferred by short peptides. *J Biol Chem* 273: 20073–20077
119 Gu Z, Harrod R, Rogers EJ, Lovett PS (1994) Antipeptidyl transferase leader peptides of attenuation-regulated chloramphenicol-resistance genes. *Proc Natl Acad Sci USA* 91: 5612–5616
120 Chittum HS, Champney WS (1995) Erythromycin inhibits the assembly of the large ribosomal subunit in growing *Escherichia coli* cells. *Curr Microbiol* 30: 273–279
121 Champney WS, Burdine R (1995) Macrolide antibiotics inhibit 50S ribosomal subunit assembly in *Bacillus subtilis* and *Staphylococcus aureus. Antimicrob Agents Chemother* 39: 2141–2144
122 Champney WS, Burdine R (1998) Macrolide antibiotic inhibition of translation and 50S ribosomal subunit assembly in methicillin-resistant *Staphylococcus aureus* cells. *Microb Drug Resis* 4: 169–174
123 Champney WS, Tober CL (2000) Specific inhibition of 50S ribosomal subunit formation in Staphylococcus aureus cells by 16-membered macrolide, lincosamide and streptogramin B antibiotics. *Curr Microbiol* 41: 126–135
124 Champney WS, Burdine R (1996) 50S ribosomal subunit synthesis and translation are equivalent targets for erythromycin inhibition in *Staphylococcus aureus. Antimicrob Agents Chemother* 40: 1301–1303
125 Champney WS, Burdine R (1998) Azithromycin and clarithromycin inhibition of 50S ribosomal subunit formation in *Staphylococcus aureus* cells. *Curr Microbiol* 36: 119–123
126 Champney WS, Tober CL (1998) Inhibition of translation and 50S ribosomal subunit formation in *Staphylococcus aureus* cells by eleven different ketolide antibiotics. *Curr Microbiol* 37: 418–425
127 Bonnefoy A, Girard AM, Agouridas Chantot JF (1997) Ketolides lack inducibility properties of MLS_B resistance phenotype. *J Antimicrob Chemother* 40: 85–90
128 Champney WS, Tober CL, Burdine R (1998) A comparison of the inhibition of translation and 50S ribosomal subunit formation in *Staphylococcus aureus* cells by nine different macrolide antibiotics. *Curr Microbiol* 37: 412–417
129 Vester B, Douthwaite S (2001) Macrolide resistance conferred by base substitutions in 23S rRNA. *Antimicrob Agents Chemother* 45: 1–12

Macrolide Antibiotics
ed. by W. Schönfeld and H. A. Kirst

Mechanisms of resistance to macrolides, lincosamides, and ketolides

Joyce A. Sutcliffe[1] and Roland Leclercq[2]

[1]*Rib-X Pharmaceuticals, 25 Science Park, Room 561, New Haven, CT 06511, USA*
[2]*Department of Microbiology, CHU, Côte de Nacre, Av. Côte de Nacre, 14033 Caen, France*

Introduction

Macrolide (M), lincosamide (L), streptogramin B(S_B), and ketolide (K) antibiotics are a structurally diverse group of antibiotics that have overlapping binding sites in the peptidyl transferase region of 23S rRNA. Some resistance determinants alter part of the common binding site, thereby reducing susceptibility to more than one of the MLS_BK antibiotics simultaneously. The incidence of strains harboring resistance determinants to macrolide-lincosamide-streptogramin (MLS_B) antibiotics has risen, especially over the past decade. Further, the microbes have collected mobile elements that help them evade the lethal effects of antibiotics. Bacterial resistance is mounted against MLS_B antibiotics on three fronts: 1) target site mutations that prevent the binding of the antibiotic to its natural cellular target (ribosome), 2) efflux of the antibiotic or alterations in the permeability barrier as a means of protection, and 3) inactivation of the antimicrobial substance. Ketolides, a novel semi-synthetic class of 14–membered macrolides, have additional binding contacts within the 50S ribosome, making them less susceptible to some of the more prevalent resistance mechanisms in pathogenic bacteria.

Interactions with the 50S subunit: target site mutations

Mutations in 23S rRNA or ribosomal proteins

Macrolide antibiotics inhibit protein synthesis through their interactions with the 50S subunit of the bacterial ribosome [1–5]. Binding near the entrance to the peptide passage channel, they appear to inhibit movement of the growing peptide chain and/or to perturb binding of the peptide moiety of the peptidyl-tRNA [6]. Mutants that are resistant to one or more of the MLS_B antibiotics because of mutations in either domain V of 23S rRNA or ribosomal proteins L4 or L22 provided genetic evidence that these antibiotics interact with the ribosome. Further, overlapping binding sites may be explained in part by similar conformations that have been defined for macrolides, lincosamides, and ketolides in recent nuclear magnetic resonance (NMR) studies [7]. Initially, A2058G was identified as conferring erythromycin resistance in yeast mitochondria, where only one rRNA operon is found [8]. Since then, there have been a plethora of strains identified with mutations in either A2058 or A2059 that confer MLS_B or ML resistance, respectively (Tab. 1) [9]. Generally, these mutations are observed in pathogens (e.g., *Mycobacterium, Brachyspira, Helicobacter, Treponema*) with one or two copies of 23S rRNA, often with each allele carrying the mutation. However, clinical strains and laboratory mutants have been identified in *Strepto-*

Table 1. 23S rRNA mutations (*E.coli* numering) that confer macrolide resistance in pathogenic bacteria

Position	Organism	Wildtype	Mutant	Reference
Δ752	*Streptococcus pneumoniae*	A	–	[13]
754	*Escherichia coli*	U	A	[29]
2032 + 2057	*Helicobacter pylori*	A/G	G/A	[196]
	Escherichia coli	G/G	A/A	[34]
2057	*Escherichia coli*	G	A	[32]
2057	*Propionibacterium acnes*	G	A	[197]
2057 + 2059	*Streptococcus pneumoniae*	G/A	A/C	[10]
2058	*Brachyspira hyodysenteriae*	A	U, G	[198]
	Escherichia coli	A	G	[34, 199]
	Helicobacter pylori	A	C, G, U	[196, 200–208]
	Propionibacterium acnes	A	G	[197]
	Propionibacterium avidum	A	G	[197]
	Propionibacterium granulosum	A	G	[197]
	Mycobacterium abscessus	A	G	[209]
	Mycobacterium avium	A	G, C, U	[210]
	Mycobacteriuam chelonae	A	G,C	[209]
	Mycobacterium intracellulare	A	G, C, U	[211]
	Mycobacterium kansasii	A	U	[212]
	Mycobacterium smegmatis	A	G	[45]
	Mycoplasma pneumoniae	A	G	[213]
	Streptococcus pneumoniae	A	G, U	[10, 12, 13]
	Treponema pallidum	A	G	[214]
2059	*Helicobacter pylori*	A	G, C, U	[196, 202–204, 215]
	Propionibacterium acnes		G	[197]
	Propionibacterium avidum		G	[197]
	Propionibacterium granulosum	A	G	[197]
	Mycobacterium abscessus	A	G, C	[209]
	Mycobacterium avium	A	C	[211]
	Mycobacterium chelonae	A	G	[209]
	Mycobacterium intracellulare	A	C	[211]
	Mycoplasma pneumoniae	A	G	[213]
	Streptococcus pneumoniae	A	G	[11]
2609	*Escherichia coli*	U	C	[30]
2611	*Escherichia coli*	C	U	[216]
2611	*Streptococcus pneumoniae*	C	G, A	[10, 12]

coccus pneumoniae that are heterozygous at these positions as well as at positions G2057 and C2611 [10–13]. In one study, a single base deletion (A752) in domain II was selected by clarithromycin passage; this pneumococcal mutant was coresistant to all macrolides and had a significant increase in its MIC to telithromycin to 4 μg/ml [13].

Mutations in L4 and L22 that confer erythromycin resistance have been documented for laboratory strains of *Escherichia coli, S. pneumoniae, Bacillus stearothermophilus*, and *Bacillus subtilis* [11–20]. In the case of clinical strains of *S. pneumoniae*, a change within a highly conserved sequence of L4 ($_{63}$KPWRQKGTGRAR$_{74}$) confers an MS phenotype [11–13]. One clinical strain from Canada had a six amino acid insert and a 500-fold increase to telithromycin, suggesting that a possible resistance mechanism to this class of compounds may be *via* mutations in ribosomal proteins [11]. Another laboratory study of mutants that arose when susceptible pneumococcal isolates were passaged with telithromycin found that changes in ribosomal protein L22 altered telithromycin susceptibility; the MIC changed from 0.008 to 0.25 μg/ml) [13]. This mutant was found to contain a combination of three mutations in the L22 gene (A93E, P91S, G83E), possibly accounting for the high number of serial passages (n = 44) required to select resistance with this antibiotic. Other point mutations in the L22 gene, G95D, P99Q, A93E, P91S, and G83E, were detected in pneumococcal strains passaged with macrolides, telithromycin, or clindamycin [12]. In an independent study, laboratory mutants of *S. pneumoniae* derived by serial passage with telithromycin also yielded L22 mutations of G95D or A97D [13]. One strain had an A97D change in L22 that resulted in an eight-fold increase to telithromycin (MIC changed from 0.006 to 0.05 μg/ml); an additional four-fold increase was seen coincident with a change at C1617T in domain III of 23S rRNA [21]. All of the mutations in ribosomal protein L22 that conferred macrolide/ketolide resistance were in the conserved carboxy-terminal region of the 114 amino acid protein. It is interesting to note that both the L4 and L22 mutations in *E. coli* perturb the three-dimensional structure of 23S rRNA at multiple sites but not at the peptidyl transferase region, as revealed by footprinting [22). The proximity of the residues in L4 or L22 is not sufficiently close in the crystal model of *Haloarcular marismortui* to envision direct contact of the antibiotics [23]. Resistance to Synercid or quinupristin/dalfopristin also can result from mutations in ribosomal protein L22 [24].

Biochemical techniques such as RNA footprinting and cross-linking studies have revealed how MLS_BK antibiotics contact the ribosome (Fig. 1) [25]. The region of involvement for 14- and 15-membered macrolides is predominantly in the peptidyl transferase region of 23S rRNA, most notably at residues A2058, A2059, A2062 (enhancement), and G2505 (*Escherichia coli* numbering) [26]. The addition of 16-membered macrolides that have a disaccharide at C-5 (tylosin, carbomycin) to 70S ribosomes protects A2058, A2059, A2062, and U2609 residues near the entrance to the peptide channel [6, 23, 27]. In addition, modification at the N1 position of residue A752 in domain II by dimethyl sulfate is enhanced in 14- and 15-membered macrolides that have cladinose at C3 [26, 28,

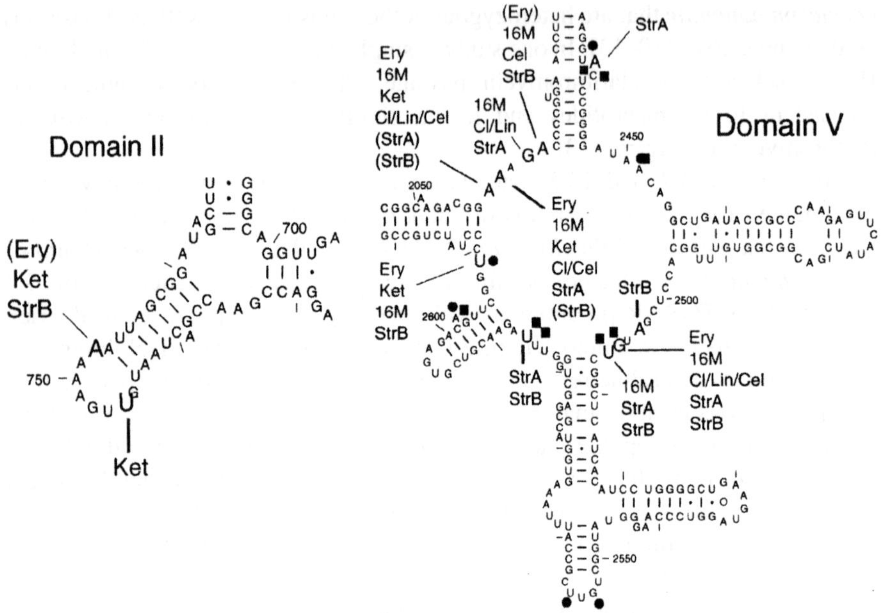

Figure 1. The peptidyl transferase region of domain V and helix 35 in domain II of 23S rRNA of *E. coli*. The nucleotides protected and enhanced (in parentheses) by MLS_BK antibiotics are indicated. Residues protected by tRNA bound in the A and P sites are marked with (●) and (■), respectively. Ery, erythromycin; 16M, 16-membered macrolides; Ket, ketolides like telithromycin and ABT-773; Cl, clindamycin; Lin, lincomycin; Cel, celesticetin; StrA, streptogramin A; StrB, streptogramin B.

29]. Removal of the cladinose and substitution by a 3-keto group as seen in the ketolide antibiotics results in a nearly 100–fold drop in drug binding affinity and loss of the A752 footprint [26, 28]. However, the addition of an extension group at C11/12 or C6 improves drug affinity, largely by protecting A752 [28, 30]. Thus, the ketolide telithromycin strongly protects A752 in addition to its interactions with A2058, A2059, U2609, and A2062 [28, 30]. A U2609C mutation in an *E. coli* strain with only one functional rRNA operon [31] mediates resistance to ketolides telithromycin and ABT-773 but changes the MIC to erythromycin only by two-fold [30]. The existence of a U754A mutation in hairpin 35 in domain II also conferred resistance to ketolides (and erythromycin) (Tab. 1) [29]. A unique footprint on the *Thermus aquaticus* ribosome was seen for telithromycin; the protected position corresponds to the *E. coli* ψ746, which could not be elucidated in footprint of *E. coli* ribosomes because of a strong reverse transcriptase stop [29]. Protection at position A752 is also afforded by 16-membered macrolides that have a mycinose moiety at position 14 [27].

Mutations at either one of the base-paired residues of G2057 and C2611 confer erythromycin resistance as well (Tab. 1) [4, 10, 12, 19, 32]. Erythromycin can still bind to A2058 and A2059 in these mutants, but higher amounts of drug are required to see equal protection [33]. In *E. coli*, the G2057A mutation conferred resistance to 14-membered macrolides and chloramphenicol but not to 16-membered macrolides, lincosamides, or streptogramin B [32]; susceptibility to 15-membered macrolides was not described. In *S. pneumoniae* mutants derived by passage with clarithromycin, there was a double mutation of G2057A and A2059C, conferring 14- and 15-membered macrolide resistance and increasing resistance to telithromycin by 16-fold [10]. *S. pneumoniae* mutants that contained a C2611G mutation derived by passage with either clarithromycin or azithromycin had a macrolide-streptogramin-resistant phenotype (MS_B) with a four-fold increase in resistance to clindamycin/lincomycin and typically higher MICs to MS_B antibiotics than did mutants containing a C2611A mutation [10, 12]. *E. coli* strains with mutations at G2032 confer an erythromycin-hypersensitive phenotype; in addition, G2032A confers resistance to clindamycin and chloramphenicol, and G2032U confers chloramphenicol resistance [34]. Erythromycin resistance also is conferred by small deletions around position 1220 in domain II of 23S rRNA [35]. Like mutations to G2057, C2611, or G2032, the deletions confer resistance by alleviating the effect of erythromycin rather than by blocking its binding.

In domain II of *E. coli* 23S rRNA, and well-conserved among most eubacteria, an open reading frame corresponding to residues 1235 through 1268 encodes a small 5 amino acid peptide (E-peptide) that confers erythromycin resistance when translated in *cis* [36, 37]. There was no cross-resistance to either clindamycin or chloramphenicol, compounds that overlap the macrolide-binding site. It is unlikely that the E-peptide actually is translated from native 23S rRNA, since the promoter is encumbered in a double-stranded helix. However, mutations to the promoter region or mutations that destabilize the helix alter the peptide's ability to confer macrolide resistance [37, 38]. Other E-peptides that confer ketolide or 14-, 15-, and 16-membered macrolide resistance have been found using a random peptide library encoding 5 or 21 amino acids [37, 39]. Among the collections of peptides, there is a strong preference for leucine or isoleucine as the third amino acid and a hydrophobic amino acid at the C-terminus. Since free E-peptides do not bind the drugs, a "bottle brush" model has been proposed to explain how translation of E-peptides interferes with the action of macrolides [39]. In this model, the newly translated peptide interacts with the macrolide molecule on the ribosome and actively displaces it from its binding site during the last translocation event. Once the antibiotic has been swept free, the ribosome is free to engage in the translation of another cellular protein, thereby permitting protein synthesis to continue.

Ribosomal methylation

In 1956, soon after the introduction of erythromycin in therapy, resistance emerged in staphylococci [40–42]. Biochemical studies demonstrated that resistance was due to methylation of the ribosomal target of the antibiotics, which yielded a broad-spectrum co-resistance to macrolides, lincosamides, and streptogramins B, the so-called MLS_B phenotype [4, 19]. The cells remained susceptible to streptogramin A antibiotics (pristinamycin IIA, virginiamycin M, dalfopristin) and to the synergistic combination of streptogramins A and B. Subsequently, the MLS_B phenotype was reported in a large number of microorganisms and was found to be encoded by a variety of *erm* (erythromycin ribosome methylase) genes. In addition to being the first recognized mechanism of resistance to erythromycin in pathogenic strains, Erm methylases are the most widespread of the resistance mechanisms to MLS_B antibiotics. Erm methylases comprise a family of highly related proteins that use S-adenosylmethionine as a methyl donor to mono- or dimethylate a single adenine residue (A2058, *E. coli* numbering) in nascent 23S rRNA. The residue, A2058, is located within a conserved region of domain V of 23S ribosomal RNA and plays a key role in the binding of MLS_B antibiotics, and when changed to C, G, or T by mutation confers erythromycin resistance (Tab. 1) [4, 10–12, 19]. As a consequence of 23S rRNA methylation, binding of erythromycin to its target is impaired. Cross-resistance between all macrolides, lincosamides, and streptogramins B (pristinamycin I, virginiamycin S, and quinupristin) occurs because of overlapping binding sites in 23S rRNA [4, 5, 9, 19, 26, 43–45].

The level of resistance conferred by ribosomal methylases to specific macrolides depends on the mode of methylation of the adenine residue and on the macrolide structure. Monomethylation or dimethylation of the adenine residue leads to two different resistant phenotypes MLS_B-I and MLS_B-II, respectively, encoded by specific *erm* genes [46]. Phenotype MLS_B-I is characterized by a high level of resistance to lincomycin, intermediate resistance to spiramycin (a 16-membered macrolide), and borderline susceptibility to tylosin (another 16-membered macrolide); phenotype MLS_B-II is defined by a high level cross-resistance to all MLS_B antibiotics. The *erm* genes in pathogenic bacteria encode the MLS_B-II phenotype and are thus responsible for frank resistance to MLS_B antibiotics. *erm* genes found in soil bacteria or producer organisms can be of either phenotype (Tab. 2). The structure of the macrolide also affects the level of resistance. For example, derivatives of 14-membered macrolides that have a cyclic C11–12 carbamate modification have the ability to bind domain II of 23S rRNA in addition to domain V. Since only A2058 is modified by methylation, these derivatives can partially overcome resistance *via* the additional interaction [29, 35]. However, in order to provide sufficient potency and spectrum for use in respiratory tract infections, the carbamate or carbazate group has to be additionally modified [47–49].

The *erm* genes

A wide range of microorganisms including Gram-positive species, phylogenetically remote Gram-negative bacteria, spirochetes, anaerobes, and macrolide producers (*Streptomyces* and *Saccharopolyspora*) express Erm methylases. Since it appears that the *erm* genes were derived from a common ancestor, possibly a macrolide producer, it is not surprising that methylation of a unique residue in 23S rRNA is performed by a diversity of Erm methylases [50]. Nearly 40 *erm* genes have been reported so far; these elements are mostly borne by plasmids and

Table 2. rRNA methylases in macrolide and lincomycin producers.

Producer microorganism	MLS Antibiotic(s) Produced	Assigned gene[a]	Original gene	Methylase function	Reference
Arthrobacter sp. (Aeromicrobium erythreum)	Erythromycin	*erm*(R)	*ermA*	Methylation	[217]
Saccharopolyspora erythraea	Erythromycin	*erm*(E)	*ermE*	Dimethylation	[218, 219]
Streptomyces thermotolerans	Carbomycin	*erm*(H)	*carB*	Monomethylation	[220]
Streptomyces mycarofaciens	Midecamycin	*erm*(I)	*mdmA*	Methylation	[53]
Streptomyces ambofaciens	Spiramycin	*erm*(O) *erm*(Z)	*srmA* *srmD*	Monomethylation Monomethylation	[58] [221]
Streptomyces fradiae	Tylosin	*erm*(S)	*ermSF* or *tlrA*	Dimethylation	[83]
Streptomyces fradiae	Tylosin	*erm*(32)	*HrB*	Monomethylation	[56]
Streptomyces fradiae	Tylosin	*erm*(N)	*tlrD*	Monomethylation	[222]
Streptomyces lincolnensis	Lincomycin	*erm*(U)	*lmrB*	Methylation	[223]
Micromonospora griseorubida	Mycinamycin	*erm*(W)	*myrB*	Methylation	[224]
Streptomyces venezuelae	Methymycin Neomethymycin Pikromycin Narbomycin	*erm*(30)[a] *erm*(31)[a]	*pikR1* *pikR2*	Methylation (putative)	[225]
Streptomyces viridochromogenes	None	*erm*(V)	*ermSV*	Monomethylation	[226]
Streptomyces caelestis	Celesticetin		*clr*	Monomethylation	[227]
Streptomyces lividans	None	*erm*(O)	*lrm*	Monomethylation	[132, 228]

[a] New gene designation according to Roberts and colleagues [2]. The class of *erm* gene is the same as the letter in parentheses.

Table 3. Distribution of *erm* genes in pathogenic bacteria, *Bacillus* and corynebacteria.

Assigned gene[a]	Original gene	Prototype host	Other bacterial hosts	Reference
erm(A)	*ermA*	*Staphylococcus aureus*	*Actinobacillus Streptococcus Enterococcus*	[229]
	ermTR	*Streptococcus pyogenes*	Group B, C, G streptococcus *S. pneumoniae*	[51]
erm(B)	*ermAM, ermAMR, ermB, ermBC, ermBP, ermIP, ermBZ1, ermBZ2, erm*(2), ermP, ermZ	*Streptococcus-Enterococcus*	*Actinobacillus Clostridium, Enterobacteriaceae, Klebsiella, Neisseria, Pediococcus, , Staphylococcus, Wolinella*	[230]
erm(C)	*ermC, ermM, ermIM*	*Staphylococcus*	*Actinobacillus, Bacillus, Eubacterium, Lactobacillus, Neisseria,Streptococcus, Wolinella*	[231]
erm(D)	*ermD, ermJ, ermK*	*Bacillus*		[82]
erm(F)	*ermF, ermFS, ermFU*	*Bacteroides*	*Actinobacillus, Clostridium, Eubacterium, Fusobacterium, Gardnerella, Haemophilus, Neisseria, Porphyromonas, Prevotella, Peptostreptococcus, Selenomonas, Streptococcus, Treponema, Veillonella, Wolinella*	[232]
erm(G)	*ermG*	*Bacillus*	*Bacteroides*	[79]
erm(Q)	*ermQ*	*Clostridium*	*Actinobacillus, Streptococcus, Wolinella*	[233]
erm(T)	*ermGT*	*Lactobacillus*		[87]
erm(X)	*ermCD, ermA, ermCX*	*Corynebacterium*		[234]
erm(Y)	*ermGM*	*Staphylococcus*		[109]

[a] New gene designation according to Roberts and colleagues [2]. The class of *erm* gene is the same as the letter in parentheses.

transposons in pathogenic bacteria [2, 4, 19]. Due to the growing number of reported genes, a nomenclature system was devised to prevent genes that are nearly identical from being assigned different letter designations [2]. *erm* genes with deduced amino acid sequences of greater than 79% difference were given separate letter designations. This new nomenclature system distinguishes 21 classes of *erm* genes and as many corresponding Erm proteins; two new ones from *Streptomyces venezuelae* are renamed in this article (Tab. 2). Macrolide resistance determinants also can be classified based on DNA-DNA hybridizations. However, the polymorphisms of DNA sequences within certain classes require careful choices of DNA probes or PCR primers to distinguish between closely related members of the same family. A specific case is *erm*(A), a rRNA methylase primarily found in staphylococci, or *erm*(TR), a member of the *erm*(A) class that has been found only in streptococci [51]. Both the original and the newly proposed names of genes will be used in this chapter.

Several *erm* genes have been characterized in macrolide and lincomycin producers (Tab. 2) and are present as protection mechanisms [52]. In the producers of erythromycin (*S. erythraea*) and midecamycin (*Streptomyces mycarofaciens*), methylase genes that dimethylate A2058 have been found [53, 54]. In *S. fradiae*, *tlrB* is found among the biosynthetic cluster of tylosin genes, and it confers resistance to tylosin but not to erythromycin in heterologous hosts like *S. lividans* [55]. Recently, the gene was determined to encode a monomethylase that modifies nucleotide G748 of helix 35 in domain II of 23S rRNA [56] and reassigned as *erm*(32) (Tab. 2) to Roberts [2]. Other homologous genes have been found, including the macrolide-resistance determinant *myrA* found in *Micromonospora griseorubida* [57]. *myrA* is 50% identical to *tlrB* and 32% similar to *rrmA* in *E. coli* at the amino acid level. The latter encodes a 23S rRNA m^1G745 methyltransferase [57]. Preliminary data suggest that *myrA* and two others (*yxjB* and the *orf* from a *Corynebacterium glutamicum* plasmid pAG1) are capable of methylating at G748 [56]. Thus, Erm(32) (TlrB) appears to be the first member of a new subclass of rRNA methyltransferases that are implicated in macrolide drug resistance.

Ribosomal methylation is often associated with other macrolide resistance genes that inactivate or efflux the antibiotic or its precursor. The methylase *erm*(O) (formerly *srmA*) may even be dispensable when other mechanisms of protection (*srm*(B) and *erm*(Z) [formerly *srmD*]) are present as in *Streptomyces ambofaciens*, the producer of spiramycin [58].

A possible role for resistance genes in antibiotic synthesis has been suspected since some of them are part of the gene cluster involved in the biosynthesis of macrolides [52, 59, 60]. Certainly, in *S. ambofaciens* at least one of the transporter pumps is involved in effluxing 2'-O-glycosyl oleandomycin extracellularly, as is discussed later in the chapter.

Although the *erm* genes are widely present in pathogenic bacteria, they are distributed in only a small number of *erm* classes (Tab. 3). Within the *erm*(B), *erm*(C), and *erm*(F) classes, the diversity is generally low (less than 5%). This is probably related to an easy interspecies exchange of genetic information. As mentioned above, a greater diversity is found in *erm*(A); however, the *erm*(A) and subclass *erm*(TR) sequences generally are conserved in the species where they were initially detected, staphylococci and beta-hemolytic streptococci, respectively. However, *erm*(A) also has been identified in *Enterococcus faecium* [61, 62], and the *erm*(TR) subclass has been identified in *S. pneumoniae* [63]. The *erm* genes are preferentially distributed in certain species, with streptococci and enterococci carrying a preponderance of *erm*(B), while *erm*(A) and *erm*(C) genes are more prevalent in staphylococci; anaerobes harbor the *erm*(F) gene (Tab. 3). Alignment of Erm methylases according to the neighbor-joining method [64] allowed the construction of a phylogenetic tree (Fig. 2). The analysis confirms that the Erm methylases are related, indicating that they are derived from a common ancestor. The methylases from producers and those from pathogenic bacteria form two distinct groups, Erm(F) being the most distant in the group of pathogenic bacteria.

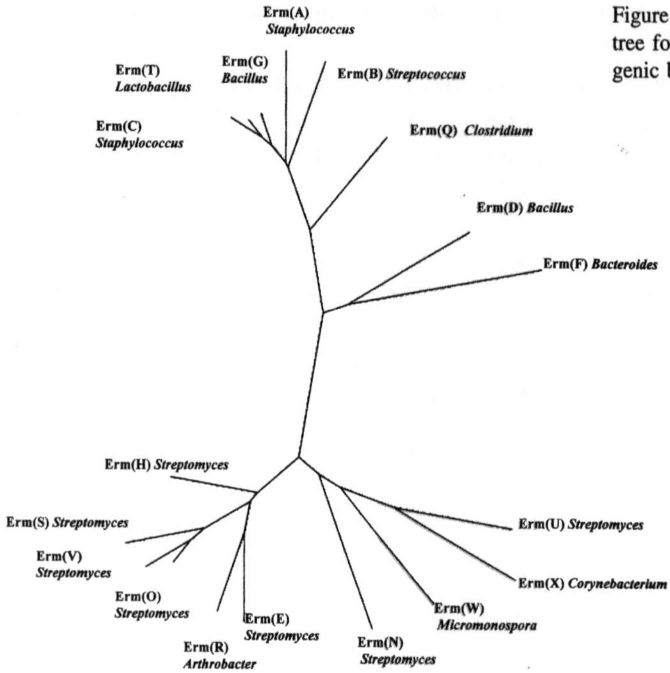

Figure 2. The phylogenetic tree for Erm proteins in pathogenic bacteria and producers.

The solution structure of Erm(B) from a clinical strain of *S. pneumoniae* was published; the catalytic domain consisting of a seven-stranded β sheet flanked by α-helices is conserved when compared with other non-Erm methyltransferases, but the C-terminal nucleic acid-binding domain has a unique RNA-recognition fold [65–67]. The crystal structure of Erm(C) complexed with S-adenosylmethione has also been published and, within the limits of the two different techniques, is not significantly different from the structure visualized by NMR [66, 67]. Taking advantage of the unique binding domain, compounds that inhibit Erm methyltransferases can be identified [68–70].

Induction mechanisms

Expression of MLS_B resistance can be constitutive or inducible. In the case of the *erm*(C) gene from staphylococcal plasmid pE194, the genetic basis for induction has been studied in detail [71, 72]. Inducible expression of the *erm*(C) determinant yields dissociated resistance to macrolides due to differences in the inducing ability of the antibiotics. The strains are resistant to 14- (clarithromycin, dirithromycin, erythromycin, and roxithromycin) and 15- (azithromycin) membered macrolides that are inducers. By contrast, non-inducer 16-membered macrolides that are available in certain countries (josamycin, midecamycin, miocamycin, rokitamycin, and spiramycin) or in veterinary practice (tylosin), commercially available lincosamides (lincomycin and clindamycin), and streptogramins B (pristinamycin I, virginiamycin S, and quinupristin) remain active. In

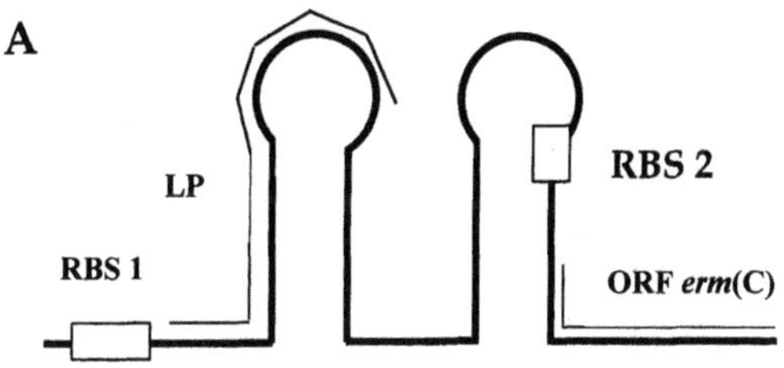

Figure 3. Conformations of an inducible *erm*(C) mRNA. A, uninduced state; B, induced state.

LP = leader peptide
RBI, RBS2 = ribosomal binding site 1, 2
ORF = open reading frame

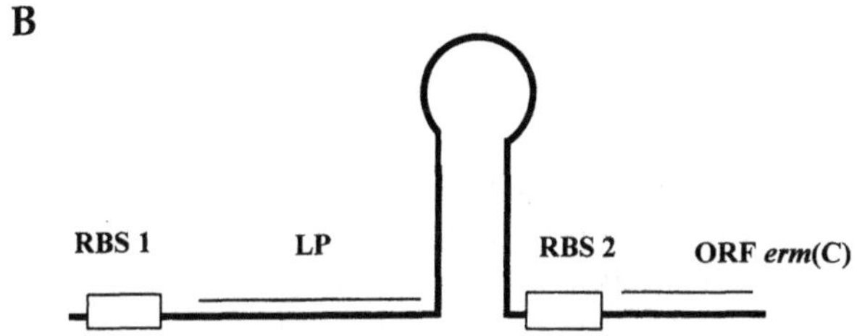

disk-diffusion tests, a D-shaped inhibition zone around disks containing a non-inducer macrolide or lincosamide can be observed, provided that a disk of erythromycin is placed nearby. However, the disk test is not always reliable in enterococci and streptococci, as inducible phenotypes can be masked [73].

Induction arises post-transcriptionally according to the model of translation attenuation [4, 71, 74]. mRNA is synthesized, but the 5' end of the mRNA has a set of four inverted repeats that sequester the initiation sequences (ribosome-binding-site and initiation codon) for the methylase by base-pairing in the absence of erythromycin (Fig. 3, conformation A). Thus, the initiation sequences are not accessible to the ribosomes for methylase translation. Induction is related to the presence of an open-reading frame encoding a short 14 amino acid peptide upstream of the *erm*(C) structural gene. In the presence of low concentrations of erythromycin, ribosomal binding of the antibiotic causes the ribosomes to stall while they are translating the leader peptide. The leader peptide sequence for *erm*(C) has been analyzed by Weisblum and colleagues; four amino acids, IFVI, are critical for induction [4, 74]. Ribosome stalling probably induces destabilization of the pairing and conformational rearrangements in the mRNA. The displacement of the stem-loop structure (Fig. 3, conformation B) would then unmask the initiation sequences for the methylase. The methylase is then synthesized by ribosomes that are not complexed to erythromycin. A third mRNA conformation has been predicted that could occur at the end of the induction process when the concentration of inducer macrolide has decreased and/ or the majority of ribosomes are methylated [74].

Of major importance is the stabilization of the mRNA that occurs during the induction process. This stabilization is an early consequence of ribosome stalling and protects the transcripts from degradation by RNases [75, 76], leading to a marked increase in the half-life of mRNA and an enhancement of enzyme synthesis. Regulation is in part due to a feedback mechanism. As the pool of methylated ribosomes increases during the process of induction, fewer ribosomes are able to stall and therefore transcripts return to the inactive conformation. In addition, it has been shown that the Erm(C) methylase from *B. subtilis* binds its own mRNA at a site that has structural similarities with the site of methylation in 23S rRNA. Thus, the methylase might block its own production when synthesized in excess [77].

Since a similar attenuator structure is found upstream of other *erm* genes, the translation attenuation model has been proposed for the inducible genes *erm*(A) of the staphylococcal transposon Tn*554*, *erm*(B) of *Streptococcus sanguis*, and *erm*(G) of *Bacillus sphaericus* [78, 79]. However, the structure of the attenuators of these genes is complex, having two control peptides (*erm*(A) and *erm*(G)) or many inverted-repeats (*erm*(B)), and the mechanism of regulation of these genes remains to be thoroughly elucidated. Unlike *erm*(C) and *erm*(D), *erm*(K) from *Bacillus licheniformis* is controlled by transcriptional attenuation [80]. Again, the structural gene is preceded by an ORF that could encode a short control peptide (19 amino acids), and a series of stem-loop structures forming hairpins has been identified. However, the two hairpins function as rho-independent terminators, with only prematurely truncated transcripts synthesized in the absence of inducer. In the presence of erythromycin, stalling of the ribosomes while translating the control peptide induces rearrangements of the secondary structure. The complete transcript is then produced. However, the analysis of the secondary structure of the transcript showed that the initiation sequences for the *erm*(D) methylase were sequestered in a hairpin, suggesting that this gene may also be regulated by translation attenuation. This hypothesis has been confirmed recently by mutagenesis experiments [81] where it appears that expression is regulated primarily by transcriptional attenuation, with a small increase in expression being attributed to translational attenuation. Translational attenuation had been shown earlier for the *erm*(D) gene from *B. licheniformis* which is essentially identical to *erm*(K) and differs only in three nucleotides [82]. Regulation by translational and transcriptional attenuation of *erm*(S) (formerly *tlrA* or *ermSF*) of *Streptomyces fradiae*, the tylosin producer, has been reported independently by two research groups [83, 84]. Constitutive MLS_B resistance can be explained by deletion of the entire attenuator, as has been shown for clinical isolates of *Staphylococcus epidermidis* and *S. aureus* containing *erm*(C) [85], and for *Enterococcus faecalis*, *Streptococus agalactiae,* and *S. pneumoniae* containing *erm*(B) [73, 86]. In addition, a point mutation in the attenuator of *erm*(T) (formerly *ermGT*) of *Lactobacillus reuteri* [87] or tandem duplications in the attenuator of *erm*(C) of *S. aureus* and *Staphylococcus equorum* [88, 89] led to constitutive resistance by decreasing the stability of the hairpin structure sequestering the initiation sequences for the methylase or by duplicating the initiation signals which are thus available for translation. Clinical isolates that are constitutively resistant to erythromycin are widespread, especially in methicillin-resistant staphylococci.

Constitutive resistance can be obtained in the laboratory at frequencies of 10^{-7} to 10^{-8} by plating inducible strains of staphylococci containing *erm*(A) or *erm*(C) genes on agar plates containing inhibitory concentrations of noninducer macrolides or lincosamides [90]. The variants display attenuator alterations similar to those reported for clinical isolates [91]. However, only rare cases of clinical failure of clindamycin therapy of infections due to inducibly resistant strains of *S. aureus* have been reported [92]. Probably, the risk for selection of constitutive resistance is the highest in infections with a heavy inoculum of staphylococcus.

Induction specificity

Regardless of class, the *erm* genes can be expressed inducibly or constitutively. However, the induction profiles differ according to the bacterial species considered. For instance, in streptococci that are inducibly resistant to erythromycin, all macrolides and lincosamides are inducers, while in inducibly resistant staphylococci only 14- or 15-membered macrolides induce. The pattern of induction does not appear to be related to the class of *erm* gene but rather to the structure of the specific attenuator that controls the expression of the *erm* gene; for a specific attenuator, the structure of the MLS_BK antibiotic determines whether a given macrolide is an inducer [93]. Although not common in clinical isolates, a strain of *E. faecalis* that contained an R7C mutation in the putative leader peptide of its *erm*(B) gene was identified that was more strongly induced by tylosin, a 16-membered macrolide, than by erythromycin [94]. It has been reported that the ketolides are poor inducers of inducible strains of streptococci and staphylococci [48, 95, 96]. It is important to note that use of non-inducers like 16-membered macrolides in the clinical environment has resulted in the selection of constitutively resistant mutants [4, 90, 97].

Some *S. pneumoniae* isolates that carry *erm*(B) were heterogeneously resistant to ketolides like HMR-3004 and telithromycin [98]. Heterogeneity was determined by population analysis and defined as a plating efficiency of ≥ 0.1% when cells were plated onto agar containing 1 µg/ml ketolide as compared with the control (absence of inducer). Among strains collected from various international sites, 41.4% of the strains [29/70] were heterogeneous, with the range of plating efficiency varying from 0.1% to 62% on agar plates containing 1 µg/ml telithromycin. The frequency of heterogeneity could not be explained by the dissemination of one or two clones as assessed by Box polymerase chain reaction (PCR). The heterogeneity trait could be transferred by genetic transformation to the standard laboratory strain R6 by selecting for resistance to erythromycin (0.5 µg/ml); *erm*(B) appears to cotransfer. All macrolide-resistant R6 transformants were heterogeneous by population analysis. Further, R6 "homoclones" that were homogeneously resistant to ketolides could be obtained by plating heterogeneous populations on 10 µg/ml telithromycin. Homoclones remained macrolide-resistant after 10 passages on ketolide-free agar plates. The clinical significance of these findings is at present unknown. It will be interesting to see if a correlation between the levels of ribosomal methylation and heterogeneity can be made. Recent work with 30 *erm*(B) clinical isolates of *S. pneumoniae* has shown that the basal levels of methylation vary from strain to strain [96].

Inactivating enzymes

Unlike target modification, inactivation of MLS_B antibiotics confers resistance to structurally related antibiotics only. Esterases, phosphotransferases, glycosyltransferases, decaylases, and formyl reductases have been identified in strains resistant to MLS_B antibiotics.

Macrolide phosphotransferases

There are early entries in the literature that show that different *Streptomyces* strains can phosphorylate 14- and 16-membered macrolide antibiotics [99-101]. High-level erythromycin resistance in gram-negative enteric bacteria also can be attributed to the synthesis of macrolide 2'-phosphotransferases that add phosphate to the 2' hydroxyl group of desosamine or mycaminose (Fig. 4). *mph*(A), *mph*(B), and *mph*(C) encode three different macrolide phosphotransferases [3, 4, 102–119]; *mph*(A) and *mph*(B) have been found in enteric bacteria, while *mph*(C), until recently, had been described only in a few strains of *S. aureus*. *mph*(A) was originally described in *E. coli* Tf418A, and *mph*(K) was described later in *E. coli*

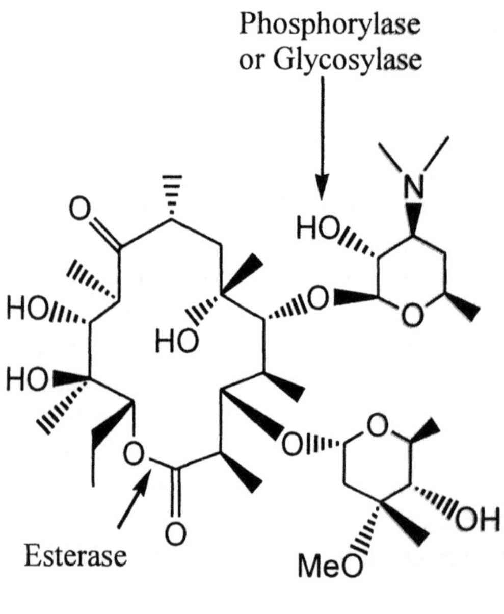

Figure 4. Scheme for inactivation of erythromycin by phosphorylases, glycosylase, or esterase.

209K. Mph(A) and Mph(K) are 98.3% identical by amino acid homology and have been folded into a single class, henceforth referred to as Mph(A) [2, 104, 110]. Mph(A) appears to be an inducible enzyme that inactivates 14- and 15-membered macrolides preferentially [114]. These proteins have weak homology overall to other phosphotransferase enzymes, but there is strong homology of two C-terminal regions that are conserved in all phosphotransferases [104, 117]. When a DNA fragment containing *mph*(A) from *E. coli* Tf481A was cloned into a recipient *E. coli* strain, the MICs to erythromycin were increased only four-fold. To get full complementation of the high-level erythromycin-resistant phenotype, another gene, *mrx*, residing downstream of *mph*(A) was required [110]. Mrx proteins from *E. coli* Tf184A and 209K are 30% and 31% identical to Tap from *Mycobacterium fortuitum,* respectively, and 20% to 30% identical to membrane efflux pumps of the major facilitator superfamily (MFS), like *mef*(A) and *tet*(V), at the protein level [104, 110, 120]. The Tap and Mrx proteins have 12 transmembrane domains and a high percentage of hydrophobic amino acids (54% and 52% for Mrx and Tap, respectively), characteristics of a membrane localization, and signature sequences that have been found in other members of the MFS. However, no evidence exists that Mrx by itself functions as an efflux pump. If *mph*(A) and *mrx* are cloned into a naïve strain of *E. coli* or *S. aureus*, macrolide resistance to 14- and 16-membered macrolides (resistance to 15-membered macrolides was not tested) is conferred in *E. coli* but not in *S. aureus* [112]. Furthermore, *mph*(A) plus *mrx* cloned into *Pseudomonas aeruginosa* express erythromycin resistance in an inducible manner [113]. It may be that the G + C contents of *mph*(A) (66%) are just too high for expression in *S. aureus* (33%) but are permitted in *E. coli* (50%).

In an earlier publication, a product using *mph*(A)-specific primers was obtained with *S. epidermidis* S1187 [118], a strain that also contains an ABC type pump, Msr(A) [121]. However, when the PCR product was sequenced from this strain, it was not homologous to *mph*(A); rather, it appeared to be a PCR artifact, as the product had homology to D-alanine-D-alanine ligase (T. Grebe and J. Sutcliffe, unpublished results).

The Mph(B) phosphotransferase has been described in *E. coli* where it inactivates 14-, 15-, and 16-membered macrolides [102, 122]. In *E. coli* strain BM2506, *mph*(B) is harbored on two plasmids, pTZ3721 (84 kb) and pTZ3723 (24 kb), both of which can be transferred conjugally to *E. coli* [102]. Site-specific mutagenesis of the gene encoding this enzyme has shown that four (at positions 200, 209, 219, 231] of the five aspartic acids in the two motifs conserved among phosphotransferases are essential for catalytic activity [117]. When *mph*(B) was introduced into a susceptible strain of *E. coli* or *S. aureus*, and expressed from its own promoter, it conferred both 14- and 16-membered macrolide resistance in *E. coli*, but only 16-membered macrolide inactivation in *S. aureus* [112]. No correlation seems to appear between the amount of enzyme expressed and the level of macrolide resistance as reflected by MIC values. Nonetheless, this suggests that *mph*(B) with a G + C content of 38% can be expressed in both Gram-positive and Gram-negative bacteria.

Until recently, the third type of phosphotransferase had been described in only a few *S. aureus* strains [109, 115, 119]. The gene from a 1971 clinical *S. aureus* strain MS8968 was shown to be on a plasmid located between *msr*(A) (previously referred to as *msrSA'*) and *erm*(Y) (previously referred to as *ermGM*), genes encoding an ABC macrolide/streptogramin B transporter and a 23S rRNA methyltransferase, respectively [109]. This gene was given the original designation of *mphBM*, but it has been renamed to conform to convention as *mph*(C) [2]. Another *S. aureus* strain, 01A1032, a 1989 isolate from the United States, also has a plasmid-encoded *mph*(C) gene that is cotranscribed as the second gene in an operon with *msr*(A) [119]. Mph(C) from strain 01A1032 differed in only 4 of 299 amino acid residues when compared with Mph(C) in strain MS8968 and is 33% and 50% identical at the amino acid level to Mph(A) and Mph(B), respectively. Recently, *mph*(C) was identified in *Stenotrophomonas maltophilia* [123]. It is 98% to 99.7% identical to the *mph*(C) genes at the amino acid level. Interestingly, when a DNA fragment containing *mph*(C) plus other genes (*e. g., bin3*, a resolvase-invertase, and *cadC/cadA*, genes encoding a regulator and an efflux pump for cadium) was cloned from *S. maltophilia* into an *E. coli acrAB* recipient, the MIC to erythromycin increased from 2 μg/ml to 32 μg/ml [123]. When DNA corresponding only to the *mph*(C) gene from *S. aureus* was cloned into a naïve *S. aureus* strain, RN4220, the MICs were not increased to erythromycin and there was no evidence of erythromycin inactivation by a radiolabeled assay [119]. One possible explanation for these results is that there is a "helper" gene on the DNA fragment from *S. maltophilia* or in the *E. coli* chromosome, but not on the *S. aureus* chromosome. Thus, it is unclear whether *mph*(C) is sufficient to confer macrolide resistance in either organism.

Pathogenic *Nocardia* spp. inactivate macrolides by a number of different mechanisms, including phosphorylation [124]. Phosphorylation of macrolides erythromycin, oleandomycin, tylosin, spiramycin, and leucomycin was observed when a cell-free extract of *Streptomyces coelicolor* was supplemented with ATP and magnesium [99, 100]. None of the genes responsible for phosphorylation has been sequenced.

Macrolide esterases

The plasmid-borne genes, *ere*(A) and *ere*(B), encode erythromycin esterases that hydrolyze the lactone of the macrocyclic template (Fig. 4). These enzymes have been found in clinical strains of *E. coli, Klebiella* spp., *Citrobacter* spp. *Proteus* spp., and *Enterobacter* spp. [2, 125–127]. In addition, *ere*(A) has been found as part of an integron cassette in *Providencia stuartii* [128]. The deduced amino acid sequence of the latter gene is 92.7% identical to that of the *ere*(A) originally described in *E. coli*. There is little apparent amino acid homology between the *ere*(A) and *ere*(B) gene products, as reflected by the low percentage of amino acid identity (~ 25%). However, the product of inactivation, hydrolyzed erythromycin, arising from either is the same [129, 130]. The product of erythromycin inactivation in *S. aureus* 01A1032 is equivalent to the detoxified product seen in *ere*(A) and *ere*(B) *E. coli* strains; however, a gene-encoding esterase activity has not been identified in this strain. Recently, in a PCR study, *ere*(B) was detected in 5 of 851 isolates (0.6%) of erythromycin-resistant *S. aureus* strains collected from 24 European hospitals; all of the isolates expressed a MLS_B constitutive phenotype and were methicillin-resistant [61]. None of this large population of *S. aureus* strains contained *ere*(A) and, of the 75 strains of macrolide-resistant *E. faecium* isolates in the study, none had either *ere* determinant. The authors did not try to detect macrolide phosphotransferases or the *erm*(TR) subclass of *erm*(A) methyltransferases; these resistance determinants may account for the resistance determinants in the 6.7% and 5.3% of the *S. aureus* and *E. faecium* strains, respectively, that did not contain *erm*(A), *erm*(B), *erm*(C), *ere*(A), *ere*(B), or *msr*(A).

A gene (ORF7) with 34% to 36% and 31% amino acid homology to *ere*(A) and *ere*(B), respectively, has been found upstream of the erythromycin biosynthetic cluster in *S. erythraea* [54]. The gene encodes a truncated esterase with a start site in the upstream IS-like element. It is possible that the intact ancestral gene played a role in self-protection.

Macrolide glycosyltransferases, deacylases, and formyl reductases

Macrolide glycosyltransferase activities have been demonstrated in 15 of 32 strains of *Streptomyces* that produced polyketide or polyether antibiotics [131]. Glycosylation of the sugar attached to position C5 in 14- and 16-membered macrolides was demonstrated originally in the nonmacrolide producer strain *S. lividans* (Fig. 4) [132, 133]. Both *S. lividans* and *Micromonospora purpurea* produce a glycosyltransferase, *mgt*, that uses UDP-glucose as a cofactor to glycosylate and inactivate 14-, 15-, and 16-membered macrolides [132, 133]. *Streptomyces antibioticus*, the producer of oleandomycin, has chosen to protect its susceptible ribosomes from oleandomycin by glycosylating the 2'-OH of desosamine intracellularly [60]. In this species, there are two enzymes produced intracellularly that can glycosylate oleandomycin, OleI and OleD. OleI prefers oleandomycin as a substrate to carbomycin, tylosin, and erythromycin, whereas OleD will glycosylate all the macrolides. Since *oleI* resides in the cluster of oleandomycin biosynthetic genes, it is likely that this gene is primarily responsible for self-protection. The detoxified compound is then exported by OleB, one of two transporters in *S. antibioticus,* and cleaved back to oleandomycin by OleR, an extracellular glycosidase. Erythromycin A can be glycosylated by *Streptomyces vendargensis* [134] but not by *S. erythraea*, despite the latter strain's ability to glycosylate avermectins and ivermectins at C4' and C4" [135]. A pathogenic strain of *Nocardia asteroides* inactivated erythromycin by glycosylation, but it could not inactivate 16-membered macrolides [124].

Deacylation of groups attached to the 4" position of 16-membered macrolides is rare, probably because the modified antibiotic is not completely inactivated. A strain of *N. asteroides* was described that removed the acyl group from rokitamycin and midecamycin, producing 3"-O-de-(*n*-propionyl)-4"-O-de-(*n*-butyryl)-rokitamycin and 4"-O-de-(*n*-propionyl)midecamycin, respectively, with 10% to 20% residual antibacterial activity [124]. The strain also reduced the formyl group attached to position 17 of the aglycone of rokitamycin and midecamycin, resulting in an inactive 18–dihydro derivative [124]. Other pathogenic *Nocarida* species, *N. brasiliensis* and *N. otitidiscaviarum,* were able to reduce the formyl group and/or phosphorylate the 2"-OH position.

Efflux of macrolides

It was originally thought that the outer membrane of Gram-negative bacteria, which exhibits low permeability to high molecular weight hydrophobic molecules (including macrolides, lincosamides, and streptogramins), was solely responsible for the intrinsic resistance [136]. With the discovery of the numerous multi-drug-resistant pumps, however, it is now recognized that certain chromosomally encoded pumps play an important role in intrinsic resistance to hydrophobic compounds. Recent experiments designed to determine the relative roles of outer membrane permeability and intrinsic pumps in *P. aeruginosa* have found that both of these mechanisms are effective alone and synergistic when combined [137, 138]. The efflux pumps that are often in part responsible for intrinsic resistance to antibiotics in many bacterial species can have unusually broad substrate specificities like the AcrAB-TolC efflux pump of *E. coli,* or they may have narrow substrate specificity like the Mef(A) pump in streptococci. In all cases, a protein residing in the cytoplasmic membrane acts alone or in concert with other proteins to pump its substrates out of the cell or the cell membrane, since recognition of a substrate at the level of the cytoplasmic membrane most likely occurs. Based on amino acid homology and membrane topology, four classes of efflux pumps can be defined.

- The resistance/nodulation/division (RND) family members are common in Gram-negative bacteria and have a subunit size of ~ 1000 amino acids encoding 12 membrane-spanning regions. There are usually three components of the pump mechanism: 1) a protein that forms a channel in the cytoplasmic membrane, 2) a linker protein that is located in the periplasm and facilitates export between the inner and outer membrane, and 3) a dedicated or generalized outer membrane porin that outwardly directs the transport of a broad array of antibiotics to the extracellular environment.
- The small multi-drug resistance (SMR) family is composed of proteins that have a subunit size of ~ 100 amino acids, with four transmembrane segments (TMS). All members of the SMR family contain a highly conserved glutamate residue within a TMS.
- Transporters (≥ 400 amino acids) that are part of the MFS span the membrane 12 or 14 times. This superfamily has been subdivided into 29 established and 5 putative MFS families based on characteristic signature sequences [139].

- Members of the ABC superfamily usually have 12 TMS and are part of a multicomponent apparatus that facilitates efflux of natural and synthetic antibacterial agents. Pumps of this superfamily are distinct from other classes in that they are fueled by ATP hydrolysis.

All but the members of the ABC superfamily are fueled by proton motive force. The SMR and RND pumps have been found exclusively in bacteria, while the other two superfamilies have memberships comprised of both procaryotes and eucaryotes.

RND pumps

In many Gram-negative species, resistance to MLS_BK antibiotics is mediated by pumps belonging to the RND superfamily. The tripartite pumps are composed of 1) a cytoplasmic membrane component (AcrB, AcrF, AmrB, MexB, MexD, MexY, and MtrD) that couples extrusion of the substrate in exchange for a proton, 2) a periplasmic protein (AcrA, AcrE, AmrA, MexA, MexC, MexY, and MtrC) that links extrusion of a molecule from the cytoplasm or inner membrane directly to 3) a component in the outer membrane that likely forms a gated channel (TolC, Omp2, OprA, OprM, OprJ, OprM, and MtrE). Recently, AcrB, which is thought to recognize its substrates largely based on hydrophobicity, was purified and reconstituted in proteoliposomes where it catalyzed the extrusion of fluorescent phospholipids in the presence of a pH gradient [140]. Erythromycin, bile salts, and cloxacillin, known substrates for the AcrAB-TolC pump, inhibited efflux, while the addition of AcrA, the periplasmic membrane fusion protein, enhanced the rate of extrusion. AcrA, a lipoprotein with a predicted length of 17 nm, promoted fusion of vesicles in the absence of mixing the intravesicular contents [140, 141]. Although many of the periplasmically localized membrane fusion proteins are lipoproteins, the acyl modification is not requisite for functioning in intact cells [141]. Recently, TolC has been crystallized as a trimer that assembles in a unique fashion to form a continuous, solvent-accessible channel that is over 140 Å long and is envisioned to span both the outer membrane and the periplasm space [142]. Although the periplasmic end of the tunnel is closed by coiled helices, interaction with the inner membrane translocase and/or the periplasmic binding protein is thought to trigger an opening of some 30 Å in diameter.

The *acrAB-tolC, acrAB-omp2*, *amrAB-oprA*, and *mexAB-oprM* genes are chromosomally encoded and expressed constitutively, providing intrinsic resistance to macrolide antibiotics for *E. coli, Haemophilus influenzae, Burkholderia pseudomallei,* and *P.aeruginosa,* respectively. Recently, *mexX* encoding a membrane fusion protein and *mexY* encoding an inner membrane pump have been described in *P. aeruginosa* that pair with either TolC in *E. coli* or OprM in *P. aeruginosa* to form another RND pump [143]. The existence of the MexXY pump components explains how a *P. aeruginosa* strain expressing OprM in the absence of *mexAB* was able to confer resistance to quinolones, erythromycin, and tetracycline [143–145]. This pump is chromosomally coded and appears to be induced by its substrates, including erythromycin [145]. Additionally, a *mexAB-oprM*-like pump has been demonstrated in *S. maltophilia* [146]. It is likely that these multi-drug-resistant pumps also provide protection against the streptogramin and lincosamide antibiotics, but these drugs are not widely tested. Other RND pumps encoded by *acrEF-tolC, mexCD-oprJ*, and *mtrCDE* found in *E. coli, P. aeruginosa,* and *Neisseria gonorrhoeae*, respectively, appear to be transcriptionally silent unless a mutation in their respective regulatory proteins, AcrS, NfxB, and MtrR, increases expression. MtrR, for example, is divergently transcribed from an operon upstream of *mtrCDE*. Clinical strains of *N. gonorrhoeae* that are erythromycin-resistant most often have a single base pair deletion in the 13-bp inverted repeat located within the promoter regions between the two operons. Other cellular components also may impact the level of resistance; indeed, higher-level resistance to erythromycin also was found to depend on the production of the full length lipooligosaccharide in gonococci [147].

SMR pumps

Several SMR family members confer resistance to erythromycin. A chromosomally encoded efflux system that has been identified in *E. coli* is *emr*(E) (also known as *mvrC* or *ebr*). Purified Emr(E) has been reconstituted in a lipid bilayer and has been shown to catalyze efflux of erythromycin and tetracycline, in addition to lipophilic monovalent cations. While it is clear that the electrochemical gradient provides the energy to fuel this pump, the oligomeric structure that constitutes a functional Emr(E) pump is not known. An SMR-type pump from *Mycobacterium tuberculosis* encoded by *mmr* is 43% identical to *emr*(E) and confers a multi-drug-resistant phenotype (including erythromycin as one of its substrates) when cloned on a multicopy plasmid into a heterologous host, *Mycobacterium smegmatis* [148]. The *mmr* gene is also present in *M. simiae, M. gordonae, M. marinum*, and *M. bovis*, but not in other mycobacterial strains; its role in conferring an erythromycin-resistant phenotype in any of its native species has yet to be determined.

MFS pumps

MFS transporters that confer macrolide resistance include the multi-drug-resistant Mdf(A) in *E. coli* [149] and the Cmr pump of *Corynebacterium glutamicum* [150]. In *E. coli*, the Mdf(A) pump confers ~ four-fold higher level of resistance to erythromycin, dyes, and other antibiotics when expressed from a multicopy plasmid. It appears that *mdf*(A) is expressed constitutively, and, when disrupted, cells become more susceptible to ethidium bromide [151]. Mdf(A) has 12 TMS segments, and TMS-1 contains a single acidic glutamate residue at position 26. The presence of an acidic residue within a TMS region has been seen with other members of MFS transporters as well as with members of the SMR family. If D26 is altered to a positively charged lysine in Mdf(A), substrate specificity for its positively charged substrates is lost [151]. The altered protein is still capable of effluxing chloramphenicol, a neutral substrate. The authors did not determine if this form of the protein was competent to efflux erythromycin, a compound that exists in both protonated (> 96%) and neutral forms at physiological pH. Recently the carboxy-terminal domain of BmrR, the repressor of the MFS multi-drug efflux protein Bmr from *B. subtilis*, has been crystallized. When purified, it forms dimers and binds aromatic cationic ligands with the same affinity as the full length BmrR. Crystal structures of the multi-drug-binding domain of BmrR and of its complex with tetraphenylphosphonium unveiled a drug-induced unfolding of an α-helix to a random coil, exposing an internal drug-binding pocket with a buried glutamate residue [152, 153]. Given that some substrates of the Bmr translocase are also recognized by BmrR, it is not unlikely that the translocase would use a similar mechanism of recognition.

The Cmr protein does not mediate a multi-drug-resistant phenotype in *C. glutamicum;* however, it mediates a multi-drug-resistant phenotype (including resistance to erythromycin) when expressed in *E. coli* on a multicopy plasmid [85]. Perhaps *cmr* is under repression in its native host.

An efflux pump, designated *mef*(A) can be found in many clinical isolates of *S. pneumoniae* and *Streptococcus pyogenes* [154–164]. Because the nucleotide sequences of *mef*(E), the original designation in *S. pneumoniae*, and *mef*(A), the original gene name in *S. pyogenes*, are 88.8% identical, the two have been reclassified into a single gene designation, *mef*(A) [2]. The Mef(A) protein was demonstrated to efflux 14- and 15-membered macrolides only, and resistance to 16-membered macrolides, clindamycin, or streptogramin B was not seen even in the presence of inducing concentrations of erythromycin [154, 156].

mef(A) has been described in a variety of other species, including *S. agalactiae; viridans* streptococci; *Streptococcus milleri; Streptococcus mitis;* Groups C, F, and G streptococci; *Micrococcus luteus;* three *Corynebacterium* spp.; and *Enterococcus* spp. [165]. More recently, the *mef*(A) gene has been described in Gram-negative clinical strains, *N. gonorrhoeae* and *Acinetobacter junii* [166]. *mef*(A) can be conjugally transferred as demonstrated in mating experiments of *S. pyogenes* and *S. pneumoniae mef*(A)$^+$ strains into their respective species [161, 167]. Two groups, working independently, have identified a transposon that encodes the *mef* gene [168, 169]. The transposon (*Tn1207*.1) described in a group of *S. pneumoniae* isolates of Italian origin carries the *mef*(A) gene sequence originally described in *S. pyogenes* [168, 169], whereas the Atlanta-derived *S. pneumoniae* isolates have *mef*(E) encoded in one of two forms of a MEGA transposon [169]. Further, the sites of integration differ between MEGA (four chromosomal locations) and Tn*1207.1* (one site). The sequences thus far have revealed what appear to be defective transposons, although Tn*1207.1* is nearly intact as a 7244-bp element. The MEGA element of either 5.4 or 5.5 kb lacks the recombinase seen upstream of the *mef-msr*(A)-like operon in *Tn1207.1.* Both transposons have the *mef* gene as the upstream gene of a bicistronic operon. The second gene in the operon has homology to *msr*(A) and is called *mel* in the MEGA transposon. It will be important to determine the contribution of the *mef* or the *mel* gene to the efflux phenotype seen in many pathogenic strains of streptococci.

Clinically, *S. pneumoniae* or *S. pyogenes* strains harboring *mef*(A) generally have MICs against clarithromycin, azithromycin and erythromycin of 1–32 μg/ml *versus* an MIC range of 0.03–0.5 μg/ml for telithromycin in *S. pneumoniae* [157, 158, 170, 171]. Occasionally, MICs to the 14- or 15-membered macrolides can be as high as 50 μg/ml [63]. The MIC ranges in *S. agalactiae* can be very different, as reported in a study from France [171]. Eighteen *S. agalactiae* isolates had a range of 0.1–1.0 μg/ml for erythromycin, 0.1–0.5 μg/ml for clarithromycin, and a more typical 1–4 μg/ml for azithromycin. There also have been reports of low MICs (1–2 μg/ml) against erythromycin in three *S. mitis* isolates from Toronto [172].

Although *mef*(A) and *mef*(E) have been reclassified as *mef*(A), it is interesting to note that of the 18 clinical *S. agalactiae* isolates from France, 17 carried the *mef*(E) sequence as published for *S. pneumoniae,* while 1 carried the *mef*(A) sequence published for *S. pyogenes*, with a single amino acid exception [171]. According to a meeting report, the *mef*(A) determinant in *E. faecium* isolates with an M phenotype was precisely the same determinant in *S. pneumoniae* [173]. The *mef* determinant in Group C streptococci was of the subclass *mef*(E) [174]. Thus, it is likely that the divergence between *mef*(A) and *mef*(E) has been recent and that the two types of *mef* genes are being horizontally spread into other microorganisms.

The existence of *S. pneumoniae* strains with both *erm*(B) and *mef*(A) has been reported [157, 167]. These strains generally have an MLS_B-resistant phenotype, but, when analyzed by PCR primers specific for the different resistance determinants or by Southern hybridization, the presence of both elements is confirmed. One clone of the "double" has recently been identified in numerous centers in South Africa accounting for nearly one-quarter of the macrolide-resistant isolates from private hospitals (Keith Klugman and Leslie McGee, unpublished findings) [235].

A gene that is 36% identical at the amino acid level to *mef*(A) has been described in multi-drug-resistant *Lactococcus lactis* strain K214 used in lactic fermentation of cheese [175]. When *mef*214 was cloned into *E. coli,* a macrolide-resistant phenotype was conferred. The role of the *mef*214 gene in its native host has recently been clarified; a new gene designated *mft*(A) (previously *mef*214) from *Lilactis* was cloned and provided glucose-dependent efflux of erythromycin and tetracycline in *E. coli* and *L. lactis* [236].

The *mef*(A) gene appears to be inducible by both 14- and 15-membered macrolides, but not by 16-membered macrolides [176]. Further, the 16-membered macrolides are poor substrates for Mef(A), as there is no change in their respective MICs in the presence of erythromycin. The ketolide telithromycin is a weak inducer and/or substrate of *mef*(A) relative to erythromycin, clarithromycin, and azithromycin as inferred by MIC differentials (50-fold *versus* 500–2000-fold, respectively) [96, 176, 177]. Induction of *mef*(A) by erythromycin A in *S. pneumoniae* was confirmed by Northern analysis using an internal *mef*(A)-

specific probe [176]. Two bands, one at 1100 bases and one at 2300 bases, were expressed in an inducible manner over 45 minutes, with no mRNA seen in the absence of erythromycin. The smaller product corresponds to the coding sequence of the *mef*(A) protein. The larger band presumably contains a second gene, most likely the *msr*(A)-like gene. These results have recently been confirmed [169].

ABC pumps

ABC transporters generally have multiple domains, two membrane-spanning domains that form a channel and two ATP-binding domains located at the cytosolic surface of the membrane or on a protein separate from the one that forms the transmembrane channel [178]. The resistance determinant in strains with a MS_B (macrolide- and inducible streptogramin B-resistant) phenotype was originally identified as *msr*(A) in *S. epidermidis*. *msr*(A) alone could confer the MS_B phenotype when cloned into a naïve strain of *S. aureus* RN4220. However, since *msr*(A) contains only two nucleotide binding domains, the putative transmembrane component of the Msr(A) pump remains elusive.

The MS_B phenotype was initially described as a PMS phenotype in *S. aureus* strains from Hungary [179]. In this study, 25.6% of the 413 hospital isolates had a MS_B phenotype. A 1993 study from England looked at the distribution of macrolide-resistance determinants in coagulase-negative staphylococci from patients with continuous ambulatory peritoneal dialysis (CAPD), blood cultures, or skin isolates from patients with acne [180]. Interestingly, *msr*(A) was the most common erythromycin-resistance determinant in strains from CAPD patients (44.4%), occurring alone in 11 or in conjunction with an *erm* determinant in 1 of 27 isolates. Ten of 28 isolates from blood cultures (35.7%) and 43 of 117 isolates from acne patients (41.0%) also harbored the *msr*(A) gene. Whether the high percentage was due to dissemination of a clone is not known.

A study of 124 macrolide-resistant *S. aureus* strains isolated in the United States between 1987 and 1994 found only 1 (0.8%) isolate with a MS_B phenotype [129]. Among 144 macrolide-resistant *S. aureus* and 150 coagulase-negative staphylococci from 32 French hospitals, 2.1% and 16% harbored *msr*(A) alone or in conjunction with *erm*(A), *erm*(C), or *lnu*(A) (lincosamide nucleotidyltransferase, formerly *linA* and *linA'*) [181]. A European study detected *msr*(A) in 13% of the *S. aureus* isolates collected from 1997 to 1998 and only in strains that were methicillin-susceptible; coagulase-negative staphylococci were not evaluated [61]. A study with 73 erythromycin-resistant *S. aureus* and 142 *S. epidermidis* strains primarily from Canada found 2.7% and 5.6% of the strains to harbor *msr*(A), respectively [182].

msr(B) from *Staphylococcus xylosus* is nearly identical to the carboxy-terminal half of *msr*(A) and has been reclassified as *msr*(A) [2, 183]. *msr*(C) is a recently described gene in *E. faecium* that has 53% identity with *msr*(A) at the nucleotide level [62, 184]. This gene is species-specific and chromosomally encoded and may be, in part, responsible for the eight-fold higher MIC_{50}s observed in "susceptible" isolates of *E. faecium versus* other enterococcal isolates [62, 184, 185]. If *msr*(C) is disrupted in *E. faecium*, there is a two- to eight-fold decrease in MICs of macrolides and quinnupristin [184]. Since *msr*(C) is found in susceptible and resistant isolates alone or in conjunction with other known resistance determinants (*erm*(B) primarily), its role in macrolide resistance remains to be clarified.

Strains that produce oleandomycin also contain homologs (*ole*(B) and *ole*(C)), carbomycin (*car*(A)), spiramycin (*srm*(B)), and tylosin (*tlr*(C)) that are part of the superfamily of ABC transporters, presumably as part of their self-protection armamenterium [186–188]. Not all these genes confer macrolide resistance when cloned into a heterologous host. *srm*(B) appears capable of conferring antibiotic resistance in *Streptomyces griseofuscus,* while *car*(A) requires additional up-stream nucleotide sequences [188]. The *tlr*(C) gene does not confer resistance to tylosin when cloned in *S. lividans*. In *S. antibioticus*, Ole(B) is part of the biosynthetic pathway, transporting the final intracellular product, oleandomycin glycosylated at the 2'-OH of desosamine, into the extracellular medium. The cloning of either the N- or C-terminal ATP-binding domains of *ole*(B) can confer oleandomycin resistance in a heterologous host [187]. The Ole(C) protein has a single membrane-spanning domain fused to an ATP-binding domain and can confer oleandomycin resistance [186].

Interestingly, *ertX*, a gene encoding a putative ABC transporter from *S. erythraea*, was cloned using PCR primers designed to a conserved region of *tlr*(C) and *car*(A) [189]. Unlike the other transporters discussed, this gene did not confer resistance to erythromycin or other 14- and 16-membered macrolides when introduced into heterologous hosts (*S. lividans* or *Streptomyces albus*) or in its native host, *S. erythraea*. Although the expression of *ertX* in *S. erythraea* was not reported, *ertX*-specific mRNA was not seen in *S. albus*.

Miscellaneous resistance determinants

Evidence for a multi-drug-resistant pump in *Campylobacter jejuni* was surmised by analysis of mutants that were obtained by passage on gradient plates containing either pefloxacin or cefotaxime [190]. Both mutants showed cross-resistance to erythromycin, chloramphenicol, tetracycline, β-lactams, and quinolones [190, 191]. The multi-drug-resistance phenotype of both strains appeared to result from the overexpression of two proteins of 55 (putative outer membrane component) and 39 kDa (putative membrane fusion component) that were absent from the outer membranes of the wild type. Although accumulation of erythromycin was not studied, comparison of the uptake of quinolones at steady state suggested that the mutants took up less compound than their parent and that the addition of carbonyl cyanide *m*-chlorophenylhydrazone (CCCP) completely eliminated the differences in uptake between mutants and parent.

A putative efflux pump *mreA* from an *S. agalactiae* strain conferred resistance to 14-, 15-, and 16-membered macrolides when cloned and expressed in *E. coli* [192]. All *E. coli* clones containing *mreA* accumulated significantly less erythromycin than did strains containing vector alone. The sequencing revealed a hydrophilic protein with no obvious homology to known transporters but with homology to *ribC*, a riboflavin kinase from *B. subtilis*. *mreA* appears to be in all isolates of *S. agalactiae* organized in the same manner as *ribC* on the *B. subtilis* chromosome, between *truB* and *arsC* [193]. The more recent investigators did not find that expression of *mreA* in a Gram-positive host, such as *E. faecalis* JH2–2 or *S. aureus* RN4220, conferred erythromycin resistance. Thus, it appears that *mreA* is a housekeeping gene and is not likely responsible for macrolide resistance in its original host strain.

Permeability in *M. tuberculosis* and *M. smegmatis* can be altered by changing the synthesis of inositol, an important component in lipoarabinomannan in the cell envelope. Mutations in *impA*, the gene-encoding inositol monophosphate phosphatase, render *M. smegmatis* more resistant to chloramphenicol, erythromycin, norfloxacin, and chenodeoxycholate but more susceptible to isoniazid and some hydrophilic β-lactams [194].

A temperature-sensitive mutant of *S. aureus* that harbors a temperature-sensitive mutation in the essential gene *yycF* (E63K) is hyper-susceptible to macrolides and lincosamides even at permissive temperature [195]. YycF is a response regulator of the two-component regulatory system *yycFG* and is conserved in Gram-positive bacteria. The hyper-susceptibility of the *yycF* mutant to ML antibiotics manifests itself most dramatically when the strain contains *erm*(C), with an MIC of 16 or 0.25 μg/ml *versus* >1 mg/ml to erythromycin and lincomycin/clindamycin HCl, respectively. However, there is little differential susceptibility to clindamycin phosphate, and the addition of phosphate (100 μM) to the medium increases lincomycin resistance to > 1 mg/ml but does not impact erythromycin susceptibility. It is unclear whether the homology of *yycF* to the *phoB* subfamily of response regulators plays a role in phosphate suppression of hyper-susceptibility. Further, the addition of 2 ng/ml of linoleic acid lowered the MICs to erythromycin a further 64-fold. In the absence of *erm*(C), the parental strain is four-fold more resistant to erythromycin than the temperature-sensitive mutant. It would be interesting to know how YycF and/or YycG abrogate resistance, especially in the presence of *erm*(C).

Conclusions

There are multiple mechanisms that confer resistance to macrolides and multiple themes are used by pathogenic bacteria. The most important resistant determinants from a Gram-positive clinical arena are the widespread Erm methylases and the Mef efflux pump. However, resistance due to the Msr(A) pump is increasing in both coagulase-negative and -positive staphylococci. In Gram-negative bacteria such as *H. influenzae and N. gonorhoeae*, intrinsic pumps of the RND family prevent ready access of the macrolides to 23S rRNA. In the atypical pathogens, target mutations in either A2058 or A2059 are found in the majority of resistant isolates. The role that 23S rRNA and ribosomal protein mutations play as the sole resistance determinant or as a part of a synergistic resistance in species like *S. pneumoniae* is not clear. Research to elucidate different resistant phenotypes will continue to play an important role in defining the structure-activity relationships of novel macrolides designed to overcome resistance.

References

1 Kaneko T, McArthur H, Sutcliffe J (2000) Recent developments in the area of macrolide antibiotics. *Exp Opin Ther Patents* 10: 403–425

2 Roberts MC, Sutcliffe J, Courvalin P, Jensen LB, Rood J, Seppala H (1999) Nomenclature for macrolide and macrolide-lincosamide-streptogramin B resistance determinants. *Antimicrob Agents Chemother* 43: 2823–2830

3 Sutcliffe J, Mueller J, Utt E (1999) Antibiotic resistance mechanisms of bacterial pathogens. In *Manual of industrial microbiology and biotechnology* (AL Demain, JE Davies, (eds)): ASM Press, Washington, D.C. 759–788

4 Weisblum B (2000) Resistance to macrolide-lincosamide-streptogramin antibiotics. In: *Gram-positive pathogens* (V Fischetti, (ed)): ASM Press, Washington, D.C. 682–698

5 Kirillov S, Porse BT, Vester B, Woolley P, Garrett RA (1997) Movement of the 3'-end of tRNA through the peptidyl transferase centre and its inhibition by antibiotics. *FEBS Lett* 406: 223–233

6 Rodriguez-Fonseca C, Amils R, Garrett RA (1995) Fine structure of the peptidyl transferase centre on 23 S-like rRNAs deduced from chemical probing of antibiotic-ribosome complexes. *J Mol Biol* 247: 224–235

7 Verdier L, Bertho G, Gharbi-Benarous J, Girault J-P (2000) Lincomycin and clindamycin conformations. A fragment shared by macrolides, ketolides and lincosamides determined from TRNOE ribosome-bound conformations. *Bioorg Med Chem* 8: 1225–1243

8 Sor F, Fukuhara H (1982) Identification of two erythromycin resistance mutations in the mitochondrial gene coding for the large ribosomal RNA in yeast. *Nucleic Acid Res* 10: 6571–6577

9 Vester B, Douthwaite S (2000) Macrolide resistance conferred by base substitutions in 23S rRNA. *Antimicrob Agents Chemother* 45: 1–12

10 Fu W, Anderson M, Williams S, Tait-Kamradt A, Sutcliffe J, Retsema J (2000) *In vitro* derived macrolide resistant *Streptococcus pneumoniae* strains have ribosomal mechanism of resistance, abst. 07–10. In Program and abstracts of the 5th International Conference on Macrolides, Azalides, Streptogramins, Ketolides, and Oxazolidinones, Seville, Spain, 65

11 Tait-Kamradt A, Davies T, Appelbaum PC, Depardieu F, Courvalin P, Petitpas J, Wondrack L, Walker A, Jacobs MR, Sutcliffe J (2000) Two new mechanisms of macrolide resistance in clinical strains of *Streptococcus pneumoniae* from Eastern Europe and North America. *Antimicrob Agents Chemother* 44: 3395–3401

12 Tait-Kamradt A, Davies T, Cronan M, Jacobs MR, Appelbaum PC, Sutcliffe J (2000) Mutations in 23S rRNA and L4 ribosomal protein account for resistance in pneumococcal strains selected *in vitro* by macrolide passage. *Antimicrob Agents Chemother* 44: 2118–2125

13 Canu A, Malbruny B, Coquemont M, Davies TA, Appelbaum PC, Leclercq R (2000) Diversity of mutations in L22, L4 ribosomal proteins and 23S ribosomal RNA in pneumococcal mutants resistant to macrolides, telithromycin, and clindamycin selected *in vitro*, abst. 1927. In Program and abstracts of the 40th Interscience Conference on Antimicrobial Agents and Chemotherapy, Toronto, Ontario, Canada, 118

14 Chittum HS, Champney WS (1994) Ribosomal protein gene sequence changes in erythromycin-resistant mutants of *Escherichia coli*. *J Bacteriol* 176: 6192–6198

15 Pardo D, Rosset R (1974) Genetic studies of erythromycin resistant mutants of *Escherichia coli*. *Mol Gen Genet* 135: 257–268

16 Schnier J, Gewitz HS, Behrens SE, Lee A, Ginther C, Leighton T (1990) Isolation and characterization of *Bacillus stearothermophilus* 30S and 50S ribosomal protein mutations. *J Bacteriol* 172: 7306–7309

17 Sharrock RA, Leighton T, Wittmann HG (1981) Macrolide and aminoglycoside antibiotic resistance mutations in the *Bacillus subtilis* ribosome resulting in temperature-sensitive sporulation. *Mol Gen Genet* 183: 538–543

18 Tipper DJ, Johnson CW, Ginther CL, Leighton T, Wittmann HG (1977) Erythromycin resistant mutations in *Bacillus subtilis* cause temperature sensitive sporulation. *Mol Gen Genet* 150: 147–159

19 Weisblum B (1995) Erythromycin resistance by ribosome modification. *Antimicrob Agents Chemother* 39: 577–585

20 Wittmann HG, Stoffler G, Apirion D, Rosen L, Tanaka K, Tamaki M, Takata R, Dekio S, Otaka E (1973) Biochemical and genetic studies on two different types of erythromycin resistant mutants of *Escherichia coli* with altered ribosomal proteins. *Mol Gen Genet* 127: 175–189

21 Sutcliffe J, Tait-Kamradt A, Walker A, Petitpas J (2000) Macrolide resistance in pneumococci: Analysis of resistant isolates obtained by passage with telithromycin, abst. 1925. In Program and abstracts of the 40th Interscience Conference on Antimicrobial Agents and Chermotherapy, Toronto, Ontario, Canada, 117

22 Gregory ST, Dahlberg AE (1999) Erythromycin resistance mutations in ribosomal proteins L22 and L4 perturb the higher order structure of 23 S ribosomal RNA. *J Mol Biol* 289: 827–834

23 Ban N, Nissen P, Hansen J, Moore PB, Steitz TA (2000) The complete atomic structure of the large ribosomal subunit at 2.4 A resolution. *Science* 289: 905–920

24 Malbruny B, Canu A, Bozdogan B, Fantin B, Leclercq R (2000) Quinupristin/Dalfopristin Resistance Mutation Reveals the Involvement of L22 Ribosomal Protein in Synergy Between Quinupristin and Dalfopristin, abst. 1928. In Program and abstracts of the 40th Interscience Conference on Antimicrobial Agents and Chemotherapy, Toronto, Ontario, Canada, 118

25 Baranov PV, Kubarenko AV, Gurvich OL, Shamolina TA, Brimacombe R (1999) The Database of Ribosomal Cross-links: an update. *Nucleic Acids Res* 27: 184–185

26 Hansen HL, Mauvais P, Douthwaite S (1999) The macrolide-ketolide antibiotic binding site is formed by structures in domain II and V of 23S ribosomal RNA. *Mol Microbiol* 31: 623–631

27 Poulsen SM, Kofoed C, Vester B (2000) Inhibition of the ribosomal peptidyl transferase reaction by the mycarose moiety of the antibiotics carbomycin, spiramycin and tylosin. *J Mol Biol* 304: 471–481

28 Douthwaite S, Hansen LH, Mauvais P (2000) Macrolide-ketolide inhibition of MLS-resistant ribosomes is improved by alternative drug interaction with domain II of 23S rRNA. *Mol Microbiol* 36: 183–193

29 Xiong L, Shah S, Mauvais P, Mankin AS (1999) A ketolide resistance mutation in domain II of 23S rRNA reveals the proximity of hairpin 35 to the peptidyl transferase centre. *Mol Microbiol* 31: 633–639

30 Mankin A (2000) Interaction of Macrolides with the Ribosome, abst. 1132. In Program and abstracts of the 40th Interscience Conference on Antimicrobial Agents and Chemotherapy, Toronto, Ontario, Canada, 534

31 Asai T, Condon C, Voulgaris J, Zaporojets D, Shen B, Al-Omar M, Squires C, Squires CL (1999) Construction and initial characterization of *Escherichia coli* strains with few or no intact chromosomal rRNA operons. *J Bacteriol* 181: 3803–3809

32 Ettayebi M, Prasad SM, Morgan EA (1985) Chloramphenicol-erythromycin resistance mutations in a 23S rRNA gene of *Escherichia coli*. *J Bacteriol* 162: 551–557

33 Douthwaite S, Aagaard C (1993) Erythromycin binding is reduced in ribosomes with conformational alterations in the 23 S rRNA peptidyl transferase loop. *J Mol Biol* 232: 725–731

34 Douthwaite S (1992) Functional interactions within 23S rRNA involving the peptidyltransferase center. *J Bacteriol* 174: 1333–1338

35 Douthwaite S, Prince JB, Noller HF (1985) Evidence for functional interaction between domains II and V of 23S ribosomal RNA from an erythromycin-resistant mutant. *Proc Natl Acad Sci USA* 82: 8330–8334

36 Tenson T, DeBlasio A, Mankin A (1996) A functional peptide encoded in the *Escherichia coli* 23S rRNA. *Proc Natl Acad Sci USA* 93: 5641–5646

37 Tenson T, Xiong L, Kloss P, Mankin AS (1997) Erythromycin resistance peptides selected from random peptide libraries. *J Biol Chem* 272: 17425–17430

38 Dam M, Douthwaite S, Tenson T, Mankin AS (1996) Mutations in domain II of 23 S rRNA facilitate translation of a 23 S rRNA-encoded pentapeptide conferring erythromycin resistance. *J Mol Biol* 259: 1–6

39 Tripathi S, Kloss PS, Mankin AS (1998) Ketolide resistance conferred by short peptides. *J Biol Chem* 273: 20073–20077

40 Chabbert Y (1956) Antagonisme in vitro entre l'erythromycine et la spiramycine. *Ann Inst Pasteur (Paris)* 90: 787–790

41 Garrod LP (1957) The erythromycin group of antibiotics. *Br Med J* 2: 57–63

42 Jones WF, Nichols RF, Finland M (1966) Development of resistance and cross-resistance *in vitro* to erythromycin, carbomycin, oleandomycin and streptogramin. *Proc Soc Experiment Biol Med* 93: 388–393

43 Fernandez-Munoz R, Monro RE, Torres-Pinedo R, Vazquez D (1971) Substrate- and antibiotic-binding sites at the peptidyl-transferase centre of *Escherichia coli* ribosomes. Studies on the chloramphenicol, lincomycin and erythromycin sites. *Eur J Biochem* 23: 185–193

44 Moazed D, Noller HF (1987) Chloramphenicol, erythromycin, carbomycin and vernamycin B protect overlapping sites in the peptidyl transferase region of 23S ribosomal RNA. *Biochimie* 69: 879-884

45 Sander P, Prammananan T, Meier A, Frischkorn K, Böttger EC (1997) The role of ribosomal RNAs in macrolide resistance. *Mol Microbiol* 26: 469-480

46 Pernodet JL, Fish S, Blondelet-Rouault MH, Cundliffe E (1996) The macrolide-lincosamide-streptogramin B resistance phenotypes characterized by using a specifically deleted, antibiotic-sensitive strain of *Streptomyces lividans*. *Antimicrob Agents Chemother* 40: 581–585

47 Capobianco JO, Cao Z, Shortridge VD, Ma Z, Flamm RK, Zhong P (2000) Studies of the novel ketolide ABT-773: transport, binding to ribosomes, and inhibition of protein synthesis in *Streptococcus pneumoniae*. *Antimicrob Agents Chemother* 44: 1562–1567

48 Denis A, Agouridas C, Auger JM, Benedetti Y, Bonnefoy A, Bretin F, Chantot JF, Dussarat A, Fromentin C, D'Ambrieres SG, Lachaud S, Laurin P, Le Martret O, Loyau V, Tessot N, Pejac JM, Perron S (1999) Synthesis and antibacterial activity of HMR 3647 a new ketolide highly potent against erythromycin-resistant and susceptible pathogens. *Bioorg Med Chem Lett* 9: 3075–3080

49 Goldman RC, Kadam SK (1989) Binding of novel macrolide structures to macrolides-lincosamides-streptogramin B-resistant ribosomes inhibits protein synthesis and bacterial growth. *Antimicrob Agents Chemother* 33: 1058–1066

50 Arthur M, Brisson-Noel A, Courvalin P (1987) Origin and evolution of genes specifying resistance to macrolide, lincosamide and streptogramin antibiotics: data and hypotheses. *J Antimicrob Chemother* 20: 783–802

51 Seppala H, Skurnik M, Soini H, Roberts MC, Huovinen P (1998) A novel erythromycin resistance methylase gene (*ermTR*) in *Streptococcus pyogenes*. *Antimicrob Agents Chemother* 42: 257–262

52 Cundliffe E (1992) Self-protection mechanisms in antibiotic producers. *Ciba Found Symp* 171: 199-208

53 Hara Q, Hutchinson CR (1990) Cloning of midecamycin (MLS)-resistance genes from *Streptomyces mycarofaciens, Streptomyces lividans* and *Streptomyces coelicolor* A3. *J Antibiot* 43: 977–991

54 Pereda A, Summers R, Katz L (1997) Nucleotide sequence of the *ermE* distal flank of the erythromycin biosynthesis cluster in *Saccharopolyspora erythraea*. *Gene* 193: 65–71

55 Fouces R, Mellando E, Diez B, Barredo JL (1999) The tylosin biosynthetic cluster from *Streptomyces fradiae*: genetic organization of the left region. *Microbiology* 145: 855–868

56 Liu M, Kirpekar F, Van Wezel GP, Douthwaite S (2000) The tylosin resistance gene *tlrB* of *Streptomyces fradiae* encodes a methyltransferase that targets G748 in 23S rRNA. *Mol Microbiol* 37: 811–820

57 Gustafsson C, Persson BC (1998) Identification of the *rrmA* gene encoding the 23S rRNA m^1G745 methyltransferase in *Escherichia coli* and characterization of an m^1G745-deficient mutant. *J Bacteriol* 180: 359-365

58 Pernodet JL, Gourmelen A, Blondelet-Rouault MH, Cundliffe E (1999) Dispensable ribosomal resistance to spiramycin conferred by *srmA* in the spiramycin producer *Streptomyces ambofaciens. Microbiology* 145: 2355–2364

59 Arisawa A, Tsunekawa H, Okamura K, Okamoto R (1995) Nucleotide sequence analysis of the carbomycin biosynthetic genes including the 3-O-acyltransferase gene from *Streptomyces thermotolerans. Biosci Biotechnol Biochem* 59: 582–588

60 Quiros LM, Aguirrezabalaga I, Olano C, Mendez C, Salas JA (1998) Two glycosyltransferases and a glycosidase are involved in oleandomycin modification during its biosynthesis by *Streptomyces antibioticus. Mol Microbiol* 28: 1177–1185

61 Schmitz FJ, Sadurski R, Kray A, Boos M, Geisel R, Kohrer K, Verhoef J, Fluit AC (2000) Prevalence of macrolide-resistance genes in *Staphylococcus aureus* and *Enterococcus faecium* isolates from 24 European university hospitals. *J Antimicrob Chemother* 45: 891–894

62 Portillo A, Ruiz-Larrea F, Zarazaga M, Alonso A, Martinez JL, Torres C (2000) Macrolide resistance genes in *Enterococcus* spp. *Antimicrob Agents Chemother* 44: 967–971

63 Syrogiannopoulos GA, Grivea IN, Tait-Kamradt A, Katopodis GD, Beratis NG, Sutcliffe J, Appelbaum PC, Davies TD (2000) Identification of *erm*(A) Erythromycin Resistance Methylase Gene in *Streptococcus pneumoniae* Isolated in Greece. *Antimicrob Agents Chemother* 45: 342–344

64 Felsenstein J (1988) Phylogenies from molecular sequences: inference and reliability. *Annu Rev Genet* 22: 521–565

65 Yu L, Petros AM, Schnuchel A, Zhong P, Severin JM, Walter K, Holzman TF, Fesik SW (1997) Solution structure of an rRNA methyltransferase (ErmAM) that confers macrolide-lincosamide-streptogramin antibiotic resistance. *Nat Struct Biol* 4: 483–489

66 Schluckebier G, Zhong P, Stewart KD, Kavanaugh TJ, Abad-Zapatero C (1999) The 2.2 A structure of the rRNA methyltransferase ErmC' and its complexes with cofactor and cofactor analogs: implications for the reaction mechanism. *J Mol Biol* 289: 277–291

67 Bussiere DE, Muchmore SW, Dealwis CG, Schluckebier G, Nienaber VL, Edalji RP, Walter KA, Ladror US, Holzman TF, Abad-Zapatero C (1998) Crystal structure of ErmC', an rRNA methyltransferase which mediates antibiotic resistance in bacteria. *Biochemistry* 37: 7103–7112

68 Clancy J, Schmieder BJ, Petitpas JW, Manousos M, Williams JA, Faiella JA, Girard AE, McGuirk PR (1995) Assays to detect and characterize synthetic agents that inhibit the ErmC methyltransferase. *J Antibiot* 48: 1273–1279

69 Hanessian S, Sgarbi PWM (2000) Design and synthesis of mimics of S-adenosyl-L-homocysteine as potential inhibitors of erythromycin methyltransferases. *Bioorg Med Chem Lett* 10: 433–437

70 Hajduk PJ, Dinges J, Schkeryantz JM, Janowick D, Kaminski M, Tufano M, Augeri DJ, Petros A, Nienaber V, Zhong P, Hammond R, Coen M, Beutel B, Katz L, Fesik SW (1999) Novel inhibitors of Erm methyltransferases from NMR and parallel synthesis. *J Med Chem* 42: 3852–3859

71 Horinouchi S, Weisblum B (1980) Posttranscriptional modification of mRNA conformation: mechanism that regulates erythromycin-induced resistance. *Proc Natl Acad Sci USA* 77: 7079-7083

72 Gryczan TJ, Grandi G, Hahn J, Grandi R, Dubnau D (1980) Conformational alteration of mRNA structure and the posttranscriptional regulation of erythromycin-induced drug resistance. *Nucleic Acids Res* 8: 6081–6097

73 Rosato A, Vicarini H, Leclercq R (1999) Inducible or constitutive expression of resistance in clinical isolates of streptococci and enterococci cross-resistant to erythromycin and lincomycin. *J Antimicrob Chemother* 43: 559-562

74 Weisblum B (1995) Insights into erythromycin action from studies of its activity as inducer of resistance. *Antimicrob Agents Chemother* 39: 797–805

75 Sandler P, Weisblum B (1989) Erythromycin-induced ribosome stall in the *ermA* leader: a barricade to 5'-to-3' nucleolytic cleavage of the *ermA* transcript. *J Bacteriol* 171: 6680–6688

76 Bechhofer DH, Dubnau D (1987) Induced mRNA stability in *Bacillus subtilis. Proc Natl Acad Sci USA* 84: 498–502

77 Denoya CD, Bechhofer DH, Dubnau D (1986) Translational autoregulation of *ermC* 23S rRNA methyltransferase expression in *Bacillus subtilis. J Bacteriol* 168: 1133–1141

78 Horinouchi S, Byeon W-H, Weisblum B (1983) A complex attenuator regulates inducible resistance to macrolides, lincosamides, and streptogramin type B antibiotics in *Streptococcus sanguis. J Bacteriol* 154: 1252–1262
79 Monod M, Mohan S, Dubnau D (1987) Cloning and analysis of *ermG*, a new macrolide-lincosamide-streptogramin B resistance element from *Bacillus sphaericus. J Bacteriol* 169: 340–350
80 Kwak JH, Choi EC, Weisblum B (1991) Transcriptional attenuation control of *erm*K, a macrolide-lincosamide- streptogramin B resistance determinant from *Bacillus licheniformis. J Bacteriol* 173: 4725–4735
81 Choi SS, Kim SK, Oh TG, Choi EC (1997) Role of mRNA termination in regulation of *ermK. J Bacteriol* 179: 2065–2067
82 Gryczan T, Israeli-Reches M, Del Bue M, Dubnau D (1984) DNA sequence and regulation of *ermD*, a macrolide-lincosamide-streptogramin B resistance element from *Bacillus licheniformis. Mol Gen Genet* 194: 349-356
83 Kamimiya S, Weisblum B (1988) Translational attenuation control of *ermSF*, an inducible resistance determinant encoding rRNA N-methyltransferase from *Streptomyces fradiae. J Bacteriol* 170: 1800–1811
84 Kelemen GH, Zalacain M, Culebras E, Seno ET, Cundliffe E (1994) Transcriptional attenuation control of the tylosin-resistance gene *tlrA* in *Streptomyces fradiae. Mol Microbiol* 14: 833–842
85 Lampson BC, Parisi JT (1986) Naturally occurring *Staphylococcus epidermidis* plasmid expressing constitutive macrolide-lincosamide-streptogramin B resistance contains a deleted attenuator. *J Bacteriol* 166: 479-483
86 Martin B, Alloing G, Mejean V, Claverys JP (1987) Constitutive expression of erythromycin resistance mediated by the *ermAM* determinant of plasmid pAM beta 1 results from deletion of 5' leader peptide sequences. *Plasmid* 18: 250–253
87 Tannock GW, Luchansky JB, Miller L, Connell H, Thode-Andersen S, Mercer AA, Klaenhammer TR (1994) Molecular characterization of a plasmid-borne (pGT633) erythromycin resistance determinant (*ermGT*) from *Lactobacillus reuteri* 100–63. *Plasmid* 31: 60–71
88 Oliveira SS, Murphy E, Gamon MR, Bastos MC (1993) pRJ5: a naturally occurring *Staphylococcus aureus* plasmid expressing constitutive macrolide-lincosamide-streptogramin B resistance contains a tandem duplication in the leader region of the *ermC* gene. *J Gen Microbiol* 139 (Pt 7): 1461–1467
89 Lodder G, Werckenthin C, Schwarz S, Dyke K (1997) Molecular analysis of naturally occuring *ermC*-encoding plasmids in staphylococci isolated from animals with and without previous contact with macrolide/lincosamide antibiotics. *FEMS Immun Med Microbiol* 18: 7–15
90 Leclercq R, Bauduret F, Soussy CJ (1989) Selection of constitutive mutants of gram-positive cocci inducible resistant to macrolides, lincosamides and streptogramins (MLS): comparison of the selective effects of the MLS. *Pathol Biol (Paris)* 37: 568–572
91 Hahn J, Grandi G, Gryczan TJ, Dubnau D (1982) Translational attenuation of *ermC*: a deletion analysis. *Mol Gen Genet* 186: 204–216
92 Watanakunakorn C (1976) Clindamycin therapy of *Staphylococcus aureus* endocarditis. Clinical relapse and development of resistance to clindamycin, lincomycin and erythromycin. *Am J Med* 60: 419-425
93 Kamimiya S, Weisblum B (1997) Induction of ermSV by 16-membered-ring macrolide antibiotics. *Antimicrob Agents Chemother* 41: 530–534
94 Oh TG, Kwon AR, Choi EC (1998) Induction of *ermAMR* from a clinical strain of *Enterococcus faecalis* by 16-membered-ring macrolide antibiotics. *J Bacteriol* 180: 5788–5791
95 Bonnefoy A, Girard AM, Agouridas C, Chantot JF (1997) Ketolides lack inducibility properties of MLS(B) resistance phenotype. *J Antimicrob Chemother* 40: 85–90
96 Zhong P, Cao Z, Hammond R, Chen Y, Beyer J, Shortridge VD, Phan LY, Pratt S, Capobianco J, Reich KA, Flamm RK, Or YS, Katz L (1999) Induction of ribosome methylation in MLS-resistant *Streptococcus pneumoniae* by macrolides and ketolides. *Microb Drug Resist* 5: 183–188
97 Saito T, Shimizu M, Mitsuhashi S (1971) Macrolide resistance in staphylococci. *Ann New York Acad Sci* 182: 267–278
98 Sutcliffe J, Tait-Kamradt A, Brennan L, Duignan J, Wondrack L, Walker A, Baima E, Mueller J (2000) Heterogeneous ketolide resistance in *erm*(B)$^+$ *Streptococcus pneumoniae* strains, abst.

1926. In Program and abstracts of the 40th Interscience Conference on Antimicrobial Agents and Chemotherapy, p. 117, Toronto, Ontario, Canada
99 Marshall VP, Cialdella JI, Baczynskyj L, Liggett WF, Johnson RA (1989) Microbial O-phosphorylation of macrolide antibiotics. *J Antibiot* 42: 132–134
100 Wiley PF, Baczynskyj L, Dolak LA, Cialdella JI, Marshall VP (1987) Enzymatic phosphorylation of macrolide antibiotics. *J Antibiot* 40: 195–201
101 Marshall VP, Liggett WF, Cialdella JI (1989) Enzymic inactivation of lincosaminide and macrolide antibiotics: divalent metal cation and coenzyme specificities. *J Antibiot* 42: 826–830
102 Katayama J, Okada H, O'Hara K, Noguchi N (1998) Isolation and characterization of two plasmids that mediate macrolide resistance in *Escherichia coli*: transferability and molecular properties. *Biol Pharm Bull* 21: 326–329
103 Katayama J, Noguchi N (1999) Nucleotide sequence of the gene cluster containing the *mphB* gene for macrolide 2'-phosphotransferase II. *Biol Pharm Bull* 22: 227–228
104 Kim S-K, Baek M-C, Choi S-S, Kim B-K, Choi E-C (1996) Nucleotide sequence, expression and transcriptional analysis of the *Escherichia coli mphK* gene encoding macrolide-phosphotransferase K. *Mol Cells* 6: 153–160
105 Kono M, O'Hara K, Ebisu T (1992) Purification and characterization of macrolide 2'-phosphotransferase type II from a strain of *Escherichia coli* highly resistant to macrolide antibiotics. *FEMS Microbiol Lett* 76: 89-94
106 Leclercq R, Courvalin P (1991) Bacterial resistance to macrolide, lincosamide, and streptogramin antibiotics by target modification. *Antimicrob Agents Chemother* 35: 1267–1272
107 Leclercq R, Courvalin P (1991) Intrinsic and unusual resistance to macrolide, lincosamide, and streptogramin antibiotics in bacteria. *Antimicrob Agents Chemother* 35: 1273–1276
108 Matsuoka M, Endou K, Kobayashi H, Inoue M, Nakajima Y (1997) A dyadic plasmid that shows MLS and PMS resistance in *Staphylococcus aureus. FEMS Microbiol Lett* 148: 91–96
109 Matsuoka M, Endou K, Kobayashi H, Inoue M, Nakajima Y (1998) A plasmid that encodes three genes for resistance to macrolide antibiotics in *Staphylococcus aureus. FEMS Microbiol Lett* 167: 221–227
110 Noguchi N, Emura A, Matsuyama H, O'Hara K, Sasatsu M, Kono M (1995) Nucleotide sequence and characterization of erythromycin resistance determinant that encodes macrolide 2'-phosphotransferase I in *Escherichia coli. Antimicrob Agents Chemother* 39: 2359-2363
111 Noguchi N, Katayama J, O'Hara K (1996) Cloning and nucleotide sequence of the *mphB* gene for macrolide 2'- phosphotransferase II in *Escherichia coli. FEMS Microbiol Lett* 144: 197–202
112 Noguchi N, Tamura Y, Katayama J, Narui K (1998) Expression of the *mphB* gene for macrolide 2'-phosphotransferase II from *Escherichia coli* in *Staphylococcus aureus. FEMS Microbiol Lett* 159: 337–342
113 Noguchi N, Katayama J (1998) Expression in *Pseudomonas aeruginosa* of an erythromycin-resistance determinant that encodes the *mphA* gene for macrolide 2'-phosphotransferase I from *Escherichia coli. Biol Pharm Bull* 21: 191–193
114 O'Hara K, Kanda T, Ohmiya K, Ebisu T, Kono M (1989) Purification and characterization of macrolide 2'-phosphotransferase from a strain of *Escherichia coli* that is highly resistant to erythromycin. *Antimicrob Agents Chemother* 33: 1354–1357
115 O'Hara K, Kawabe T, Taniguchi K, Nakamura A, Sawai T (1997) A new macrolide 2'phosphotransferase in *E. coli*, abst. C-67. In Program and abstracts of the 37th Interscience Conference on Antimicrobial Agents and Chemotherapy p. 57, Toronto, Ontario, Canada
116 O'Hara K, Yamamoto K (1996) Reaction of roxithromycin and clarithromycin with macrolide-inactivating enzymes from highly erythromycin-resistant *Escherichia coli. Antimicrob Agents Chemother* 40: 1036–1038
117 Taniguchi K, Nakamura A, Tsurubuchi K, Ishii A, O'Hara K, Sawai T (1999) Identification of functional amino acids in the macrolide 2'- phosphotransferase II. *Antimicrob Agents Chemother* 43: 2063–2065
118 Sutcliffe J, Grebe T, Tait-Kamradt A, Wondrack L (1996) Detection of erythromycin-resistant determinants by PCR. *Antimicrob Agents Chemother* 40: 2562–2566
119 Cheng J, Grebe T, Wondrack L, Courvalin P, Sutcliffe J (1999) Characterization of genes involved in erythromycin resistance in a clinical strain of *Staphylococcus aureus,* abst. 837. In

Program and abstracts of the 39th Interscience Conference on Antimicrobial Agents and Chemotherapy. p. 114, San Francisco, CA

120 Ainsa JA, Blokpoel MC, Otal I, Young DB, De Smet KA, Martin C (1998) Molecular cloning and characterization of Tap, a putative multidrug efflux pump present in *Mycobacterium fortuitum* and *Mycobacterium tuberculosis. J Bacteriol* 180: 5836–5843

121 Ross JI, Farrell AM, Eady EA, Cove JH, Cunliffe WJ (1989) Characterisation and molecular cloning of the novel macrolide-streptogramin B resistance determinant from *Staphylococcus epidermidis. J Antimicrob Chemother* 24: 851–862

122 Taniguchi K, Nakamura A, Tsurubuchi K, Ishii A, O'Hara K, Sawai T (1999) Appearance in Japan of highly macrolide-resistant *Escherchia coli* producing macrolide 2'-phosphotransferace II. *Microbios* 97: 137–144

123 Alonso A, Sanchez P, Martinez JL (2000) *Stenotrophomonas maltophilia* D457R contains a cluster of genes from Gram-positive bacteria involved in antibiotic and heavy metal resistance. *Antimicrob Agents Chemother* 44: 1778–1782

124 Yazawa K, Mikami Y, Sakamoto T, Ueno Y, Morisaki N, Iwasaki S, Furihata K (1994) Inactivation of the macrolide antibiotics erythromycin, midecamycin, and rokitamycin by pathogenic *Nocardia* species. *Antimicrob Agents Chemother* 38: 2197–2199

125 Arthur M, Autissier D, Courvalin P (1986) Analysis of the nucleotide sequence of the *ereB* gene encoding the erythromycin esterase type II. *Nucleic Acids Res* 14: 4987–4999

126 Ounissi H, Courvalin P (1985) Nucleotide sequence of the gene *ereA* encoding the erythromycin esterase in *Escherichia coli. Gene* 35: 271–278

127 Arthur M, Andremont A, Courvalin P (1987) Distribution of erythromycin esterase and rRNA methylase genes in members of the family *Enterobacteriaceae* highly resistant to erythromycin. *Antimicrob Agents Chemother* 31: 404–409

128 Plante I, Roy PH (1998) Sequencing and PCR mapping of integrons reveals a novel combination of resistance genes and an *ereA* gene cassette in the multiresistant strain *Providencia stuartii* 1723. *GenBank accession number X03988*

129 Wondrack L, Massa M, Yang BV, Sutcliffe J (1996) Clinical strain of *Staphylococcus aureus* inactivates and causes efflux of macrolides. *Antimicrob Agents Chemother* 40: 992–998

130 Barthelemy P, Autissier D, Gerbaud G, Courvalin P (1984) Enzymic hydrolysis of erythromycin by a strain of *Escherichia coli.* A new mechanism of resistance. *J Antibiot* 37: 1692–1696

131 Sasaki J, Mizoue K, Morimoto S, Omura S (1996) Microbial glycosylation of macrolide antibiotics by *Streptomyces hygroscopicus* ATCC 31080 and distribution of a macrolide glycosyl transferase in several *Streptomyces* strains. *J Antibiot* 49: 1110–1118

132 Jenkins G, Cundliffe E (1991) Cloning and characterization of two genes from *Streptomyces lividans* that confer inducible resistance to lincomycin and macrolide antibiotics. *Gene* 108: 55–62

133 Cundliffe E (1992) Resistance to macrolides and lincosamides in *Streptomyces lividans* and to aminoglycosides in *Micromonospora purpurea. Gene* 115: 75–84

134 Kuo MS, Chirby DG, Argoudelis AD, Cialdella JI, Coats JH, Marshall VP (1989) Microbial glycosylation of erythromycin A. *Antimicrob Agents Chemother* 33: 2089-2091

135 Schulman M, Doherty P, Arison B (1993) Microbial conversion of avermectins by *Saccharopolyspora erythraea*: glycosylation at C-4' and C-4". *Antimicrob Agents Chemother* 37: 1737–1741

136 Nikaido H (1998) Antibiotic resistance caused by gram-negative multidrug efflux pumps. *Clin Infect Dis* 27 Suppl 1: S32–S41

137 Germ M, Yoshihara E, Yoneyama H, Nakae T (1999) Interplay between the efflux pump and the outer membrane permeability barrier in fluorescent dye accumulation in *Pseudomonas aeruginosa. Biochem Biophys Res Commun* 261: 452–455

138 Li XZ, Zhang L, Poole K (2000) Interplay between the MexA-MexB-oprM multidrug efflux system and the outer membrane barrier in the multiple antibiotic resistance of *Pseudomonas aeruginosa. J Antimicrob Chemother* 45: 433–436

139 Saier J, M.H., Beaty JT, Goffeau A, Harley KT, Heijne WHM, Huang S-C, Jack DL, Jahn PS, Lew K, Liu J, Pao SS, Paulsen IT, Tseng T-T, Virk PS (1999) The major facilitator superfamily. *J Mol Microbiol Biotechnol* 1: 257–279

140 Zgurskaya HI, Nikaido H (1999) Bypassing the periplasm: reconstitution of the AcrAB multidrug efflux pump of *Escherichia coli*. *Proc Natl Acad Sci USA* 96: 7190–7195
141 Zgurskaya HI, Nikaido H (1999) AcrA is a highly asymmetric protein capable of spanning the periplasm. *J Mol Biol* 285: 409-420
142 Koronakis V, Sharff A, Koronakis E, Luisi B, Hughes C (2000) Crystal structure of the bacterial membrane protein TolC central to multidrug efflux and protein export. *Nature* 405: 914–919
143 Mine T, Morita Y, Kataoka A, Mizushima T, Tsuchiya T (1999) Expression in *Escherichia coli* of a new multidrug efflux pump, MexXY, from *Pseudomonas aeruginosa*. *Antimicrob Agents Chemother* 43: 415–417
144 Zhao Q, Li XZ, Srikumar R, Poole K (1998) Contribution of outer membrane efflux protein OprM to antibiotic resistance in *Pseudomonas aeruginosa* independent of MexAB. *Antimicrob Agents Chemother* 42: 1682–1688
145 Masuda N, Sakagawa E, Ohya S, Gotoh N, Tsujimoto H, Nishino T (2000) Contribution of the MexX-MexY-oprM efflux system to intrinsic resistance in *Pseudomonas aeruginosa*. *Antimicrob Agents Chemother* 44: 2242–2246
146 Zhang L, Li XZ, Poole K (2000) Multiple antibiotic resistance in *Stenotrophomonas maltophilia*: involvement of a multidrug efflux system. *Antimicrob Agents Chemother* 44: 287–293
147 Lucas CE, Hagman KE, Levin JC, Stein DC, Shafer WM (1995) Importance of lipooligosaccharide structure in determining gonococcal resistance to hydrophobic antimicrobial agents resulting from the *mtr* efflux system. *Mol Microbiol* 16: 1001–1009
148 De Rossi E, Branzoni M, Cantoni R, Milano A, Riccardi G, Ciferri O (1998) *mmr*, a *Mycobacterium tuberculosis* gene conferring resistance to small cationic dyes and inhibitors. *J Bacteriol* 180: 6068–6071
149 Edgar R, Bibi E (1997) MdfA, an *Escherichia coli* multidrug resistance protein with an extraordinarily broad spectrum of drug recognition. *J Bacteriol* 179: 2274–2280
150 Jager W, Kalinowski J, Puhler A (1997) A *Corynebacterium glutamicum* gene conferring multidrug resistance in the heterologous host *Escherichia coli*. *J Bacteriol* 179: 2449-2451
151 Edgar R, Bibi E (1999) A single membrane-embedded negative charge is critical for recognizing positively charged drugs by the *Escherichia coli* multidrug resistance protein MdfA. *EMBO J* 18: 822–832
152 Zheleznova EE, Markham P, Edgar R, Bibi E, Neyfakh AA, Brennan RG (2000) A structure-based mechanism for drug binding by multidrug transporters. *Trends Biochem Sci* 25: 39-43
153 Zheleznova EE, Markham PN, Neyfakh AA, Brennan RG (1999) Structural basis of multidrug recognition by BmrR, a transcription activator of a multidrug transporter. *Cell* 96: 353–362
154 Tait-Kamradt A, Clancy J, Cronan M, Dib-Hajj F, Wondrack L, Yuan W, Sutcliffe J (1997) *mefE* is necessary for the erythromycin-resistant M phenotype in *Streptococcus pneumoniae*. *Antimicrob Agents Chemother* 41: 2251–2255
155 Sutcliffe J, Tait-Kamradt A, Wondrack L (1996) *Streptococcus pneumoniae* and *Streptococcus pyogenes* resistant to macrolides but sensitive to clindamycin: a common resistance pattern mediated by an efflux system. *Antimicrob Agents Chemother* 40: 1817–1824
156 Clancy J, Petitpas J, Dib-Hajj F, Yuan W, Cronan M, Kamath AV, Bergeron J, Retsema JA (1996) Molecular cloning and functional analysis of a novel macrolide- resistance determinant, *mefA*, from *Streptococcus pyogenes*. *Mol Microbiol* 22: 867–879
157 Johnston NJ, De Azavedo JC, Kellner JD, Low DE (1998) Prevalence and characterization of the mechanisms of macrolide, lincosamide, and streptogramin resistance in isolates of *Streptococcus pneumoniae*. *Antimicrob Agents Chemother* 42: 2425–2426
158 Klugman KP, Capper T, Widdowson CA, Koornhof HJ, Moser W (1998) Increased activity of 16-membered lactone ring macrolides against erythromycin-resistant *Streptococcus pyogenes* and *Streptococcus pneumoniae*: characterization of South African isolates. *J Antimicrob Chemother* 42: 729-734
159 Limia A, Jimenez ML, Delgado T, Sanchez I, Lopez S, Lopez-Brea M (1998) Phenotypic characterization of erythromycin resistance in strains of the genus *Streptococcus* isolated from clinical specimens. *Rev Esp Quimioter* 11: 216–220
160 Setchanova L, Tomasz A (1999) Molecular characterization of penicillin-resistant *Streptococcus pneumoniae* isolates from Bulgaria. *J Clin Microbiol* 37: 638–648

161 Kataja J, Huovinen P, Skurnik M, Seppala H (1999) Erythromycin resistance genes in group A streptococci in Finland. The Finnish Study Group for Antimicrobial Resistance. *Antimicrob Agents Chemother* 43: 48–52

162 Orden B, Perez-Trallero E, Montes M, Martinez R (1998) Erythromycin resistance of *Streptococcus pyogenes* in Madrid. *Pediatr Infect Dis J* 17: 470–473

163 Perez-Trallero E, Urbieta M, Montes M, Ayestaran I, Marimon JM (1998) Emergence of *Streptococcus pyogenes* strains resistant to erythromycin in Gipuzkoa, Spain. *Eur J Clin Microbiol Infec Dis* 17: 25–31

164 de Azavedo JC, Yeung RH, Bast DJ, Duncan CL, Borgia SB, Low DE (1999) Prevalence and mechanisms of macrolide resistance in clinical isolates of group A streptococci from Ontario, Canada. *Antimicrob Agents Chemother* 43: 2144–2147

165 Kataja J, Seppala H, Skurnik M, Sarkkinen H, Huovinen P (1998) Different erythromycin resistance mechanisms in group C and group G streptococci. *Antimicrob Agents Chemother* 42: 1493–1494

166 Luna VA, Cousin S, Jr., Whittington WL, Roberts MC (2000) Identification of the conjugative mef gene in clinical *Acinetobacter junii* and *Neisseria gonorrhoeae isolates. Antimicrob Agents Chemother* 44: 2503–2506

167 Luna VA, Coates P, Eady EA, Cove JH, Nguyen TT, Roberts MC (1999) A variety of gram-positive bacteria carry mobile *mef* genes. *J Antimicrob Chemother* 44: 19-25

168 Santagati M, Iannelli F, Oggioni MR, Stefani S, Pozzi G (2000) Characterization of a genetic element carrying the macrolide efflux gene *mef*(A) in *Streptococcus pneumoniae. Antimicrob Agents Chemother* 44: 2585–2587

169 Gay K, Stephens DS (2001) Structure and dissemination of a chromosomal insertion element encoding macrolide efflux in *Streptococcus pneumoniae J Infect Dis* 184: 56–65

170 Brennan L, Duignan J, Petitpas J, Anderson M, Fu W, Retsema J, Rainville J, Smyth D, Su W, Sutcliffe J (1998) CP-544372: MIC90 studies and killing kinetics against key respiratory tract pathogens, abst. F-124. In Program and abstracts of the 38th Interscience Conference on Antimicrobial Agents and Chemotherapy p. 264, San Diego, California USA

171 Arpin C, Daube H, Tessier F, Quentin C (1999) Presence of *mefA* and *mefE* Genes in *Streptococcus agalactiae. Antimicrob Agents Chemother* 43: 944–946

172 Poutanen SM, de Azavedo J, Willey BM, Low DE, MacDonald KS (1999) Molecular characterization of multidrug resistance in *Streptococcus mitis. Antimicrob Agents Chemother* 43: 1505–1507

173 Fraimow H, Knob C (1997) Amplification of macrolide efflux pumps *msr* and *mef* from *Enterococcus faecium* by polymerase chain reaction. In 98th General Meeting of the American Society for Microbiology p. 22, American Society for Microbiology, Miami Beach, Florida

174 Arpin C, Canron MH, Noury P, Quentin C (1999) Emergence of *mefA* and *mefE* genes in beta-haemolytic streptococci and pneumococci in France. *J Antimicrob Chemother* 44: 133–134

175 Perreten V, Schwarz F, Boeglin M, Cresta L, Dawen G, Teuber M (1997) Antibiotic resistance spread in food. *Nature* 389: 801–802

176 Sutcliffe J (1999) Resistance to macrolides mediated by efflux mechanisms. *Curr Opin Investig Drugs* 1: 403–412

177 Rosato A, H. V, Bonnefoy A, Chantot JF, Leclercq R (1998) A new ketolide, HMR 3004, active against streptococci inducibly resistant to erythromycin. *Antimicrob Agents Chemother* 42: 1392–1396

178 Jones PM, George AM (1999) Subunit interactions in ABC transporter: towards a functional architecture. *FEMS Microbiol Lett* 179: 187–202

179 Janosi L, Nakajima Y, Hashimoto H (1990) Characterization of plasmids that confer inducible resistance to 14-membered macrolides and streptogramin type B antibiotics in *Staphylococcus aureus. Microbiol Immunol* 34: 723–735

180 Eady EA, Ross JI, Tipper JL, Walters CE, Cove JH, Noble WC (1993) Distribution of genes encoding erythromycin ribosomal methylases and an erythromycin efflux pump in epidemiologically distinct groups of staphylococci. *J Antimicrob Chemother* 31: 211–217

181 Lina G, Quaglia A, Reverdy ME, Leclercq R, Vandenesch F, Etienne J (1999) Distribution of genes encoding resistance to macrolides, lincosamides, and streptogramins among staphylococci. *Antimicrob Agents Chemother* 43: 1062–1066

182 Martineau F, Picard FJ, Lansac N, Menard C, Roy PH, Ouellette M, Bergeron MG (2000) Correlation between the resistance genotype determined by multiplex PCR assays and the antibiotic susceptibility patterns of *Staphylococcus aureus* and *Staphylococcus epidermidis*. *Antimicrob Agents Chemother* 44: 231–238

183 Milton ED, Hewitt CL, Harwood CR (1992) Cloning and sequencing of a plasmid-mediated erythromycin determinant from *Staphylococcus xylosus*. *FEMS Microbiol Lett* 97: 141–147

184 Singh KV, Malathum K, Murray BE (2001) Disruption of an *Enterococcus faecium* species-specific gene, a homologue of acquired macrolide resistance genes of staphylococci, is associated with an increase in macrolide susceptibility. *Antimicrob Agents Chemother* 45: 263–266

185 Neu HC (1993) *Activity of macrolides against common pathogens in vitro*, Arnette, Blackwell, Paris, France

186 Rodríguez AM, Olano C, Vilches C, Méndez C, Salas JA (1993) *Streptomyces antibioticus* contains at least three oleandomycin-resistance determinants, one of which shows similarity with proteins of the ABC-transporter superfamily. *Mol Microbiol* 8: 571–582

187 Olano C, Rodríguez AM, Méndez C, Salas JA (1995) A second ABC transporter is involved in oleandomycin resistance and its secretion by *Streptomyces antibioticus*. *Mol Microbiol* 16: 333–343

188 Schoner B, Geistlich M, Rosteck JP, Rao RN, Seno E, Reynolds P, Cox K, Burgett S, Hershberger C (1992) Sequence similarity between macrolide-resistance determinants and ATP-binding transport proteins. *Gene* 115: 93–96

189 O'Neill MP, Eady EA, Radford A, Baumberg S, Cove JH (1995) The use of PCR to isolate a putative ABC transporter from *Saccharopolyspora erythraea*. *FEMS Microbiol Lett* 131: 189-195

190 Charvalos E, Tselentis Y, Hamzehpour Mm, Köhler T, Pechere J-C (1995) Evidence for an efflux pump in multidrug-resistant *Campylobacter jejuni*. *Antimicrob Agents Chemother* 39: 2019–2022

191 George AM (1996) Multidrug resistance in enteric and other gram-negative bacteria. *FEMS Microb Lett* 139: 1–10

192 Clancy J, Dib-Hajj F, Petitpas JW, Yuan W (1997) Cloning and characterization of a novel macrolide efflux gene, *mreA*, from *Streptococcus agalactiae*. *Antimicrob Agents Chemother* 41: 2719-2723

193 Gervais C, Leclercq R (1999) The macrolide resistance gene *mreA* is ubiquitous in this bacterial species, abst. 840. In Program and abstracts of the 39th Interscience Conference on Antimicrobial Agents and Chemotherapy, p. 115, San Franscisco, California

194 Parish T, Liu J, Nikaido H, Stoker NG (1997) A *Mycobacterium smegmatis* mutant with a defective inositol monophosphate phosphatase gene homolog has altered cell envelope permeability. *J Bacteriol* 179: 7827–7833

195 Martin PK, Li T, Sun D, Biek DP, Schmid MB (1999) Role in cell permeability of an essential two-component system in *Staphylococcus aureus*. *J Bacteriol* 181: 3666–3673

196 Hulten K, Gibreel A, Skold O, Engstrand L (1997) Macrolide resistance in *Helicobacter pylori*: mechanism and stability in strains from clarithromycin-treated patients. *Antimicrob Agents Chemother* 41: 2550–2553

197 Ross JI, Eady EA, Cove JH, Jones CE, Ratyal AH, Miller YW, Vyakrnam S, Cunliffe WJ (1997) Clinical resistance to erythromycin and clindamycin in cutaneous propionibacteria isolated from acne patients is associated with mutations in 23S rRNA. *Antimicrob Agents Chemother* 41: 1162–1165

198 Karlsson M, Fellstrom C, Heldtander MU, Johansson KE, Franklin A (1999) Genetic basis of macrolide and lincosamide resistance in *Brachyspira (Serpulina) hyodysenteriae*. *FEMS Microbiol Lett* 172: 255–260

199 Vester B, Garrett RA (1987) A plasmid-coded and site-directed mutation in *Escherichia coli* 23S RNA that confers resistance to erythromycin: implications for the mechanism of action of erythromycin. *Biochimie* 69: 891–900

200 Wang G, Taylor DE (1998) Site-specific mutations in the 23S rRNA gene of *Helicobacter pylori* confer two types of resistance to macrolide-lincosamide-streptogramin B antibiotics. *Antimicrob Agents Chemother* 42: 1952–1958

201 Wang G, Jiang Q, Taylor DE (1998) Genotypic characterization of clarithromycin-resistant and -susceptible *Helicobacter pylori* strains from the same patient demonstrates existence of two unrelated isolates. *J Clin Microbiol* 36: 2730–2731

202 Stone GG, Shortridge D, Versalovic J, Beyer J, Flamm RK, Graham DY, Ghoneim AT, Tanaka SK (1997) A PCR-oligonucleotide ligation assay to determine the prevalence of 23S rRNA gene mutations in clarithromycin-resistant *Helicobacter pylori*. *Antimicrob Agents Chemother* 41: 712–714
203 Occhialini A, Urdaci M, Doucet-Populaire F, Bebear CM, Lamouliatte H, Megraud F (1997) Macrolide resistance in *Helicobacter pylori*: rapid detection of point mutations and assays of macrolide binding to ribosomes. *Antimicrob Agents Chemother* 41: 2724–2728
204 van Doorn LJ, Debets-Ossenkopp YJ, Marais A, Sanna R, Megraud F, Kusters JG, Quint WG (1999) Rapid detection, by PCR and reverse hybridization, of mutations in the *Helicobacter pylori* 23S rRNA gene, associated with macrolide resistance. *Antimicrob Agents Chemother* 43: 1779-1782
205 Debets-Ossenkopp YJ, Brinkman AB, Kuipers EJ, Vandenbroucke-Grauls CM, Kusters JG (1998) Explaining the bias in the 23S rRNA gene mutations associated with clarithromycin resistance in clinical isolates of *Helicobacter pylori*. *Antimicrob Agents Chemother* 42: 2749-2751
206 Debets-Ossenkopp YJ, Sparrius M, Kusters JG, Kolkman JJ, Vandenbroucke-Grauls CM (1996) Mechanism of clarithromycin resistance in clinical isolates of *Helicobacter pylori*. *FEMS Microbiol Lett* 142: 37–42
207 Taylor DE, Ge Z, Purych D, Lo T, Hiratsuka K (1997) Cloning and sequence analysis of two copies of a 23S rRNA gene from *Helicobacter pylori* and association of clarithromycin resistance with 23S rRNA mutations. *Antimicrob Agents Chemother* 41: 2621–2628
208 Versalovic J, Osato MS, Spakovsky K, Dore MP, Reddy R, Stone GG, Shortridge D, Flamm RK, Tanaka SK, Graham DY (1997) Point mutations in the 23S rRNA gene of *Helicobacter pylori* associated with different levels of clarithromycin resistance. *J Antimicrob Chemother* 40: 283–286
209 Wallace RJ, Jr., Meier A, Brown BA, Zhang Y, Sander P, Onyi GO, Bottger EC (1996) Genetic basis for clarithromycin resistance among isolates of *Mycobacterium chelonae* and *Mycobacterium abscessus*. *Antimicrob Agents Chemother* 40: 1676–1681
210 Nash KA, Inderlied CB (1995) Genetic basis of macrolide resistance in *Mycobacterium avium* isolated from patients with disseminated disease. *Antimicrob Agents Chemother* 39: 2625–2630
211 Meier A, Kirschner P, Springer B, Steingrube VA, Brown BA, Wallace RJ, Jr., Bottger EC (1994) Identification of mutations in 23S rRNA gene of clarithromycin-resistant *Mycobacterium intracellulare*. *Antimicrob Agents Chemother* 38: 381–384
212 Burman WJ, Stone BL, Brown BA, Wallace J, R.J., Bottger EC (1998) AIDS-related *Mycobacterium kansasii* infection with initial resistance to clarithromycin. *Diagn Microbiol Infect Dis* 31: 369-371
213 Lucier TS, Heitzman K, Liu SK, Hu PC (1995) Transition mutations in the 23S rRNA of erythromycin-resistant isolates of *Mycoplasma pneumoniae*. *Antimicrob Agents Chemother* 39: 2770–2773
214 Stamm LV, Bergen HL (2000) A point mutation associated with bacterial macrolide resistance is present in both 23S rRNA genes of an erythromycin-resistant *Treponema pallidum* clinical isolate. *Antimicrob Agents Chemother* 44: 806–807
215 van Doorn LJ, Debets-Ossenkopp YJ, Marais A, Megraud F, Kusters JG, Quint WGV (1999) Rapid detection of mutations in the 23S rRNA gene associated with macrolide resistance in *Helicobacter pylori* by PCA and reverse hybridization. In 39th Annual International Conference on Antimicrobial Agents and Chemotherapy p. 263, American Society for Microbiology, Washington, DC, San Francisco, California
216 Vannuffel P, Di Giambattista M, Morgan EA, Cocito C (1992) Identification of a single base change in ribosomal RNA leading to erythromycin resistance. *J Biol Chem* 267: 8377–8382
217 Roberts AN, Hudson GS, Brenner S (1985) An erythromycin-resistance gene from an erythromycin-producing strain of *Arthrobacter* sp. *Gene* 35: 259-270
218 Uchiyama H, Weisblum B (1985) N-Methyl transferase of *Streptomyces erythraeus* that confers resistance to the macrolide-lincosamide-streptogramin B antibiotics: amino acid sequence and its homology to cognate R-factor enzymes from pathogenic bacilli and cocci. *Gene* 38: 103–110
219 Bibb MJ, Janssen GR, Ward JM (1985) Cloning and analysis of the promoter region of the erythromycin resistance gene (*ermE*) of *Streptomyces erythraeus*. *Gene* 38: 215–226

220 Epp JK, Burgett SG, Schoner BE (1987) Cloning and nucleotide sequence of a carbomycin-resistance gene from *Streptomyces thermotolerans. Gene* 53: 73–83

221 Pernodet JL, Blondelet-Rouault MH, Guerineau M (1993) Resistance to spiramycin in *Streptomyces ambofaciens,* the producer organism, involves at least two different mechanisms. *J Gen Microbiol* 139: 1003–1011

222 Gandecha AR, Cundliffe E (1996) Molecular analysis of *tlrD*, an MLS resistance determinant from the tylosin producer, *Streptomyces fradiae. Gene* 180: 173–176

223 Peschke U, Schmidt H, Zhang HZ, Piepersberg W (1995) Molecular characterization of the lincomycin-production gene cluster of *Streptomyces lincolnensis* 78–11. *Mol Microbiol* 16: 1137–1156

224 Inouye M, Morohoshi T, Horinouchi S, Beppu T (1994) Cloning and sequences of two macrolide-resistance-encoding genes from mycinamicin-producing *Micromonospora griseorubida. Gene* 141: 39-46

225 Xue Y, Zhao L, Liu HW, Sherman DH (1998) A gene cluster for macrolide antibiotic biosynthesis in *Streptomyces venezuelae*: architecture of metabolic diversity. *Proc Natl Acad Sci USA* 95: 12111–12116

226 Fujisawa Y, Weisblum B (1981) A family of r-determinants in *Streptomyces* spp. that specifies inducible resistance to macrolide, lincosamide, and streptogramin type B antibiotics. *J Bacteriol* 146: 621–631

227 Calcutt MJ, Cundliffe E (1990) Cloning of a lincosamide resistance determinant frm *Streptomyces caelestis*, the producer of celesticetin, and characterization of the resistance mechanism. *J Bacteriol* 172: 4710–4714

228 Jenkins G, Zalacain M, Cundliffe E (1989) Inducible ribosomal RNA methylation in *Streptomyces lividans,* conferring resistance to lincomycin. *J Gen Microbiol* 135: 3281–3288

229 Murphy E, Huwyler L, de Freire Bastos MdC (1985) Transposon Tn*554*: complete nucleotide sequence and isolation of transposition-defective and antibiotic-sensitive mutants. *EMBO J* 4: 3357–3365

230 Shaw JH, Clewell DB (1985) Complete nucleotide sequence of macrolide-lincosamide-streptogramin B-resistance transposon Tn*917* in *Streptococcus faecalis. J Bacteriol* 164: 782–796

231 Horinouchi S, Weisblum B (1982) Nucleotide sequence and functional map of pE194, a plasmid that specifies inducible resistance to macrolide, lincosamide, and streptogramin type B antibiotics. *J Bacteriol* 150: 804–814

232 Rasmussen JL, Odelson DA, Macrina FL (1986) Complete nucleotide sequence and transcription of *ermF*, a macrolide-lincosamide-streptogramin B resistance determinant from *Bacteroides fragilis. J Bacteriol* 168: 523–533

233 Berryman DI, Lyristis M, Rood JI (1994) Cloning and sequence analysis of *ermQ*, the predominant macrolide-lincosamide-streptogramin B resistance gene in *Clostridium perfringens. Antimicrob Agents Chemother* 38: 1041–1046

234 Serwold-Davis TM, Groman NB (1988) Identification of a methylase gene for erythromycin resistance within the sequence of a spontaneously deleting fragment of *Corynebacterium diphtheriae* plasmid pNG2. *FEMS Microbiol Lett* 46: 7–14

235 McGee L, Klugmann KP, Wasas A, Capper T, Brink A (2001) Serotype 19f multiresistant pneumococcal clone harboring two erythromycin resistance determinants (*erm*(B) and *erm*(A)) in South Africa. *Antimicrob Agents Chemother* 45: 1595–1598

236 Perreten V, Schwarz FV, Teuber M, Levy SB (2001) Mdt(A), a new efflux protein conferring multiple antibiotic resistance in *Lactococcus lactis* and *Escherichia coli. Antimicrob Agents Chemother* 45: 1109–1114

Index

MIX
Papier aus verantwortungsvollen Quellen
Paper from responsible sources
FSC® C105338

If you have any concerns about our products,
you can contact us on
ProductSafety@springernature.com

In case Publisher is established outside the EU,
the EU authorized representative is:
Springer Nature Customer Service Center GmbH
Europaplatz 3, 69115 Heidelberg, Germany

Printed by Libri Plureos GmbH
in Hamburg, Germany